Medical Coding
Practice and Review

Marsha S. Diamond, CPC, CPC-H

Department Chair
Health Information Technology
Central Florida College
Orlando, Florida

National Advisory Board Member
American Academy of Professional Coders
Salt Lake City, Utah

Senior Consultant/Auditor
Medical Audit Resource Services, Inc.
Orlando, Florida

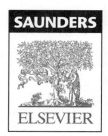

SAUNDERS

ELSEVIER

D1226029

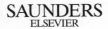

SAUNDERS
ELSEVIER

11830 Westline Industrial Drive
St. Louis, Missouri 63146

Publishing Director: Andrew M. Allen
Executive Editor: Susan Cole
Developmental Editor: Beth LoGiudice
Publishing Services Manager: Patricia Tannian
Designer: Paula Ruckenbrod
Producer: Cindy Ahlheim

Working together to grow
libraries in developing countries

www.elsevier.com | www.bookaid.org | www.sabre.org

ELSEVIER   BOOK AID
International   Sabre Foundation

Printed in the United States of America

Last digit is the print number: 9   8   7   6   5   4   3   2   1

INTRODUCTION

The office notes and worksheets found in this supplement serve as additional practical exercises to accompany *Mastering Medical Coding,* Third Edition. Instructors and students may use these exercises for additional practical application of ICD-9-CM and CPT-4 coding. Each exercise provides data representing real-life patient chart notes.

These exercises have been divided into the following coding sections: Evaluation and Management, Surgery, and Radiology. These exercises concentrate on only those applications that typically require an operative report or dictated report rather than computer-driven interpretations and reports. The breakdown of exercises along with their corresponding textbook chapters is as follows:

	Text Chapters (ICD-9-CM)	*Text Chapters (CPT-4)*
Section One Evaluation and Management	2, 3, 4, 5, 6	10
Section Two Surgery		
Integumentary Exercises	2, 3, 4, 5, 6	12
Musculoskeletal Exercises	2, 3, 4, 5, 6	12
Respiratory Exercises	2, 3, 4, 5, 6	12
Cardiovascular Exercises	2, 3, 4, 5, 6	12
Gastrointestinal Exercises	2, 3, 4, 5, 6	12
Genitourinary Exercises	2, 3, 4, 5, 6	12
Nervous System Exercises	2, 3, 4, 5, 6	12
Eye Exercises	2, 3, 4, 5, 6	12
Ear Exercises	2, 3, 4, 5, 6	12
Section Three Radiology	2, 3, 4, 5, 6	13

The exercises may be done after the completion of the corresponding textbook chapters.

All these exercises can also be used for application in pathology, anesthesia, and medicine. Simply extract the additional descriptors from CPT-4 to assign codes. Instructors can also use additional exercises from the testbank found in the Instructor's Manual accompanying the textbook.

Marsha S. Diamond

CONTENTS

EVALUATION
AND MANAGEMENT

EXERCISE 1

Level I

OFFICE NOTE

Chief complaint: _____

Date: _____

Vital signs: BP_____ P_____ R_____

History:

SUBJECTIVE: This 74-year-old white female new patient with a history of polymyalgia presented after suddenly noticing and developing discomfort superficially at the right medial calf on the right lower extremity. She has noticed a knot and a swelling there and is concerned about a possible blood clot. She has a history of significant pulmonary conditions and has been the subject of multiple episodes of pneumonia. She states that she has not had any increased chest pain or shortness of breath.

Exam:

Pulse 81. Respiratory rate 18. Blood pressure 127/76. The patient is not out of breath. Her lungs are clear. Her heart is regular. Evaluation of the right calf shows a superficial clot right over a blood vessel on the medial surface of the calf approximately 1/3 of the way down from the tibial plateau. There is no leaking of fluid down the leg underneath the skin, and the calf muscle itself is flabby and not swollen.

Diagnosis/assessment:

IMPRESSION: Superficial blood vessel rupture, right lower extremity.

PLAN: We asked her to ice the area for the next couple of days and then apply heat to the area. We warned her of possible tracking of blood down the skin toward the ankle. We have given her antiembolic thigh-high stockings that she is to wear for the next 3–7 days, and she is to continue on her aspirin as before. She is to follow up with her primary care doctor on Thursday, to be monitored for potential complications to deep system. She is to return for any chest pain, shortness of breath, or evidence of infection in that area.

Maurice Doater, MD

Patient name: _____

Date of service: _____

GODFREY MEDICAL ASSOCIATES
1532 Third Avenue, Suite 120 • Aldon, FL 77713 • (407) 555-4000

EXERCISE 2

Level II

EMERGENCY ROOM RECORD

Name:		Age:	ER physician:
		DOB:	

Allergies/type of reaction:	Usual medications/dosages:
No known drug allergies.	Aspirin, metoprolol, Lopressor, Lanoxin, Prevacid, Coumadin, isosorbide, K-Dur, lisinopril, Lasix, hydrocodone prn for leg pain, Metamucil.

Triage/presenting complaint:

Initial assessment:

SUBJECTIVE: 73-year-old brought in by family. He comes in with episodes of coughing up blood in the morning—a few red clots. Patient has a history of nasopharyngeal carcinoma. Was given radiation therapy followed by chemotherapy according to patient. Patient states that he had similar episode a long time ago when he was diagnosed with pulmonary congestion. Was put in the hospital at that time. Recently had an extensive evaluation earlier this year for his

Time	T	P	R	BP	Other:					

Medication orders:

Lab work:

Labs show PT 20, INR 2.78 (therapeutic). CBC shows WBC 5.9, hemoglobin 11.8, hematocrit 33.2, platelet 162. Comprehensive metabolic panel showed glucose of 135, BUN 34, creatinine 1.4. Amylase is 147, CPK 39. Liver function within normal limits, troponin 0.

X-ray:

Chest x-ray shows some degree of cardiomegaly, no pleural effusion. No pulmonary congestion. No mass or infiltrates seen.

Physician's report:

PHYSICAL EXAMINATION: Alert and oriented times three. Does not appear to be in any acute distress. T. 97.4, P. 75, R. 16, BP in the range of 89/53 asymptomatic, saturating 94% on room air.

HEENT: PERRLA, EOMI. Anicteric sclerae. Throat clear.

CHEST: Clear. A few basal crackles.

ABDOMEN: Soft, nontender.

EXTREMITIES: No edema, no cyanosis.

I advised patient to return to the clinic immediately if any further episodes or if he develops any dizziness or increased tiredness or notices any black, tarry stool or hematemesis. Discussed with Dr. Doate regarding patient condition. Will schedule for a CT scan of chest abdomen to look for any reason for elevated amylase. Patient to follow up with Dr. Seers in the next couple of days after the above tests are done. Will also give pain medication, Percocet 1 mg, PO tid to qid for his back pain. Patient was discharged from the ER in stable condition.

Diagnosis:	Physician sign/date
ASSESSMENT: Hemoptysis, apparently no evidence of current bleeding at this time. His blood pressure I have checked in the previous reports and as per patient also; it usually runs low. He otherwise is totally asymptomatic, no evidence of hematemesis or melena. The episodes of hemoptysis were in the morning; hasn't repeated again yet.	*Nancy Caully* MD

Discharge	Transfer	Admit	Good	Satisfactory	Other:

GODFREY REGIONAL HOSPITAL
123 Main Street • Aldon, FL 77714 • (407) 555-1234

Continued

EMERGENCY ROOM RECORD

Name:	Age:	ER physician:
	DOB:	

Allergies/type of reaction:	Usual medications/dosages:

Triage/presenting complaint:

Initial assessment: chest, including CT scanning, etc., which was negative for any mass. Patient states this morning he coughed and saw a couple clots that he spitted out. Denies any fever or chills. No respiratory problem otherwise, no shortness of breath. Patient does feel tired. He has an appointment to see his primary care doctor in the next couple of days for repeat upper endoscopy. No fever, no chills. No urinary symptoms, no joint swelling. No hematemesis, no melena.

Time	T	P	R	BP	Other:					

Medication orders:

Lab work:

X-ray:

Physician's report:

Diagnosis:	Physician sign/date
	Nancy Caully MD

Discharge	Transfer	Admit	Good	Satisfactory	Other:

GODFREY REGIONAL HOSPITAL
123 Main Street • Aldon, FL 77714 • (407) 555-1234

Continued

EMERGENCY ROOM RECORD

| Name: | Age: | ER physician: |
| | DOB: | |

Allergies/type of reaction: **Usual medications/dosages:**

Triage/presenting complaint:

Initial assessment: Appetite has been fairly good; eating OK.
PAST MEDICAL HISTORY: Esophageal cancer, hypertension, atrial fibrillation, peptic ulcer disease.

| Time | T | P | R | BP | Other: | | | | | |

Medication orders:

Lab work:

X-ray:

Physician's report:

Diagnosis: **Physician sign/date**

Maurice Doater, MD

Discharge   Transfer   Admit   Good   Satisfactory   Other:

GODFREY REGIONAL HOSPITAL
123 Main Street • Aldon, FL 77714 • (407) 555-1234

EXERCISE 3

Level II

EMERGENCY ROOM RECORD

Name:	Age:	ER physician:
	DOB:	

Allergies/type of reaction:	Usual medications/dosages:
Penicillin and Naprosyn.	Lanoxin, 125 mg qd; isosorbide 30 mg half tablet qd; Lasix 20 mg one tablet bid; Lotensin 5 mg qd; aspirin one tablet qd; Plavix 75 mg po qd.

Triage/presenting complaint: 86-year-old was brought in for chest pain that was relieved with oxygen. Patient stated it was in the range of 5. By the time she got to the ER, the pain had completely resolved. During this time she was given some nitro that completely resolved the pain. Denies any nausea or vomiting at this time.
PAST MEDICAL HISTORY: CHF, angina, hypertension, and peripheral vascular disease.

Initial assessment:

Time	T	P	R	BP	Other:					

Medication orders:

Lab work: CBC shows WBC 7.8, hemoglobin 10.0, hematocrit 131.7, platelets 302. Metabolic panel showed glucose 120, BUN 20, creatinine 1.1, CPK 95. ALT is 117, AST 82, troponin 0, CPK 95.

X-ray: X-rays show cardiomegaly with no evidence of any infiltrate or pleural effusion.

Physician's report:

PHYSICAL EXAMINATION: Alert and oriented times three. At the time of examination, patient is chest-pain-free. T. 98.0, P. 89, R. 24, BP 128/69, saturating 99% on 3 liters.
HEENT: PERRLA, EOMI. Anicteric sclerae. Throat clear.
CHEST: Bilaterally clear with a few basilar crackles.
CARDIOVASCULAR: S1, S2 normal.
ABDOMEN: Soft, nontender.
EXTREMITIES: No edema, no cyanosis.
CNS: Grossly intact with no focal deficit.
PLAN: Increase isosorbide to 30 mg po qd and increase Lasix to 40 mg po qd. Follow up with primary care physician for the next couple of days. If the pain presents, return to the clinic to seek medical attention or come back to the emergency room.

Patient was discharged in stable condition.

Diagnosis:	Physician sign/date
ASSESSMENT: CHF, angina.	*Robert Rai MD*

Discharge	Transfer	Admit	Good	Satisfactory	Other:

GODFREY REGIONAL HOSPITAL
123 Main Street • Aldon, FL 77714 • (407) 555-1234

EXERCISE 4

Level II

OFFICE NOTE

Date:		Vital signs:	T	R
Chief complaint:			P	BP

SUBJECTIVE: Esther is an 83-year-old patient who was brought in after she had an episode of "tingling all over" and some dizziness "as if I were going to pass out." By the time she arrived here, the sensation had resolved. Upon review of the ambulance crew description of how they found her, they stated that she was oriented and cooperative, sitting in a chair. Skin was warm and dry, and she didn't have any difficulties with speech or weakness. She did have initial blood pressure of 200/100 and then, en route, she was lowered to 138/64. She was sating 100% on 1 liter.

While here, Esther has had resolution of her symptoms as described above. She was not complaining of any pain. She

Examination:

REVIEW OF SYSTEMS: It is equivocal whether she has had a low-grade fever at home or not, since she didn't take her temperature. She has had some chills and generalized weakness and malaise as above. Energy is very poor; appetite has been well maintained, and she usually sleeps very well. Vision: no blurred vision or diplopia.

HEENT: No facial pressures, sore throat, rhinorrhea, or earache.

RESPIRATORY: Denies cough, sputum production, or hemoptysis. No pleuritic chest pain.

CARDIOVASCULAR: As above.

GASTROINTESTINAL SYSTEM: No further episodes of nausea or vomiting; no hematemesis, no early satiety, no dysphagia. Denies any changes in bowel habits. No melena or hematochezia. No abdominal pain.

GENITOURINARY SYSTEM: No dysuria, frequency, or hematuria. The remainder is negative.

PHYSICAL EXAMINATION: Very pleasant elderly lady who appears frail. She is fully oriented and cooperative. Initial

Impression:

Elderly lady presenting with resolved episode of diffuse tingling, unclear etiology. No focal findings on examination; no evidence of disease on x-rays or labs. Importantly, she has chronic dyspnea with minimal exertion.

Plan:

We discussed extensively with the patient and her son what the present situation brings up. I do not think that we are going to come up with the answer of why she is so short of breath for so long, and it certainly doesn't seem to be the main concern. The shortness of breath may be due to numerous factors, and these should be worked up on an outpatient basis.

The patient was advised to take an extra potassium tablet daily for two days and to drink plenty of fluids. They were also advised to call tomorrow to make an appointment with her physician for follow-up. She may need further work-up, as her weakness and dyspnea have been persistent for so long.

We reviewed all of these labs and chest x-rays with them. They agreed that the present problem has resolved and chronic problem needs to be worked up later. They feel comfortable trying it at home and will return if needed.

	Patient name:
	DOB:
	MR/Chart #:

GODFREY REGIONAL OUTPATIENT CLINIC
3122 Shannon Avenue • Aldon, FL 77712 • (407) 555-7654

Continued

OFFICE NOTE

Date:	Vital signs: T R
Chief complaint:	P BP

felt better than she had at home. After interviewing her for a while, it was obvious that she has been feeling very weak for quite some time, and that this is an ongoing problem. She also has felt dyspnea with minimal exertion, which she had experienced after her surgery two years ago. She also states that yesterday she had an episode or two of vomiting clear material. She states she didn't have any accompanying diarrhea. This resolved later in the evening, and today she didn't have any and was able to eat well.

PAST MEDICAL HISTORY: CAD, SP CABG. Patient does not recall having had an acute myocardial infarction.

Examination:

BP was 160/82; prior to discharge it was 148/74. She was sating 100% on 3 liters per nasal cannula. Temperature 98.1, pulse was in the 70s, regular; and monitor showed a normal sinus rhythm. Respiratory rate was normal. There were no difficulties with speech. HEENT: no facial asymmetries, no pallor, no jaundice. Hydration is fairly well maintained, although her lips are a little dry. PERRL, EOMI, no nystagmus. Oral examination is unremarkable. NECK: supple without lymphadenopathy or thyromegaly; no JVD noted, symmetric carotid upstrokes bilaterally. CHEST: lungs—respiration is quite shallow. EXTREMITIES: no edema. NEUROLOGICAL: is actually intact with mental status as above; no meningeal signs; CN 2-12 intact; motor strength is 4/4 in all four extremities, DTRs are 11 at bicipital and patellar levels; no sensory deficits elicited.

LABS AND X-RAYS: Chest x-ray (portable) revealed heart of normal size, no infiltrates or effusions, and the surgical changes consistent with her CABG. I do not see other major differences with previous chest x-ray from over two years ago. EKG showed a normal sinus rhythm with a rate of 80 beats per minute. LAFB, incomplete RBBB, and diffuse IVCD.

Impression:

Plan:

Patient name:
DOB:
MR/Chart #:

GODFREY REGIONAL OUTPATIENT CLINIC
3122 Shannon Avenue • Aldon, FL 77712 • (407) 555-7654

Continued

OFFICE NOTE

| Date: | Vital signs: | T | R |
| Chief complaint: | | P | BP |

Breast carcinoma SP lumpectomy. On tamoxifen, approximately a year ago. Hypothyroidism; on replacement. History of TIA some time ago that was worked up with carotid Dopplers. Unclear at this time what these rendered, but she was advised to take an aspirin a day.

MEDICATIONS: Tamoxifen, Synthroid, metoprolol, ASA, HCTZ, and potassium supplements.

ALLERGIES: None known.

Examination:

Labs showed glucose of 118, BUN 21, creatinine 0.7. All electrolytes were normal with potassium of 3.7; CK was 77, troponin 0, WBC count was 4.8 with normal differential, and hemoglobin and hematocrit were 12.8 and 35.6, respectively. Platelet count 251.

Impression:

Plan:

Patient name:

DOB:

MR/Chart #:

GODFREY REGIONAL OUTPATIENT CLINIC
3122 Shannon Avenue • Aldon, FL 77712 • (407) 555-7654

Level I

OFFICE NOTE

Date:	Vital signs:	T	R
Chief complaint:		P	BP

77-year-old comes in with pain in all the limbs, specifically the left elbow that has become swollen and tender. Patient has past history of gout in both ankles. States that the left elbow is swollen and has difficulty bending his arm. Unsure if he fell down. States that when he woke up this morning, his mattress was on the other side of the room and he was sleeping on the floor. Patient comes in with his nephew who confirms the above finding. Patient also has recently begun remembering events a little

Examination:

Alert and oriented times three; does not appear to be in any acute distress, does not appear to be dehydrated. T. 99.1, P. 49, R. 20, BP 137/88, saturating 97% on room air.

HEENT: PERRLA, EOML. Anicteric sclerae. Throat clear.

CHEST: Clear.

ABDOMEN: Soft, nontender.

EXTREMITIES: No edema, no cyanosis. Left elbow is swollen and tender.

LABS AND X-RAYS: CBC shows WBC 11.4, hemoglobin 16.1, hematocrit 46.5, platelets 149. X-rays of the left elbow do not show any specific fracture; however, questionable area of the left medial epicondyle. Either it has bony spur or is slightly moved away.

Impression:

ASSESSMENT: Most likely gouty arthritis.

Plan:

Will start on Celebrex 100 mg po bid. 15 tablets were given from the clinic. Also patient does not appear to take care of himself on a regular basis, and he does require some degree of assistance. Will get County Services involved for his health care. Patient advised to follow up with family physician in the next couple of days and was discharged from the clinic in stable condition.

	Patient name:
	DOB:
	MR/Chart #:

GODFREY REGIONAL OUTPATIENT CLINIC
3122 Shannon Avenue • Aldon, FL 77712 • (407) 555-7654

Continued

OFFICE NOTE

Date:	Vital signs:	T	R
Chief complaint:		P	BP

differently; however, is able to provide a history consistently without any problems.
MEDICATIONS: Cardura, Toprol, nitro, Lanoxin, and Coumadin.
ALLERGIES: No known drug allergies.

Examination:

Impression:

Plan:

Willen Obst MD

Patient name:
DOB:
MR/Chart #:

GODFREY REGIONAL OUTPATIENT CLINIC
3122 Shannon Avenue • Aldon, FL 77712 • (407) 555-7654

E X E R C I S E   6

Level I

OFFICE NOTE

Chief complaint: _____

Date: _____

Vital signs: BP_____   P_____   R_____

History:

Jason is a 27-year-old man who comes in because of persistent bleeding from his gums. He had four wisdom teeth removed earlier today by his dentist: two on the lower jaw and two on the upper jaw. This was done because of significant pain the patient was experiencing.

Interestingly, the reason why Jason is bleeding so much is because he is on Coumadin. His last INR was 2.9. His anticoagulation is secondary to aortic valve replacement secondary to endocarditis, which was performed a few years ago. He follows up with another physician for this purpose and he has been doing very well since.

Exam:

He appears as a healthy young man, in no distress, afebrile; BP is 138/98.

HEENT: no pallor or jaundice. Hydration is well maintained. Oral examination reveals soaked gauze that patient was holding between his teeth. When these were removed, there were obviously four opened sockets with very soft clot in the bottom ones and oozing from the upper ones. Otherwise, there were no abnormalities.

NECK: supple without lymphadenopathies.

CHEST: lungs—CTA. Heart regular rate and rhythm. 2-3/6 systolic ejection murmur and a click are heard, no gallops or tachycardia.

LOWER EXTREMITIES: no edema.

NEUROLOGICAL: intact.

Diagnosis/assessment:

IMPRESSION: Persistent slow bleed SP teeth extraction times four secondary to anticoagulation.

PLAN: We will recheck his PT and INR. If it is certainly above 2.7 or 2.8, we may need to give him some vitamin K today until the clots are formed and oozing from the sockets is decreased. Then he should restart his Coumadin. Will await the test results to make any further decisions. This was explained to the patient.

ADDENDUM: The patient's PT and INR were a little bit higher, although not super-therapeutic. His INR was 3.06. At this time, we have suggested the following:
A. Vitamin K 5 mg IM now.
B. Hold Coumadin tomorrow morning.
C. Continue to apply pressure to the sockets.
D. If he continues to have problems with oozing and bleeding the following day, he needs to still hold his Coumadin and come back here to have everything rechecked. He showed understanding and agreement.

Steny Kreitt, MD

Patient name: _____

Date of service: _____

GODFREY MEDICAL ASSOCIATES
1532 Third Avenue, Suite 120 • Aldon, FL 77713 • (407) 555-4000

EXERCISE 7

Level II

OFFICE NOTE

Date:	Vital signs:	T	R
Chief complaint:		P	BP

S: Patient presents complaining of bilateral leg aches and left knee pain. He states that this has been bothering him off and on for a long period of time. He has had CVAs in the past. He has diabetes mellitus and alcoholic liver disease. He was sent up to Atlanta about 1–2 weeks ago with alcoholic encephalopathy. They treated him there for a few days and were able to send him home. He has mitral regurgitation and atrial fibrillation. He did have a heart cath about two years ago. He has had a couple CVAs in the past. Current medications are as listed on his ER sheet. He has no known allergies. He states that off and on for the last month his left knee has been painful for him, as have his legs through the upper legs and lower legs. It tends to be fairly nondescript.

Physical examination:

O: On examination, his left knee has a joint effusion and some mild decreased range of motion. Right knee is normal except for some arthritic changes but no effusion. His left knee is not warm to the touch. It is not erythematous. He has scattered areas of tenderness over his thighs and calves. It does not seem to be focused into any one region. There is a little bit of ankle edema but this is fairly typical for him. He has no evidence of respiratory distress at this time and has no other complaints in regards to his heart or lungs.

Assessment:

A: Arthritis, left knee with mild joint effusion; does not appear to be a septic knee. Scattered muscle aches and tenderness, probably related to deconditioning and his chronic health issues.

Plan:

P: Recommended exercise as much as he possibly can. Use Tylenol in limited amounts for his pain. Suggested using approximately half the usual dose of Tylenol, whatever strength he has. Discussed repeatedly and in detail how to split the recommended dose in half for each dose and for total daily requirements, and to try and get by on as little as he can. We discussed the metabolism of Tylenol to the liver and the fact that his liver doesn't "burn it up" as fast as it should. Discussed other procedures that

| Patient name: |
| DOB: |
| MR/Chart #: |

GODFREY REGIONAL OUTPATIENT CLINIC
3122 Shannon Avenue • Aldon, FL 77712 • (407) 555-7654

Continued

OFFICE NOTE

| Date: | Vital signs: | T | R |
| Chief complaint: | | P | BP |

Physical examination:

Assessment:

Plan:

can be done for the knee such as aspiration injection with cortisone, but did not recommend it at this time. We will have him reassessed on a prn basis if any problems arise or if he seems to be worsening. Discussed his care at home. His wife does take care of him and they felt they could handle it at home. We offered hospitalization but the patient did not feel that this would be necessary.

Stary Kractt, MD

Patient name:

DOB:

MR/Chart #:

GODFREY REGIONAL OUTPATIENT CLINIC
3122 Shannon Avenue • Aldon, FL 77712 • (407) 555-7654

EXERCISE 8

Level I

OFFICE NOTE

Chief complaint: _____

Date: _____

Vital signs: BP_____ P_____ R_____

History:

S: This is a 65-year-old gentleman complaining of epistaxis. He has had it intermittently for a week and a half. It is on the right side today. He was actually just in hospital in another city, and was here last month. He has diabetes, hypertension, atrial fibrillation, mitral regurgitation, cirrhosis related to alcoholism, coronary artery disease with previous MI, previous CVA, congestive heart failure, and renal insufficiency. He isn't on any blood thinners other than aspirin. He is on numerous medications that are listed.

Exam:

O: On exam his pressure is not bad. He has a little dried scab of blood in the left nostril so I didn't touch that. On the right side he had just some oozing from the septum that looked raw. I did put a little epinephrine on a cotton swab in there, left it on for awhile, and removed it, and I used a little silver nitrate to cauterize that side of the septum. He is to use a little Vaseline in the left side. He has been on an Atrovent nasal spray for a drippy nose with eating. I told him that this could be causing his problem as it does cause drying and is a known side effect, so he should stop that. He can continue to use his saline nasal spray. He was stable at discharge.

Diagnosis/assessment:

Willen Obst MD

Patient name: _____

Date of service: _____

GODFREY MEDICAL ASSOCIATES
1532 Third Avenue, Suite 120 • Aldon, FL 77713 • (407) 555-4000

Level I

OFFICE NOTE

Chief complaint: _____

Date: _____

Vital signs: BP_____ P_____ R_____

History:

S: 83-year-old female presents with difficulty swallowing since noon lunch. She states she had a few bites of some leftover ribs when she had difficulty swallowing. She states she has been unable to get anything down; even saliva comes back up. She has been gagging and vomiting all afternoon. She has had burning in her throat. She has been coughing up a lot of thick phlegm. She has had no prior history of ulcers or gastric problems. She currently takes Prinivil and Norvasc for hypertension, Glucotrol for diabetes, and is on three different eye drops for glaucoma. She is allergic to penicillin.

Exam:

O: On physical exam, her conjunctivae are injected and she is overdue for some drops, she states. Her pupils are equal, round, and reactive. TMs nondistended. Nasopharynx noncongested. Posterior pharynx is nonerythematous. Oropharynx without lesion. Lung sounds are clear. Heart is regular and without murmur. Abdomen is soft. There is no tenderness noted. Pressing in the epigastric area, however, increases the patient's symptoms in the mid chest where she feels this stuck food. Shortly, after pressing on her abdomen, she was given a glass of water, was able to swallow, and the water did go down and her symptoms resolved.

Diagnosis/assessment:

A: Dysphagia, suspect esophageal stricture.

P: Patient started on Protonix 40 mg, one po qd. She will fill that prescription tomorrow and call a specialist's office for evaluation for EGD, as most likely she has an esophageal stricture that will need to be dilated.

Felix Warden MD

Patient name: _____
Date of service: _____

GODFREY MEDICAL ASSOCIATES
1532 Third Avenue, Suite 120 • Aldon, FL 77713 • (407) 555-4000

EXERCISE 10

Level II

OFFICE NOTE

Date:	Vital signs:	T		R	
Chief complaint: Food reaction		P		BP	

S: This is a soon to be 66-year-old woman who says that since she was in her 30s, she would have some reaction when she ate certain foods, and this happened yesterday. It has been the same each time. She had eaten at some kind of church dinner but she says when she eats processed foods like Chicken McNuggets or something else, she will get a sensation that she has too much electrical activity in her head. The closest I can get as far as a description is some pressure, and then she feels her heart flip-flops and she feels funny. This happened yesterday so she came in early this morning to have things evaluated since she now has high blood pressure. Other than hypertension, she

Examination:

O: On exam, this is an older woman who is in no distress. Her pressure was a little high to begin with, but it did come down and I think she was partly a little bit anxious. Her O2 sats were fine. Pulse was stable. Eyes showed no papilledema. Neck had good carotid upstrokes without bruits. No nuchal rigidity. Lungs were clear. Heart is regular without any murmurs noted. Abdomen is negative. She moves all her extremities fine. Motor and sensory is intact. An EKG looks unremarkable.

Impression:

A: Vague symptoms. I can't exclude that she couldn't have some kind of weird reaction to MSG. It also may be just anxiety related with blood pressure elevation and palpitations.

Plan:

P: Discussion. She should continue on her Diovan. Her pressure at 174/93 actually isn't much higher than when she was in the clinic last. She was given an Rx for Lopressor 50 mg to take one a day when she has these episodes, #30 with a couple of refills. She will return if there are other problems. She was stable at discharge. She also had blood gases done that were normal.

	Patient name:
	DOB:
	MR/Chart #:

GODFREY REGIONAL OUTPATIENT CLINIC
3122 Shannon Avenue • Aldon, FL 77712 • (407) 555-7654

Continued

OFFICE NOTE

| Date: | Vital signs: | T | R |
| Chief complaint: Food reaction | | P | BP |

denies any other acute problems. She is on Diovan for her blood pressure once a day. She also has fibromyalgia. She has a codeine allergy. On review of systems, no HEENT complaints. Respiratory: negative. Cardiac: just this flip-flop sensation. No history of exertional or other kind of cardiac symptoms. GI: negative. GU: negative.

Examination:

Impression:

Plan:

Jdr Palermo

Patient name:

DOB:

MR/Chart #:

GODFREY REGIONAL OUTPATIENT CLINIC
3122 Shannon Avenue • Aldon, FL 77712 • (407) 555-7654

EXERCISE 11

Level I

OFFICE NOTE

Date:	Vital signs:	T	R
Chief complaint:		P	BP

S: This 62-year-old female with longstanding asthma/COPD was seen last week by her usual physician and diagnosed with bronchitis/pneumonia and started on Levaquin. She took it two days and stated it made her sick to her stomach, so she stopped it. She has now been off of antibiotics for five days. She complains of increased wheezing and cough productive of green sputum. She has been more short of breath and she presents for evaluation.

Examination:

O: On exam, she is afebrile. Temp is 97. Pulse is 92. Respirations are 20. Blood pressure 119/88. O2 sats are 95% on room air. She is alert and oriented 3 3. She is in no obvious distress and only mildly dyspneic at rest. Pupils equal, round, and reactive. Conjunctivae noninjected. TMs nondistended and nonerythematous. Right TM is a little injected. Ear canals are without lesion. Nasopharynx is noncongested with septum midline. Posterior pharynx is mildly erythematous. Neck reveals no lymphadenopathy. Lung sounds revealed diffuse, coarse, expiratory wheezes throughout both lungs. Heart sounds are distant and regular without murmur. Abdomen is obese, soft, and nontender. Extremities are without cyanosis. There is no edema. She was given albuterol with Atrovent nebulization. Her dyspnea improved but she continues to have coarse wheezes. She was given Solu-Medrol 125 mg IM. Chest x-ray shows a questionable early right lower lobe infiltrate. She has a white count of 10,200 with normal differential. Hemoglobin is 14.1. Platelets are 281.

Impression:

A: 1. Early acute right lower lobe pneumonia. 2. Exacerbation of COPD/asthma.

Plan:

P: She is given Zithromax Z-Pak as directed, since she did not tolerate the Levaquin. She will use her albuterol neb. at home as needed. She is also given a Medrol dose pack, which she will start later this afternoon. She will follow up in the clinic if she is not improving over the next 3–4 days.

Jay Carson MD

Patient name:

DOB:

MR/Chart #:

GODFREY REGIONAL OUTPATIENT CLINIC
3122 Shannon Avenue • Aldon, FL 77712 • (407) 555-7654

EXERCISE 12

Level I

OFFICE NOTE

Date:	Vital signs:	T	R
Chief complaint: Right hand injury		P	BP

HISTORY: This is a 44-year-old gentleman who was going to ride his horse. He had his hand in the bridle when the horse jerked up, and he injured his right middle and ring fingers with a deformity. He has a little blood coming around the nail too.

He is on Paxil. No other health problems. No allergies.

Physical examination:

O: On exam he has obvious deformities probably due to fractures of his right middle and ring finger. I am not sure if it is at the DIP joint or in the mid-phalanx at this point. He can feel to touch distally, but he isn't moving because of the pain. His little finger and ring finger are not really tender; color, movement, and sensation are intact in those. Color was good in the middle and ring finger too. X-rays show comminuted fractures with displacement impacting of his mid-phalanx of the ring and middle fingers.

Assessment:

A: Comminuted fractures of the mid-phalanx of the right middle and ring fingers.

Plan:

P: A hand surgeon was in the building, so I showed him the x-rays. He suggested just straightening the fingers out under some anesthesia and putting a volar splint on and then having him [the patient] see either himself or another hand surgeon after two days. That will allow the swelling to go down. I did do a digital block with just under 5 cc in each finger, of 2% lidocaine after a Betadine prep. After good anesthesia, each finger was grasped, pulled on the longitudinal aspect, and straightened out. With middle finger there was a fair amount of clunking but it did straighten out nicely. He was then put in a volar splint from the mid forearm with the wrist slightly in hyperextension and out past the fingers, the middle and ring fingers. Ace wrap was applied. He is to leave this on until he is rechecked. He can elevate

Patient name:
DOB:
MR/Chart #:

GODFREY REGIONAL OUTPATIENT CLINIC
3122 Shannon Avenue • Aldon, FL 77712 • (407) 555-7654

Continued

OFFICE NOTE

Date:	Vital signs:	T	R
Chief complaint: Right hand injury		P	BP

Physical examination:

Assessment:

Plan:

the arm. He was given Tylenol #3 to use 1 to 2 q4h prn for pain, #30. He still had good color in the fingers. Sensation was not present because of anesthesia from the digital block. If he has any numbness that develops in his ring or little finger, he will loosen the bandages. He was stable at discharge, and he will need to bring his x-rays with him to see the hand surgeon or orthopedist.

Maurice Doates, MD

Patient name:

DOB:

MR/Chart #:

GODFREY REGIONAL OUTPATIENT CLINIC
3122 Shannon Avenue • Aldon, FL 77712 • (407) 555-7654

EXERCISE 13

Level II

OFFICE NOTE

Chief complaint: _____

Date: _____

Vital signs: BP_____   P_____   R_____

History:

S: New patient presents complaining of right upper tooth pain. She noticed through the night that she developed swelling and pain. It has been bothering her a little bit, but now it seems to have suddenly worsened overnight. It has been occurring for the last week or two, and she has been waiting to get in to see a dentist.

Exam:

O: On examination, her right upper molars are tender to palpation. She has swelling at the jaw line in this region and some spasm in the masseter muscles.

Diagnosis/assessment:

A: Abscessed tooth.

P: Appointment with dentist recommended. Keflex 500 mg tid x 10 days. Tylenol #3 one to two q4h prn #20, and recheck with dentist to have this further assessed, or sooner with us if pain seems to be progressing before she can get in to see the dentist.

Jay Carson MD

Patient name: _____

Date of service: _____

GODFREY MEDICAL ASSOCIATES
1532 Third Avenue, Suite 120 • Aldon, FL 77713 • (407) 555-4000

EXERCISE 14

Level I

OFFICE NOTE

Date:	Vital signs:	T	R
Chief complaint:		P	BP

S: 28-year-old gentleman presents with a severe sore throat; is unable to even swallow Tylenol at this time because his throat is so sore. He has had fever and chills today.

Physical examination:

O: On exam, his temp is 98.2. Pulse is 95. Respirations are 20. Blood pressure is 144/23. He is lying on the cot in the exam room with his coat over his shoulders and a blanket over that. He is in moderate distress from his sore throat and he has a muffled sounding voice. His TMs are nondistended and nonerythematous. Conjunctivae are noninjected. Pupils are equal, round, and reactive. Nasopharynx: noncongested with septum midline. Posterior pharynx is very erythematous with large tonsillar hypertrophy and white and yellow exudate seen in the tonsillar crypts. Neck reveals lymphadenopathy along the cervical chain. Lung sounds are clear. Heart is regular rate and rhythm without murmur.

Assessment:

A: Acute tonsillitis/pharyngitis.

Plan:

P: Patient is given Bicillin CR 1.2 milliunits IM. He will rest and take Tylenol as needed for fever, drink plenty of fluids, and follow up if worsening occurs over the course of the next 24 hours or if not improving in the next two days.

William Obst MD

Patient name:
DOB:
MR/Chart #:

GODFREY REGIONAL OUTPATIENT CLINIC
3122 Shannon Avenue • Aldon, FL 77712 • (407) 555-7654

EXERCISE 15

Level II

EMERGENCY ROOM RECORD

Name:	Age:	ER physician:
	DOB:	

Allergies/type of reaction:	Usual medications/dosages:
He has no allergies.	Prednisone, 5 mg, one-half bid; methotrexate 0.6 cc once a week; Protonix 40 mg qd; Celebrex 100 mg po bid; Lanoxin 0.125 mg qd; folic acid 1 mg daily; and Ditropan XL 5 mg daily.

Triage/presenting complaint:

NURSING HOME ADMIT
CHIEF COMPLAINT: Confusion.

HISTORY: This is an 86-year-old gentleman who has had problems with confusion over the last few months related to low sodium. Yesterday he became disoriented and began talking inappropriately, but had no other focal neurologic symptoms. He needed to be fed and would just

Initial assessment:

Time	T	P	R	BP	Other:					

Medication orders:

Lab work:

X-ray:

Physician's report:

REVIEW OF SYSTEMS: Mental status is abnormal, as noted above, with the confusion. HEENT: No acute complaints. Respiratory: no cough or shortness of breath noted. Cardiac: negative for symptoms. GI: no nausea or vomiting. He has been eating okay other than trouble self-feeding yesterday. GU: bladder incontinence, which was not improved by the Ditropan XL. Endocrine is negative. Neurologic: some microvascular cerebrovascular disease noted on previous MRI and CT. Also had a carotid Duplex scan that showed no stenosis. Psychiatric: has been unremarkable.

PHYSICAL EXAM: On exam his blood pressure was a little elevated. It has been normal in the past, so that will just be observed. He is smiling, but he is disoriented to real place and time. He has difficulty following directions. He definitely has an abnormal mental status exam. Answers questions inappropriately. Initially couldn't raise up his left hand per my request, I think due to lack of comprehension. Later, when he was ready to go to the nursing home, he was able to do this, but he was moving it spontaneously. His pulse is regular today. It looked like he was in a sinus rhythm. He has a history of a bundle branch block. Respirations were unlabored and he was afebrile. Ears are negative. Pupils are equal and reactive. Extraocular eye movements: intact; fundus looks unremarkable. Oropharynx is unremarkable. Neck: no adenopathy or thyromegaly. He has referred murmurs. Lungs are clear today. Heart is regular with a systolic murmur. Upper sternal border is just slightly to the apex. He had an echocardiogram in the past that showed mild aortic stenosis and regurgitation and mild mitral regurgitation. Abdomen: no masses, organomegaly, or bruits or tenderness. GU: Rectal wasn't done. Upper extremities: spontaneous movement. He had trouble following directions, so it was hard to tell if he had any slight weakness on one side or the other. He had trouble walking, so we didn't really stand him. Lower extremities: just a little bit of pedal edema. Pedal pulses: present. He did move both feet, but he has had weakness too.

Diagnosis:	Physician sign/date
ASSESSMENT: Confusion; abnormal mental status; suspect he has frontal lobe ischemic event. PLAN: His wife cannot take care of him. He doesn't need acute hospital care, so he will be	

Discharge	Transfer	Admit	Good	Satisfactory	Other:

GODFREY REGIONAL HOSPITAL
123 Main Street • Aldon, FL 77714 • (407) 555-1234

Continued

EMERGENCY ROOM RECORD

Name:		Age:	ER physician:
		DOB:	

Allergies/type of reaction:	Usual medications/dosages:
	The wife does not feel it is helping with his bladder control. He used to be on Megace, but his wife says that she brought in all the pills he is on, and that was not enclosed. Tobacco: none for 10 years. Alcohol: none.

Triage/presenting complaint: chew his food and chew his food; this behavior occurred fairly suddenly yesterday and it's still present, and she [his wife] thought he looked odd, so she brought him to the emergency room. He has not been sick recently. No fever, chills, sore throat, or other complaints. PAST MEDICAL HISTORY: Coronary artery disease; episodic atrial fibrillation; rheumatoid arthritis; peptic ulcer disease with positive pylori serology.

Initial assessment:

Time	T	P	R	BP	Other:					

Medication orders:

Lab work:

X-ray:

Physician's report:

His white count was normal, as was his hemoglobin. His BMP was normal. Sodium was 135. A dig. level was fine, and his urine was negative.

Diagnosis:	Physician sign/date
admitted to the nursing home on his present medications except for the Ditropan XL since that was not of benefit. If his blood pressure elevation does not resolve, he will need to be on blood pressure pills also.	

Discharge   Transfer   Admit   Good   Satisfactory   Other:

GODFREY REGIONAL HOSPITAL
123 Main Street • Aldon, FL 77714 • (407) 555-1234

Continued

EMERGENCY ROOM RECORD

Name:		Age:	ER physician:
		DOB:	

Allergies/type of reaction: | **Usual medications/dosages:**

Triage/presenting complaint: | PREVIOUS SURGERIES: Bilateral cataracts; herniorrhaphy; bilateral total knee arthroplasties; meniscectomy of the right knee prior to that; hemorrhoidectomy; TURP; excision of a squamous cell skin cancer, left scalp; basal cell skin cancer from his right ear.

Initial assessment:

Time	T	P	R	BP	Other:					

Medication orders:

Lab work:

X-ray:

Physician's report:

Diagnosis:	Physician sign/date

Discharge   Transfer   Admit   Good   Satisfactory   Other:

GODFREY REGIONAL HOSPITAL
123 Main Street • Aldon, FL 77714 • (407) 555-1234

Continued

EMERGENCY ROOM RECORD

Name:		Age:	ER physician:
		DOB:	

Allergies/type of reaction:	Usual medications/dosages:

Triage/presenting complaint:	FAMILY HISTORY: Father died at age 65 of complications from an MI. Mother died in her 90s of old age. He had a brother die of a cerebral aneurysm. One sister deceased from breast cancer.

SOCIAL HISTORY: He is married and lives with his wife. They have just one child. No grandchildren.

Initial assessment:

Time	T	P	R	BP	Other:					

Medication orders:

Lab work:

X-ray:

Physician's report:

Diagnosis:	Physician sign/date
	Nancy Cauley MD

Discharge	Transfer	Admit	Good	Satisfactory	Other:

GODFREY REGIONAL HOSPITAL
123 Main Street • Aldon, FL 77714 • (407) 555-1234

EXERCISE 16

Level I

EMERGENCY ROOM RECORD

Name:	Age:	ER physician:
	DOB:	

Allergies/type of reaction:	Usual medications/dosages:

Triage/presenting complaint:

S: This is an 84-year-old white female who became suddenly unresponsive. She was witnessed to go down. The attendant at her nursing home immediately called 911. Upon arrival, the ambulance personnel stated that she appeared to be in a fine fibrillation. She was shocked and went

Initial assessment:

O: Upon arrival, she was noted to have excellent pulses with CPR in progress. Rhythm appeared to be initially PEA. This degenerated into asystole. CPR was commenced. We gave one more milligram of epinephrine and this again developed some electrical activity of a very wide complex, but no pulse was generated with this. Because of the extremely poor prognosis with this situation, we opted to cease CPR, having gone through the protocol and generating only PEA.

Time	T	P	R	BP	Other:					

Medication orders:

Lab work:

X-ray:

Physician's report:

P: The patient does have cancer and therefore is not a candidate for organ donation. We inquired about autopsy. I stated that I felt there was no reason that this would need to be done, and the family and the attendant at her nursing home concurred. She has no first-degree relatives, only nieces and nephews. Many of them were present at this time. All lines and tubes were discontinued.

Diagnosis:	Physician sign/date
A: Probable cause of death: acute MI.	

Discharge	Transfer	Admit	Good	Satisfactory	Other:

GODFREY REGIONAL HOSPITAL
123 Main Street • Aldon, FL 77714 • (407) 555-1234

Continued

EMERGENCY ROOM RECORD

Name:		Age:	ER physician:
		DOB:	

Allergies/type of reaction:	Usual medications/dosages:

Triage/presenting complaint: into an asystole, was run through the asystole protocol, and was able to be revived to a PEA but with full-dose atropine and epinephrine 34 and pacing. The best rhythm that could be obtained was a pulseless electrical activity.

Initial assessment:

Time	T	P	R	BP	Other:					

Medication orders:

Lab work:

X-ray:

Physician's report:

Diagnosis:	Physician sign/date
	Robert Rai MD

Discharge	Transfer	Admit	Good	Satisfactory	Other:

GODFREY REGIONAL HOSPITAL
123 Main Street • Aldon, FL 77714 • (407) 555-1234

Level I

OFFICE NOTE

Date:	Vital signs:	T		R	
Chief complaint:		P		BP	

S: Patient presents complaining of headache and dizziness. She woke in the middle of the night and had an episode of dizziness for about 15 minutes. She didn't sleep very well the rest of the night, and this morning she has had a headache on the left-hand side at the occiput and temporal region. She had a stroke in September where she lost half her vision and her right side became numb. This was very transient. She questions whether her left eye might be a little bit blurry but notices no other neurologic symptoms. The vertigo has completely resolved. She has a history of labyrinthitis and a hospitalization for this.

Physical examination:

O: On examination, neurologically, she appears to be intact. Romberg is very steady. Eyes: PERRLA. EOM normal. Ears appear clear. Normal strength upper and lower extremities.

Assessment:

A: Episode of vertigo, possibly labyrinthitis or possibly Ménière's disease, as she did describe a little bit of a pulsatile tinnitus at the time.

Plan:

P: Recommended observation for now. Discussed the headaches as likely being related to tension headaches and to use symptomatic treatment for this. We discussed having meclizine around to use for vertigo, and if she notices any worsening symptoms then she should be reevaluated.

Felix Warden MD

	Patient name:
	DOB:
	MR/Chart #:

GODFREY REGIONAL OUTPATIENT CLINIC
3122 Shannon Avenue • Aldon, FL 77712 • (407) 555-7654

EXERCISE 18

Level II

OFFICE NOTE

Date:	Vital signs:	T	R
Chief complaint:		P	BP

S: Patient presents to the office complaining of increasing shortness of breath. He was having gradually increasing shortness of breath over a long period of time. He had an angiogram a couple of years ago, and he states that his dyspnea has been present since that time. He also has had some episodes of mild chest tightness when he exerts himself, but as soon as he rests, it goes away fairly quickly. He has not been taking his furosemide. He has been taking his other medications as prescribed. He has not seen anybody for this for about two years. He usually follows with a cardiologist for his heart. He has a history of severe coronary artery disease, and the patient states that he has an ejection fraction of about 40 percent.

Examination:

O: On examination, patient appears mildly dyspneic as he arrives. His chest has a few bibasilar crackles. Heart regular rate and rhythm. No rubs, murmurs, or gallops are noted. Heart sounds are somewhat distant. He has a large chest. Abdomen is obese, soft, and nontender. Extremities 1 to 2+ edema at his ankles. We gave him Lasix 20 IV and obtained labs. His EKG showed no acute changes. His chest x-ray showed an enlarged heart but not a lot of fluid in his lung fields. Remainder of his labs were within acceptable limits.

Impression:

A: CHF.

Plan:

P: Patient has stated that the cardiologists have told him that there is not anything more that they can do for his coronary artery disease. We did discuss possibly starting him on a beta blocker for his CHF, but I would recommend follow-up with Cardiology before this is considered. The patient stated he would arrange a follow-up appointment with Cardiology to have this further assessed. We recommended strongly that he go ahead and start his Lasix, 40 mg daily, as prescribed previously. He hasn't been taking this for a very long period of time, with reason being that he doesn't like to void afterwards. We will discharge him to home, and we will have him reassessed on a prn basis if he has increasing dyspnea. Did recommend staying in a cool environment, maintaining adequate hydration, taking his furosemide regularly along with his other medications, and trying to rest as much as possible.

Jay Corm MD

	Patient name:
	DOB:
	MR/Chart #:

GODFREY REGIONAL OUTPATIENT CLINIC
3122 Shannon Avenue • Aldon, FL 77712 • (407) 555-7654

Level I

OFFICE NOTE
_____

Date/time
_____

CHIEF COMPLAINT: Shortness of breath

S:

This is an older gentleman, 79 years old, with COPD, coronary artery disease, and hypertension who had a recent illness and was on Levaquin and prednisone. He has just been off that for a short period of time, and over the last couple of days, he has had more shortness of breath. He has a dry nonproductive cough. No fever, chills, or sore throat. Chest is sore from coughing. No peripheral edema. No angina or other symptoms. Health problems as above. Medications are as listed in his ER record. He is allergic to penicillin.

O:

On exam, 98.9 temp. He is on oxygen chronically. Throat is negative. He has no JVD and no adenopathy. Lungs: He has some bilateral expiratory wheezing and a few rales in the right base. Heart sounds mildly irregular. I don't hear any murmur. Abdomen negative. No peripheral edema. Chest x-ray, I think, shows mostly fibrotic changes.

A:

LRI with an exacerbation of COPD.

P:

He has a nebulizer. He was given Solu-Medrol, 100 mg IV, and Kenalog, 60 mg IM, to boost the steroids. He was given one dose of Levaquin with an Rx for #9 of them at 500 mg one qd. He should return if there is worsening. He was stable at discharge.

Felix Warden MD

GODFREY REGIONAL HOSPITAL
123 Main Street • Aldon, FL 77714 • (407) 555-1234

EXERCISE 20

Level II

OFFICE NOTE

Chief complaint: _____

Date: _____

Vital signs: BP_____ P_____ R_____

History:

S: 76-year-old gentleman presents with a nosebleed. He was seen here this past week for a left nostril epistaxis. It was cauterized, and he has had no problems until today. He started to get a nosebleed about an hour ago, and does not seem to be improving despite pressure.

Exam:

O: On physical exam, he is bleeding extensively from the left nostril. Pressure was applied for 20 minutes. Blood continued to ooze. The area in the left nostril was packed with Neo-Synephrine–soaked cotton pledgets. These were left in for 15 to 20 minutes and the bleeding slowed significantly. Further exam revealed obvious cauterization to the inferior medial nares on the left side over the septum and inferior inspect of the nares. There is active bleeding from the area of prior cauterization.

Diagnosis/assessment:

A: Epistaxis, left nostril.

P: Further silver nitrate was used for cauterization of the bleeding area, and a small amount of cellulose strip was applied to the area, with good clotting noted and no further bleeding. A Merocel nasal tampon was then inserted, and he will return in two days for removal of this. He will return if he has any further bleeding that is not stopped with some minor pressure to the nares.

Willem Obst MD

Patient name: _____

Date of service: _____

GODFREY MEDICAL ASSOCIATES
1532 Third Avenue, Suite 120 • Aldon, FL 77713 • (407) 555-4000

Level I

OFFICE NOTE

Date:	Vital signs:	T	R
Chief complaint:		P	BP

SUBJECTIVE: This 38-year-old man presents with drainage from his right little finger. The patient suffered an injury to the back of his right fingers in an accident 7 days ago. He had the skin partially peeled off, and it has been healing slowly. The other fingers seem to have healed well, but he still has some drainage right at the PIP joint of the little finger. It is sort of orange and reddish, and he is a little concerned about it. He has not noticed a lot of redness or swelling in the area.

Examination:

OBJECTIVE: Temperature 97.8, pulse 64, respiratory 16, BP 102/60.

Shows patient to be alert. The right hand shows good pulses, sensation, and capillary refill. The patient has full range of motion of each finger, including the little finger. At the PIP joint of the back of the little finger, there is an open area with some serosanguineous discharge. No pus is noted. No swelling is noted. No red streaks are noted.

Impression:

Right little finger serosanguineous discharge.

Plan:

Patient was told that this is fairly normal and that it will take time for the joint to heal. He was to rest it and to use soap and water on it. He was to follow up with his physician in 7–10 days if it had not healed. He was to return or see his physician sooner if he developed any redness, swelling, or pus and was discharged home in stable condition.

	Patient name:
	DOB:
	MR/Chart #:

GODFREY REGIONAL OUTPATIENT CLINIC
3122 Shannon Avenue • Aldon, FL 77712 • (407) 555-7654

Continued

OFFICE NOTE

Date:	Vital signs:	T	R
Chief complaint:		P	BP

Past medical history—Smoker
Current medications—Vicodin
Allergies—None
Last tetanus shot was two years ago.

Examination:

Impression:

Plan:

Maurice Doater, MD

Patient name:

DOB:

MR/Chart #:

GODFREY REGIONAL OUTPATIENT CLINIC
3122 Shannon Avenue • Aldon, FL 77712 • (407) 555-7654

EXERCISE 22

Level I

OFFICE NOTE

Date:	Vital signs:	T	R
Chief complaint:		P	BP

SUBJECTIVE: This 43-year-old woman new patient presents complaining of a migraine headache. The patient states that she woke up a little after midnight and started vomiting. She has not been able to keep anything down and rates her pain as an 8 on a 1–10 scale. The pain is behind her right eye and she has photophobia. These are her typical migraine headache problems. Patient has been seen multiple times over the last couple of months for these types of migraine headaches.

Past medical history—Migraine headaches.

Current medications—See nurse's list.

Allergies—See list.

Physical examination:

OBJECTIVE: Temperature 99.1, pulse 64, respiratory 12, BP 116/82.

Shows patient to be alert. HEENT shows pupils equal, round, and reactive to light and accommodation extraocular motion intact. Patient has normal nasal and oral mucosa. Neck is supple without adenopathy. Lungs are clear. Heart is regular rate and rhythm. Abdomen is soft with positive bowel sounds. She is tender diffusely. Extremities show full range of motion. Neurologically, the cranial nerves are grossly intact. The patient has good strength and sensation in all extremities. Normal gait. Glasgow Coma Scale of 15.

Assessment:

Migraine headache.

Plan:

The patient had a saline-lock IV started and was given 10 mg of IV Reglan and 6 mg of IV morphine. She did require another 2 mg of IV morphine, but her headache was much improved. She felt that she could go home and sleep. She was instructed to return if her headache worsened or if she developed any new symptoms.

Felix Wander M

	Patient name:
	DOB:
	MR/Chart #:

GODFREY REGIONAL OUTPATIENT CLINIC
3122 Shannon Avenue • Aldon, FL 77712 • (407) 555-7654

EXERCISE 23

Level II

EMERGENCY ROOM RECORD

Name:		Age:	ER physician:
		DOB:	

Allergies/type of reaction:	Usual medications/dosages:
Aspirin, codeine, and opiates.	

Triage/presenting complaint:

SUBJECTIVE: This 45-year-old woman presents by ambulance unresponsive. The patient reportedly sat down to eat dinner and ate a couple bits of potato. She then seemed to doze off and was snoring. People tried to wake her but they found her to be unresponsive. An ambulance was called, and upon their arrival, they noted her blood sugar to read low. The patient is a known diabetic and on Glucovance and Avandia. They were unable to arouse her and tried to

Initial assessment:

Time	T	P	R	BP	Other:					

Medication orders:

Lab work:

Labs show white blood count of 13,400 with hematocrit of 32.4 and MCV of 71.3. Normal electrolytes, BUN, creatinine, and a glucose of 109. Urine analysis is unremarkable.

X-ray:

Physician's report:

OBJECTIVE: Temperature 97, pulse 76, respiratory 24, blood pressure 18/74. Oxygen saturation is 92 percent on room air.

PHYSICAL EXAM: Shows patient to be unresponsive to even painful stimuli. She will not open her eyes and is snoring. She is breathing well on her own. HEENT shows pupils equal, round, and reactive to light and accommodation extraocular motion intact. Patient has normal nasal and oral mucosa. Neck is supple without adenopathy. Lungs are clear with good breath sounds in all four quadrants. Heart is regular rate and rhythm. Abdomen is soft, nontender with positive bowel sounds. Extremities show pre-tibular edema. Neurologically, the patient was initially unresponsive and snoring. After receiving 1 amp of D-50, she did awaken and returned to her normal state according to her friends.

Diagnosis:	Physician sign/date
ASSESSMENT: 1. Low blood sugar. 2. Microcytic anemia. 3. Possible sleep apnea. PLAN: The patient is not usually on a strict diabetic diet, and her medications have been	

Discharge	Transfer	Admit	Good	Satisfactory	Other:

GODFREY REGIONAL HOSPITAL
123 Main Street • Aldon, FL 77714 • (407) 555-1234

Continued

EMERGENCY ROOM RECORD

Name:		Age:	ER physician:
		DOB:	

Allergies/type of reaction: **Usual medications/dosages:**

Triage/presenting complaint:

give her a little Gluco paste in the mouth. They suctioned her and kept her on oxygen. The patient continued to be unresponsive and was brought to the emergency room.

Past medical history—mental retardation, depression, diabetes.
Current medications—See list.

Initial assessment:

Time	T	P	R	BP	Other:					

Medication orders:

Lab work:

X-ray:

Physician's report:

Diagnosis:	Physician sign/date

adjusted for that type of diet. However, the patient has come up to this area and is now on a fairly strict diet. She probably has not been receiving enough calories and so her blood sugar has become quite low.
She had an IV started and received 1 amp of D-50. She did awaken and became much more alert and responsive. Her friends here state that she is pretty much back to her normal status.

| Discharge | Transfer | Admit | Good | Satisfactory | Other: |

GODFREY REGIONAL HOSPITAL
123 Main Street • Aldon, FL 77714 • (407) 555-1234

Continued

EMERGENCY ROOM RECORD

Name:		Age:	ER physician:
		DOB:	

Allergies/type of reaction:	Usual medications/dosages:

Triage/presenting complaint:

Initial assessment:

Time	T	P	R	BP	Other:					

Medication orders:

Lab work:

X-ray:

Physician's report:

Diagnosis:	Physician sign/date
Her blood count is mildly low and microcytic. This is probably a chronic condition. The patient also appears to be very sleepy at times and may be having some problems with sleep apnea, given her obesity and snoring respirations. A physician from her area is present and will talk to her local doctor about readjusting her medications and doing further work-up for the anemia and sleep apnea problems. She was discharged home in stable condition.	Robert Rai MD

Discharge	Transfer	Admit	Good	Satisfactory	Other:

GODFREY REGIONAL HOSPITAL
123 Main Street • Aldon, FL 77714 • (407) 555-1234

EXERCISE 24

Level I

OFFICE NOTE

Chief complaint: _____

Date: _____

Vital signs: BP_____   P_____   R_____

History:

This 50-year-old man developed epigastric pain radiating into his back 3 days ago after drinking about one six-pack of beer. That night he developed the hiccoughs and did a lot of belching. The next day he slept. Yesterday he felt improved and today he feels much improved. For the past 2 days, there has been no abdominal pain. His appetite has been poor. There has been no nausea or vomiting. His bowel function is regular. He has a history of alcohol abuse with abnormal liver function test. He also has psychiatric illness. He has had no surgery. His regular medications include Xanax and Zyprexa. He is allergic to sulfa.

Exam:

REVIEW OF SYSTEMS: He denies chest pain or palpitations. He has no cough or shortness of breath. There has been no dysuria or increased urinary frequency.

EXAMINATION: Reveals the patient to be alert. He is afebrile. Eyes are clear. Tympanic membranes appear normal. There is no nasal congestion. Mouth is moist. Throat reveals no redness or swelling. The neck is supple with no adenopathy. There is no heart murmur. Lungs are clear. The abdomen is soft and nontender. Bowel tones are active. Lab data include hemoglobin of 16.3; white count is 12,500. Chemistry panel includes calcium of 8.1, albumin is 3.4, bilirubin is 3.4, alkaline phosphatase is 202, AST 212, ALT 102, and sodium 126. Other values are within normal limits. Amylase is 75, CK is 117, and troponin is 0.3. Chest x-ray appears normal. EKG shows sinus rhythm with no acute change.

Diagnosis/assessment:

DIAGNOSIS:
1. Abdominal pain resolved
2. Abnormal liver function test probably secondary to alcoholism

DISPOSITION: Patient is to stay on a light diet. He admits to drinking about 1 six-pack of beer daily and was encouraged to stop drinking alcohol, which he has been able to do in the past. If he develops recurrent abdominal pain, vomiting, fever, or any other problem, he is to return to the office. Otherwise, he will follow up at the VA next week as scheduled. He was given copies of his lab reports.

Jay Corman MD

Patient name: _____

Date of service: _____

GODFREY MEDICAL ASSOCIATES
1532 Third Avenue, Suite 120 • Aldon, FL 77713 • (407) 555-4000

EXERCISE 25

Level II

EMERGENCY ROOM RECORD

| Name: | Age: | ER physician: |
| | DOB: | |

| Allergies/type of reaction: | Usual medications/dosages: |
| None. | Allegra, prednisone, potassium, Prilosec, stool softener, Niferex, Lotensin, Carafate, dapsone, Pamelor, and insulin. |

Triage/presenting complaint:

SUBJECTIVE: This 67-year-old woman presents by ambulance after 2 occurrences of unresponsive episodes. The patient is usually in a nursing home but is visiting a relative. The patient usually goes to bed around 9:00 p.m., but they have been keeping her up tonight and they were getting her to the bathroom at 1:00 this morning. While sitting on the toilet, the patient suddenly became unresponsive and started having a little bit of twitching of her right arm.

Initial assessment:

Time	T	P	R	BP	Other:					

Medication orders:

Lab work:

Laboratories show a normal urinalysis with a white blood count of 14,700 with only 4 bands. Hematocrit is 4.6 with essentially normal electrolytes, BUN, and creatinine. Glucose was 150. CPK was less than 20 and troponin was less than 0.3.

X-ray:

A chest x-ray shows some mild increased heart size and some possible vasculature changes but is pretty much unremarkable.

Physician's report:

OBJECTIVE: Temperature 95.3, pulse 103, respirations 16, and blood pressure 116/66. Oxygen saturation 91% on room air.

PHYSICAL EXAM: Shows patient to be alert. She does not appear in any distress. HEENT shows pupils equal, round, and reactive to light and accommodation. Extraocular motion intact. The patient has normal oral and nasal mucosa. Neck is supple. The lungs are clear with some slight upper airway wheezes. Heart is regular rate and rhythm. Abdomen is soft, nontender with positive bowel sounds. Extremities all show red patches on her legs, which seem to be fading. She does have 11 pretibial edema. EKG shows a sinus tachycardia with no ischemic changes.

| Diagnosis: | Physician sign/date |
| ASSESSMENT: Syncopal episodes

PLAN: The patient usually goes to bed around 9:00 p.m. and takes several medications at night. This includes the Pamelor that makes her very sleepy. I do not feel that the patient had a | |

| Discharge | Transfer | Admit | Good | Satisfactory | Other: | |

GODFREY REGIONAL HOSPITAL
123 Main Street • Aldon, FL 77714 • (407) 555-1234

Continued

EMERGENCY ROOM RECORD

Name:		Age:	ER physician:
		DOB:	

Allergies/type of reaction:	Usual medications/dosages:

Triage/presenting complaint: They were unable to hold her up on the toilet, and after a couple of minutes, she seemed to come around and was completely alert again. They called the ambulance, and upon its arrival, the ambulance personnel noted that she had an unresponsive episode with a very fine tremor of her right arm, which lasted only about a minute. She again became completely responsive afterwards. Her blood sugar was checked and noted to be normal at the scene. She does

Initial assessment:

Time	T	P	R	BP	Other:					

Medication orders:

Lab work:

X-ray:

Physician's report:

Diagnosis:	Physician sign/date

seizure episode, since she did not have any postictal state. I feel it most likely they got her up onto the toilet and that she had a vaso vagal reaction with a short syncopal episode. The patient was mildly hypotensive according to the ambulance personnel, but her blood pressure had come up well in the emergency room. She has been alert and was kept in the emergency

Discharge   Transfer   Admit   Good   Satisfactory   Other:

GODFREY REGIONAL HOSPITAL
123 Main Street • Aldon, FL 77714 • (407) 555-1234

Continued

EMERGENCY ROOM RECORD

Name:		Age:	ER physician:
		DOB:	

Allergies/type of reaction:	Usual medications/dosages:

Triage/presenting complaint: not appear to have any postictal state, and her blood pressure in the ambulance was initially around a systolic of 80. The patient denies any pain and feels completely back to normal in the emergency room. She is acting normally according to her relatives.

Initial assessment:

Time	T	P	R	BP	Other:					

Medication orders:

Lab work:

X-ray:

Physician's report:

Diagnosis:	Physician sign/date

room for over 2 hours. She did not have any more episodes and felt well. She was given an albuterol nebulizer treatment because of the slight wheezes in her lungs, and her oxygen saturation came up to 94% on room air. I feel her elevated white blood count is secondary to the prednisone that she has recently started on because of the rash on her legs. She remained

Discharge   Transfer   Admit   Good   Satisfactory   Other:

GODFREY REGIONAL HOSPITAL
123 Main Street • Aldon, FL 77714 • (407) 555-1234

Continued

EMERGENCY ROOM RECORD

Name:		Age:	ER physician:
		DOB:	

Allergies/type of reaction: **Usual medications/dosages:**

Triage/presenting complaint: Past medical history: Stroke in August 4 years ago, causing left-sided weakness; myocardial infarction 2 years ago; and diabetic.

Initial assessment:

Time	T	P	R	BP	Other:					

Medication orders:

Lab work:

X-ray:

Physician's report:

Diagnosis: **Physician sign/date**

stable in the emergency room, and the family will take her home and have her rest. They were to follow her usual schedule more closely. She was to return if she had any further problems. The patient was discharged home in stable condition.

Nancy Cauley, MD

Discharge   Transfer   Admit   Good   Satisfactory   Other:

GODFREY REGIONAL HOSPITAL
123 Main Street • Aldon, FL 77714 • (407) 555-1234

EXERCISE 26

Level I

OFFICE NOTE

Chief complaint: _____

Date: _____

Vital signs: BP_____ P_____ R_____

History:

SUBJECTIVE: This 69-year-old white female presents after developing left back pain. She feels as if it has come forward somewhat but is indistinct in the anterior part of the chest. The patient states that it is worse after movement and today it began after sleep. She felt it may or may not go into the left arm. It is not associated with diaphoresis, nausea, vomiting, cough, or pleuritic chest pain. She states that the pain is actually in the back. The patient is a smoker and has hypertension. She says she has had her cholesterol checked in the past and it was felt to be normal. There is a positive family history of MI in her brother and there is no diabetes.

Exam:

Temperature 98.8, pulse 76, respiratory 20, blood pressure 175/101. Patient is not in any acute distress. The ears are clear. The throat is clear. The neck is supple. The lungs are clear. The heart is regular. The abdomen is soft, and having the patient sit up, there is perivertebral knot that I can actually push on and elicit the pain on the left side, parallel to the scapula off the vertebral column. She states that this is the discomfort that she is having and this reproduces the pain acutely. Lab work includes white count 10.7, hemoglobin 13.2, hematocrit 39, platelet count 3.6, CK 36; troponin is less then 0.3, sodium 141, potassium 3.3, BUN 15, creatinine 0.7, glucose 88; LFTs are within normal limits. Her chest x-ray shows COPD but no acute pulmonary disease. Her EKG is read as normal sinus rhythm. I do not see any unusual T waves.

Diagnosis/assessment:

IMPRESSION: Muscle strain upper left back

PLAN: She is to take 2 Advil 3 times a day for the next 7 days as needed. We have discussed the application of heat to the area with a heating pad or a heat patch to be used as directed. We have given her some Vicodin for relief of the discomfort, 1/2 to 1 pill po q4h prn for severe pain. We have asked her to follow up with her usual physician in 48 hours as needed. She is to return for any worsening symptoms.

Stany Knartt MD

Patient name: _____

Date of service: _____

GODFREY MEDICAL ASSOCIATES
1532 Third Avenue, Suite 120 • Aldon, FL 77713 • (407) 555-4000

E X E R C I S E 2 7

Level I

OFFICE NOTE

Chief complaint: _____

Date: _____

Vital signs: BP_____ P_____ R_____

History:

This 69-year-old woman was shopping this afternoon when she developed some lower abdominal cramping. She had a bowel movement and appeared to pass some red blood that she estimates at 2–3 teaspoons. She has no abdominal pain at this time. There has been no nausea or vomiting. Four days ago, she was started on iron for upcoming knee surgery. She has a history of acid peptic disease with prior upper GI bleeds. She also has hypertension. Her medications are as listed. She states that she occasionally takes an ibuprofen. She is allergic to penicillin.

Exam:

REVIEW OF SYSTEMS: She denies chest pain or palpitations. There has been no cough or shortness of breath. She has no dysuria or increased urinary frequency. She is a nonsmoker. She does not drink alcohol.

EXAMINATION: Reveals an alert, pleasant woman. Eyes are clear. Tympanic membranes appear normal. There is no nasal congestion. Mouth is moist. Throat reveals no redness or swelling. The neck is supple with no adenopathy. There is no heart murmur. Lungs are clear. The abdomen is soft and nontender. There is no mass. Bowel tones are active. There is a small amount of red blood on the perianal skin. Digital exam reveals good sphincter tone. There is no rectal mass or fissure palpable. Anoscopy shows a small amount of red blood in the anal canal, but no active bleeding or a bleeding site was seen. She is noted to have formed stool that does not appear black or grossly bloody. Lab data includes hemoglobin of 12.7. White count is 9,100.

Diagnosis/assessment:

DIAGNOSIS: Rectal bleeding probably secondary to anal irritation from iron-induced constipation.

DISPOSITION: She is to stop the iron for the next several days and take Surfak bid. She is also to increase her intake of fluids and fiber. If she develops continued rectal bleeding, abdominal pain, vomiting, or any other problem, she is to return to the office. Otherwise, in 2 days she will make telephone contact with her usual physician who was called and agreed with the above plan.

Maurice Doater, MD

Patient name: _____

Date of service: _____

GODFREY MEDICAL ASSOCIATES
1532 Third Avenue, Suite 120 • Aldon, FL 77713 • (407) 555-4000

EXERCISE 28

Level I

OFFICE NOTE

Date:	Vital signs:	T	R
Chief complaint:		P	BP

SUBJECTIVE: This 70-year-old white female apparently fell backwards in a parking lot and hit the crown of her head against a car license plate. She has a 2.5 cm laceration at the crown of the occiput. She had triple-shunted hydrocephalus with surgery in February. She feels that this was not a seizure but more of a misstep. Tetanus shot was 3–4 years ago.

Examination:

Temperature 98. Pulse 90. Respiratory rate 20. Blood pressure 129/68. The site is cleaned and anesthetized with 2 cc 1 percent lidocaine with adequate anesthesia. Three 5-0 Ethilon interrupted sutures are placed to bring the skin together. The edges are well approximated. Patient tolerated the procedure well.

Impression:

2.5 cm scalp laceration

Plan:

Patient is to follow up in 7 days for removal of the stitches or sooner, should they become infected.

William Obst MD

	Patient name:
	DOB:
	MR/Chart #:

GODFREY REGIONAL OUTPATIENT CLINIC
3122 Shannon Avenue • Aldon, FL 77712 • (407) 555-7654

EXERCISE 29

Level I

OFFICE NOTE

Date:	Vital signs:	T	R
Chief complaint:		P	BP

S: Arvin is here for assessment of a laceration. He is a 19-year-old who was involved in a motor vehicle accident approximately 2 hours prior to arrival. He says he was a passenger in the front seat of a car. He was not wearing a seatbelt and was sleeping when the car went into a ditch and hit an approach. He was then thrown forward and hit his head very forcefully on the dashboard. He is not certain if he lost consciousness or not. In any event, he sustained a gaping laceration just inferior to his left eyebrow. He is up to date on his tetanus immunization.

Physical examination:

O: Temperature 95. Pulse 70. Respirations 20. Blood pressure 110/64. In general, Arvin is alert, responsive, smells of alcohol, nontoxic appearing, and in no acute distress. Skin: There is a 3-centimeter total length laceration noted just inferior to the left eyebrow in the upper eye socket. It is quite gaping and fairly deep. It is an L-shaped configuration. No other injuries noted of the head.

HEENT: EOMI without nystagmus. PERRLA.

Assessment:

A: Laceration with layered repair.

Plan:

P: The wound was prepped with Betadine and anesthetized with 1% epinephrine. Four 4-0 Vicryl sutures were placed subcutaneously in the muscle layer to help bring together the edges of the wound. The wound edges were then approximated using eight 5-0 Ethilon sutures. The patient tolerated the procedure well. He was instructed in wound care and to return in a week for suture removal or prn before that if there are any other difficulties.

Maurice Doater, MD

Patient name:
DOB:
MR/Chart #:

GODFREY REGIONAL OUTPATIENT CLINIC
3122 Shannon Avenue • Aldon, FL 77712 • (407) 555-7654

EXERCISE 30

Level I

OFFICE NOTE

Date:	Vital signs: T R
Chief complaint: Back pain. Passed out.	P BP

S: This is a 73-year-old woman who has had back pain since September, and it has been very bad the last couple of days. She woke up this morning with severe back pain, tried going down some stairs, and she got lightheaded. Her husband feels she may have passed out doing this. Therefore they called an ambulance. She does not have chest pain, trouble breathing, or other neurological symptoms. She had fallen off a step in September, and she had had a sort of constant pain in the low back since then, but it has recently been worse as noted above for the past couple of days. She doesn't have pain that goes

Examination:

O: On exam, her vital signs are stable. She is alert and orientated. She has good carotid upstrokes. Lungs are clear. Heart sounds fairly regular, and I don't hear any murmurs. Abdomen is nontender. She has a little bit of tenderness over her right greater trochanter. She says she has pain in this area when she lies on that side. There is a little bit of lower back palpatory tenderness. Straight leg raising is negative. Motor and sensory is intact. Pulses are good. Reflexes are normal. X-rays of her back show anterior slippage of L4 on 5 but no compression fractures.

Impression:

A: Vasovagal episode secondary to acute back pain.

Plan:

P: Discussion. She has a little slippage of the spine vertebrae that is probably causing her back problems. I am not sure how long this slippage has been there. She was given Toradol, 60 mg IM, that gave her some relief, so she was dispensed with Toradol, 10 mg q6h prn pain #30. She should follow up with her physician regarding her back problems.

	Patient name:
	DOB:
	MR/Chart #:

GODFREY REGIONAL OUTPATIENT CLINIC
3122 Shannon Avenue • Aldon, FL 77712 • (407) 555-7654

Continued

OFFICE NOTE

Date:	Vital signs:	T	R
Chief complaint: Back pain. Passed out.		P	BP

into her legs, numbness in the legs, or bladder dysfunction. She has been taking ibuprofen, two twice a day. She had had a headache also from the fall. Medical history includes atrial fibrillation and depression. She is on Lanoxin and Effexor also. She doesn't have allergies. No heart disease other than atrial fibrillation. No diabetes or high blood pressure. Review of systems is otherwise negative.

Examination:

Impression:

Plan:

Willem Obst MD

Patient name:

DOB:

MR/Chart #:

GODFREY REGIONAL OUTPATIENT CLINIC
3122 Shannon Avenue • Aldon, FL 77712 • (407) 555-7654

EXERCISE 31

Level II

OFFICE NOTE

Date:	Vital signs:	T		R	
Chief complaint:		P		BP	

SUBJECTIVE: This 76-year-old woman new patient presents complaining of pain in her left knee. The patient states that she has been having pain in her knee for the last couple of weeks and has had pain in the past. She actually had injections in the left knee for arthritis in January/February of this year. Over the last couple of weeks, she has been having pain off and on, but it became much worse last night. She states that she was at a party last night and had to go up and down stairs frequently. Her knee has become more swollen and painful. She denies any pain in the calf but does have occasional pain

Examination:

OBJECTIVE: Temperature 99.2, pulse 88, respirations 22, blood pressure 170/99.

Shows patient to be alert. The left leg shows good pulses, sensation, and capillary refill in the foot. The patient has good range of motion of the toes and at the ankle. She has pain with full extension and flexion but is able to move the knee fairly well. There is some mild swelling across the knee but no erythema. It is not warm to the touch. She is tender over the top of the knee, more on the lateral aspect than the medial aspect. She does have some tenderness behind the knee, but no cord can be felt. The calf is nontender to palpation and it has a negative Homans' sign. X-rays of the left knee show no fracture. Minimal arthritic changes.

Impression:

Left knee pain

Plan:

It is not clear what is causing the patient's pain, but I feel that a cartilage problem may be the culprit. She was instructed to rest the knee as much as possible and to limit walking. She is to try and take some aspirin as needed and was given some Vicodin to use as needed for pain. She was to follow up with her usual physician to determine if she needs to have the knee injected again or if she needs to see an orthopedic surgeon. She is able to walk on the knee and was discharged home in stable condition.

	Patient name:
	DOB:
	MR/Chart #:

GODFREY REGIONAL OUTPATIENT CLINIC
3122 Shannon Avenue • Aldon, FL 77712 • (407) 555-7654

Continued

OFFICE NOTE

Date:	Vital signs:	T	R
Chief complaint:		P	BP

running down the front of her leg. She denies any numbness of the toes.

Past medical history: Spinal surgery for slipped disk. Injection in left knee. Bladder suspension.

Current medications: aspirin, Aleve, Tylenol, urinary medication.

Allergies: penicillin and labetalol.

Examination:

Impression:

Plan:

Stony Kratt, MD

Patient name:

DOB:

MR/Chart #:

GODFREY REGIONAL OUTPATIENT CLINIC
3122 Shannon Avenue • Aldon, FL 77712 • (407) 555-7654

EXERCISE 32

Level II

OFFICE NOTE

Chief complaint: _____

Date: _____

Vital signs: BP_____ P_____ R_____

History:

SUBJECTIVE: This 77-year-old white female presents to the office for the first time with actually two complaints. She has been having some pubic pressure and increased urinary frequency, which she has noted for the last day without fever. She has a long-standing history of bladder problems and recurrent UTIs and has been treated successfully both with sulfa drugs and fluoroquinolones in the past. She is allergic to Macrodantin. She has not been vomiting or having any unusual fevers. Today, however, she had noticed a large amount of blood after going to the bathroom to urinate. She states that she does have a history of external hemorrhoids and has had a colonoscopy in the past, which was said to be normal 3 years ago. She has not been losing any weight. She is being presently evaluated for angina and is on Coumadin for having a past CVA. She will be having a treadmill test on Wednesday.

Exam:

Patient is not in acute distress. Temperature 97.9, pulse 86, respiratory 18, blood pressure 160/88. The conjunctivae are not pale, and the patient has good facial color. Lungs are clear. The heart is regular. The abdomen is overweight. Bowel sounds are present; unable to palpate any masses. Rectally, the patient has thrombosed external hemorrhoid that looks like it had recently bled. There is no blood in this area at the present time, and there is no active bleeding noted. Anoscopy is performed, and some stool noted at the end of the anoscope; a cotton swab is placed and stool sample is taken. This is found to be heme-negative. Lab work showed white count 10.9, hemoglobin of 13.3, platelet count of 286, INR of 3.0, and urine consistent with a urinary tract infection.

Diagnosis/assessment:

IMPRESSION:
1. External hemorrhoidal bleeding has stopped on its own.
2. UTI

PLAN: Patient is given instructions in hemorrhoidal care and is started on Anusol-HC of 1 prn bid 5–7 days as needed; 14 are given without a refill. We have asked her also to use Tucks as needed. We have in addition started her on Bactrim DS, 1 po bid for 7 days, and have asked her to follow up with her usual physician in 7–10 days. We have explained to her that she may need repeat colonoscopy and that she should discuss this with her physician. She should return for any worsening bleeding.

Maurice Doaters, MD

Patient name: _____

Date of service: _____

GODFREY MEDICAL ASSOCIATES
1532 Third Avenue, Suite 120 • Aldon, FL 77713 • (407) 555-4000

EXERCISE 33

Level II

OFFICE NOTE

Date:	Vital signs:	T	R
Chief complaint:		P	BP

77-year-old white male presents to the office with a history of intermittent feeling of shortness of breath at rest. The patient has recently been treated for stomach discomfort and has been using what sounds like acid reflux medications without effect; in fact, they have made him feel worse. Did not notice any blood in his stools. The patient states that the shortness of breath seems to increase when he takes a deep breath and that there is minimal, at best, pressure in the chest. Patient denies having any chest pain, denies any chest pressure, feels comfortable at the present time, and feels much better since

Examination:

Temperature 97.8, pulse 77, respiratory rate 24, blood pressure 204/108 initially with an O2 saturation of 98%. Rechecking blood pressure dropped to 165/91, and patient does not appear in any acute distress and does not appear in severe respiratory distress. EOMI PERRL. The throat is clear. The neck is supple. I do not see any JVD. There are some crackles noted on the right side greater than the left. There is a faint hint of an S3 but it is intermittent. The abdomen is soft and nontender. Bowel sounds are hypoactive. There is 2+ lower extremity edema on the right side. The left side has a prosthesis. Neurologically, the patient is intact. He is in good spirits. Lab work shows a white count of 6.7, hemoglobin of 11.5, hematocrit 33.6, platelet count 138; sodium is 142, potassium 4.8, BUN is 40, and creatinine is consistent with hospitalization in January. His glucose is 135, his CK is 56, his troponin is 0.3, and his dig is 0.8. His chest x-ray shows some slight increase in fluid on the right side. I do not see any curly B lines. Patient does have a large heart and evidence of chronic CHF, as well as COPD. The

Impression:

CHF, mild

Plan:

We have given him an extra 20 mg of po Lasix right now and have asked him to start taking 1 full pill of Lasix daily until he sees his usual physician on Friday. We have given him copies of his lab work and have asked his wife to check on him through the night to make sure that he is doing OK. Should he have any change, develop increased shortness of breath, or if he develops chest pain, he is to go to the emergency room.

	Patient name:
	DOB:
	MR/Chart #:

GODFREY REGIONAL OUTPATIENT CLINIC
3122 Shannon Avenue • Aldon, FL 77712 • (407) 555-7654

Continued

OFFICE NOTE

Date:	Vital signs:	T	R
Chief complaint:		P	BP

coming to the office. The patient does have a history of significant cardiomegaly, mild diabetes, and a history of catheterization in 1990. He claims he has not smoked since 1970. The patient has a history of amputation of the lower extremity 3 years ago. The patient denies any anginal equivalence in the left arm, burning in the throat, jaw pain, or numbness down either arm.

Examination:

ECG shows normal sinus rhythm with a primary AV block and LVH with ventricular strain consistent with prior ECGs.

Impression:

Plan:

Jay Corm MD

Patient name:

DOB:

MR/Chart #:

GODFREY REGIONAL OUTPATIENT CLINIC
3122 Shannon Avenue • Aldon, FL 77712 • (407) 555-7654

EXERCISE 34

Level I

OFFICE NOTE

Chief complaint: _____

Date: _____

Vital signs: BP_____ P_____ R_____

History:

This 85-year-old woman tripped on some steps and fell, injuring the anterior aspects of both knees. She denies head injury or injury to the neck, back, or chest. She has a history of heart disease. Her medications are as listed and include Coumadin. There is no allergy to medicine.

Exam:

Reveals an alert, pleasant elderly woman. There is swelling and ecchymosis of the anterior aspects of both knees. There is tenderness, particularly on the left. Function and sensation of both feet are intact. X-rays of both knees show a nondisplaced fracture of the left patella.
TREATMENT COURSE: A knee immobilizer was applied to the left leg.

Diagnosis/assessment:

DIAGNOSIS: Non-displaced fracture of left patella

DISPOSITION: She is to wear her immobilizer and elevate the leg with ice. She was given Vicodin that she may take every 4 hours as needed. If she develops increased pain or any other problems, she is to go to the emergency room. She is to see Dr. Connelly on Wednesday.

Patient name:_____

Date of service: _____

GODFREY MEDICAL ASSOCIATES
1532 Third Avenue, Suite 120 • Aldon, FL 77713 • (407) 555-4000

EXERCISE 35

Level I

OFFICE NOTE

Date:		Vital signs:	T		R	
Chief complaint:			P		BP	

SUBJECTIVE: This 85-year-old female new patient presents complaining of blood in her urine. The patient states that she started noticing the blood in her urine last night and it seemed to get quite dark. It has since cleared but she is concerned. She has not had any burning or pain with urination and denies any recent weight loss or illness.

Past medical history: High blood pressure, coronary artery bypass grafting 3 3 six years ago, hysterectomy seven years ago for some type of tumor, which later required radiation therapy, and a pulmonary embolism.

Current medications: Lotensin, warfarin, Zocor, and a depression medication.

Allergies: Possibly Fragmin.

Physical examination:

OBJECTIVE: Temperature 97.6, pulse 78, respirations 18, and blood pressure 176/80.

PHYSICAL EXAM: Shows patient to be alert. She does not appear in any acute distress. HEENT shows pupils equal, round, and reactive to light and accommodation. Extraocular motion intact. The patient has normal oral and nasal mucosa. Neck is supple without adenopathy. The lungs are clear with good breath sounds in all four quadrants. Heart is regular rate and rhythm. Abdomen is soft, nontender, with positive bowel sounds. Back shows no spinal or CVA tenderness. Rectal exam shows heme-negative stool. No hemorrhoids are noted. A urinalysis shows 25 to 50 red blood cells with no white blood cells or bacteria. White blood count is 5.7 with hematocrit of 38.2. INR is 3.0.

Assessment:

Hematuria of unknown cause.

Plan:

The patient does have a history of hysterectomy for a cancer, and it is possible that she may have a bladder tumor. It seems to be clearing at this point, and we will contact her usual physician so that she can follow up with him on an outpatient basis. She is to return if she starts having any pain or worsening of her symptoms. She was to see her physician later this week.

Jay Carson MD

Patient name:
DOB:
MR/Chart #:

GODFREY REGIONAL OUTPATIENT CLINIC
3122 Shannon Avenue • Aldon, FL 77712 • (407) 555-7654

EXERCISE 36

Level I

OFFICE NOTE

Date:	Vital signs:	T	R
Chief complaint: Swollen, painful right leg		P	BP

S: This new patient is a 63-year-old gentleman who, about a week ago, had problems with pain in his right elbow. He developed swelling in his right elbow, as well as swelling in the right knee and calf with some discomfort. He saw his usual physician who felt he had tendinitis. He presented because he has had increased pain and swelling in his calf, and it hurts to bear weight. He has also noticed a little bit of bruising down below his ankle. There is no history of injury. He is on Celebrex, 200 mg daily, as of Wednesday. His health problems are significant for cervical dystonia for which he gets Botox periodically, and he also takes Clonopin and Flexeril. He has no allergies. He has no history of high blood pressure, diabetes, heart disease, GI disease, or urinary problems. He hasn't had any fever, chills, or other symptoms.

Physical examination:

O: He is afebrile. On exam of his elbow, he has just slight loss of full extension, but otherwise good stipulation, pronation. Elbow is nontender, and there is no warmth or redness. Exam of the right knee reveals a little swelling around the knee; it is not hot or red. The popliteal spaces feel symmetrical. He also has pain with squeezing of the calf with some edema in the lower extremity, but not much in the foot. Squeezing the calf is tender and Homans' sign is tender also. Concern was DVT versus Baker's cyst. He was sent for Doppler study, and it showed no DVT, but did confirm a Baker's cyst.

Assessment:

A: Right Baker's cyst

Plan:

P: Discussion. He should use ice, continue with the Celebrex, and follow up with his usual physician to discuss what he would like to do further about the symptomatic problem.

Stony Knatt, MD

Patient name:
DOB:
MR/Chart #:

GODFREY REGIONAL OUTPATIENT CLINIC
3122 Shannon Avenue • Aldon, FL 77712 • (407) 555-7654

EXERCISE 37

Level I

OFFICE NOTE

Date:	Vital signs:	T		R	
Chief complaint:		P		BP	

SUBJECTIVE: This 86-year-old white male with a history of significant COPD presents with chest discomfort and coughing. This began 2 days ago and has become increasingly worse. He states that he has a severe pain with coughing and he can't get the phlegm out; when he does cough, the pain in his chest is worse, and when he is resting, he has no discomfort. He had not been having any fevers, and he does state that he has a tenacious sputum. He is allergic to penicillin and sulfa. He has steroid-dependent COPD.

Physical examination:

Patient does not appear in any acute distress. Temperature is 97.5, pulse 86, respiratory 24, blood pressure 149/84. Oxygen saturation is 94 percent on 2 liters per minute. The ears have wax on the left; right ear is clear. The throat is pink and dry. The patient is not in respiratory distress with breathing. His lungs have diminished breath sounds bilaterally. Rare crackles in the bases. His white count is 8.6, hemoglobin 12.1, platelet 187. Chest x-ray shows no acute pulmonary disease when compared to films from December.

Assessment:

IMPRESSION: Bronchitis with pleurisy.

Plan:

Since the patient is on a steroid at present, it will be inappropriate to treat him with a non-steroidal. Because of his discomfort with his cough, we will go ahead and start him on Tylenol #3,1 po q6h prn severe cough only. We have given him 5 and gave him another prescription for 8. He has Tessalon pearls at home, and I have asked him to use as directed by his physician. If he is having trouble with the cough, then he is to use the Tylenol with codeine, but he is not to use it every 6 hours, only as needed. We have started him on Levaquin at 500 mg p.o. QD, and we have given him a 7-day course. We have asked him to follow up with his primary care doctor in 3 days. He is to return for any worsening symptoms.

Willem Obt MD

Patient name:
DOB:
MR/Chart #:

GODFREY REGIONAL OUTPATIENT CLINIC
3122 Shannon Avenue • Aldon, FL 77712 • (407) 555-7654

EXERCISE 38

Level I

OFFICE NOTE

Date:	Vital signs:	T	R
Chief complaint:		P	BP

HISTORY: This 86-year-old woman slipped in the shower and fell, injuring her right wrist last evening. During the night she rolled out of the bed and seemed to re-injure the wrist. This morning she has increased pain and swelling. She has a history of heart disease with a pacemaker and hypertension. Her medications are as listed. There is no allergy to medicine.

Physical examination:

Reveals an alert, pleasant elderly woman. There is swelling and tenderness of the right wrist. The skin is intact. Function and sensation of the right hand are intact. X-rays of the right wrist show a non-displaced fracture of the distal radius. There is good capillary refill.

TREATMENT COURSE: A short-arm fiberglass splint was applied.

Assessment:

DIAGNOSIS: Non-displaced fracture to distal right radius

Plan:

DISPOSITION: She is to leave the splint in place. She will elevate the wrist with ice. She may take Tylenol as needed. She was given Darvocet that she may take for more severe pain. If she develops increased pain, weakness, or numbness of the hand or any other problems, she is to go to the emergency room; otherwise, in about 10 days she will follow up with her usual physician.

Jay Coram MD

Patient name:
DOB:
MR/Chart #:

GODFREY REGIONAL OUTPATIENT CLINIC
3122 Shannon Avenue • Aldon, FL 77712 • (407) 555-7654

EXERCISE 39

Level I

EMERGENCY ROOM RECORD

Name:	Age:	ER physician:
	DOB:	

Allergies/type of reaction:	Usual medications/dosages:

Triage/presenting complaint:	HISTORY: This 86-year-old woman was seen in this ER five days ago with a fractured right radius. Her splint has become loose and is irritating her arm. Her medications are as listed. There is no allergy to medicine. The splint was removed. There is ecchymosis of the distal forearm. The skin is intact.

Initial assessment:

Time	T	P	R	BP	Other:					

Medication orders:

Lab work:

X-ray:

Physician's report:

TREATMENT COURSE: A fiberglass short-arm splint was reapplied.

Diagnosis:	Physician sign/date
Fracture, right radius. DISPOSITION: She is to keep the splint clean and dry. If she develops increased pain or any other problem, she is to go to the emergency room; otherwise, she plans to follow up with her regular physician next week after returning home.	*Nancy Caully* MD
Discharge Transfer Admit Good Satisfactory Other:	

GODFREY REGIONAL HOSPITAL
123 Main Street • Aldon, FL 77714 • (407) 555-1234

Level II

OFFICE NOTE

Date:	Vital signs:	T	R
Chief complaint:		P	BP

SUBJECTIVE: This 87-year-old white male with a history of a PE and a DVT and recently treated in May presents after 3 episodes of emesis and low blood pressure at a nursing home. In review of his recent chart, it seems as if his blood pressure varies anywhere from 80 to 120. He has not been having any fevers, and the patient himself offers no complaints. He is on digitalis. The patient denies any chest pain, shortness of breath, or abdominal discomfort. He has been able to pass gas, and while here, he has been able to drink fluids.

Examination:

Temperature is 97.8, respiration is 18, blood pressure 84/56 lying down and 86/58 when sitting up. His pulse remains unchanged at 62. Patient is perfectly alert. His lungs are clear. His heart is regular. His abdomen is soft, and I do not appreciate any pulsatile mass or abdominal mass in the belly. Rectal exam shows unformed almost watery stool, and it is heme-negative. There is no lower extremity swelling. His skin color is pink in the face, and he seems alert and is using both hands to drink water. White count is 7.9, hemoglobin 11.1, platelet count 266, his amylase is 147, his sodium is 129, potassium is 4.1, BUN 66 and 2.5; these are consistent with previous lab values from May except for the sodium. Glucose is 106, his chloride is 89; his urine is clear without evidence of ketones or blood.

Impression:

Vomiting; possible gastroenteritis.

Plan:

Liberal use of fluids recommended. Follow up in 1 to 2 days. We have obtained a dig level, which is less than 0.3. We have asked the nursing home to contact his usual physician with that result.

Felix Warden MD

Patient name:
DOB:
MR/Chart #:

GODFREY REGIONAL OUTPATIENT CLINIC
3122 Shannon Avenue • Aldon, FL 77712 • (407) 555-7654

EXERCISE 41

Level I

OFFICE NOTE

Date:	Vital signs:	T	R
Chief complaint:		P	BP

HISTORY: This 88-year-old new patient was lifting a pan, which fell on her right hand. She does have osteoporosis. Her medications are as listed. Her allergies are also as listed.

Physical examination:

Reveals an alert, pleasant elderly woman. There is ecchymosis and tenderness of the base of the proximal phalanx of the right middle finger. The skin is intact. Motion of the finger is limited. Sensation is intact. There is good capillary refill. X-rays of the right hand show no fracture.

Assessment:

DIAGNOSIS: Contusion, right hand.

Plan:

DISPOSITION: She is to elevate the hand with ice. She may take ibuprofen as needed. If she develops increased pain or any other problem she is to follow up with her usual physician.

Maurice Doater, MD

	Patient name:
	DOB:
	MR/Chart #:

GODFREY REGIONAL OUTPATIENT CLINIC
3122 Shannon Avenue • Aldon, FL 77712 • (407) 555-7654

EXERCISE 42

Level I

OFFICE NOTE

Date:	Vital signs:	T	R
Chief complaint:		P	BP

SUBJECTIVE: This 88-year-old woman presents complaining of feeling that her pessary has slipped. The patient states that she was wiping herself after urinating when she felt it a little funny. She feels that it has slipped down a little bit, but has not had any problems urinating or any prolapse of her bladder. She did have some problems lubricating the area today. No unusual discharge. She states that it was just cleaned and reinserted three days ago.
Past medical history—Hard of hearing, depression, and breast cancer.
Current medications—See nurse's notes.
Allergies—penicillin, Macrodantin, and sulfa.

Examination:

OBJECTIVE: Pulse 64, respirations 16, and blood pressure 160/86.
Shows patient to be alert. The abdominal exam shows the abdomen to be soft, nontender with positive bowel sounds. Pelvic exam shows the pessary to be back into the vaginal area with no unusual discharge or redness. It can be felt to be in fairly good position and will not push back at all.

Impression:

ASSESSMENT: Irritation from the pessary.

Plan:

It is not clear what type of pessary the patient uses, but it does feel different to her. It is possible it has slipped somewhat or it is in a slightly different location than she is used to. She was told to watch for any pain or problems with urination and to return if she had any of these problems. She was to continue to try to use her lubricant and to follow up with her usual physician in the next 1 to 2 days if she still felt that it just wasn't right. She was discharged home in stable condition.

Felix Wardin M

	Patient name:
	DOB:
	MR/Chart #:

GODFREY REGIONAL OUTPATIENT CLINIC
3122 Shannon Avenue • Aldon, FL 77712 • (407) 555-7654

EXERCISE 43

Level II

OFFICE NOTE

Date:	Vital signs:	T	R
Chief complaint:		P	BP

HISTORY: This 90-year-old man who is a resident of a nursing home presents with a 2-day history of intermittent left lateral chest pain, which varies with respiration. He has an occasional nonproductive cough but denies increased shortness of breath. There has been no injury to the chest. He has a history of coronary artery disease with congestive heart failure and COPD. His medications are as listed. He is allergic to Vancenase.

Physical examination:

REVIEW OF SYSTEMS: He denies anterior chest pain or palpitations. His appetite has been good. He has no abdominal pain. His bowel function is regular. He had a large bowel movement today. There has been no dysuria or increased urinary frequency.

EXAMINATION: Reveals the patient to be afebrile. He is alert. Eyes are clear. Tympanic membranes appear normal. There is no nasal congestion. Mouth is moist. Throat reveals no redness or swelling. The neck is supple with no adenopathy. There is no heart murmur. Lungs are clear. The abdomen is soft and nontender. There is no chest wall tenderness. There is 1+ pitting edema of both lower legs. There is no calf tenderness. Lab data include hemoglobin of 12.5; white count is 6300. Chemistry panel includes a BUN of 29 and other values are within normal limits. D–dimer is positive. ECG shows what appears to be atrial fibrillation with a ventricular rate on right of 56. There are no acute changes. Chest x-ray shows COPD but no active pulmonary disease.

Assessment:

DIAGNOSIS: Pleuritic left chest pain

Plan:

DISPOSITION: He is to continue his regular medications. He may take Tylenol as needed. If he develops increased pain, shortness of breath, fever, or any other problem, he is to go to the emergency room; otherwise, he will follow up with his usual physician next week regarding further evaluation. The above was discussed with patient and his son.

Jay Corzine MD

	Patient name:
	DOB:
	MR/Chart #:

GODFREY REGIONAL OUTPATIENT CLINIC
3122 Shannon Avenue • Aldon, FL 77712 • (407) 555-7654

Level I

OFFICE NOTE

Chief complaint: _____

Date: _____

Vital signs: BP_____ P_____ R_____

History:

SUBJECTIVE: This 92-year-old man presents complaining of a rash. The patient was sent over from a nursing home because he started having a rash on his face and on both thighs. He started with this rash 2 to 3 days ago, but it seems to be getting a little worse on the face today. The patient states that he is not having any pain or itching in the areas and has not had any fevers. Denies any difficulty breathing or shortness of breath.

Past medical history: Dementia, anemia, TURP, and hard of hearing.

Current medications: Paxil, Metamucil, and vitamin B12.

Allergies: none.

Exam:

OBJECTIVE: Temperature 97.1, pulse 70, respirations 18, and blood pressure 190/84.

PHYSICAL EXAM: Shows patient to be alert. He seems to be answering questions fairly well. HEENT shows pupils equal, round, and reactive to light and accommodation. Extraocular motion intact. The patient has normal oral and nasal mucosa. There is a pink ring around the eyes and on the sides of the cheeks and down onto just below the mouth. It is slightly swollen. Neck is supple without adenopathy. The lungs are clear. Heart is regular rate and rhythm. Abdomen is soft, nontender with positive bowel sounds. Extremities all show good range of motion and pulses. The skin only shows the rash on the face and also a deep red rash that is flat on both anterior thighs. These are large rashes with a large red patch. They do not have any areas of tenderness. Laboratories show white blood count of 5.5 with hematocrit of 32.8.

Diagnosis/assessment:

ASSESSMENT: Rash of unknown etiology

PLAN: The patient does not appear to be itching at the area, and I do not feel it is an allergic type of reaction. It appears to be more of an edema on the face but not on the legs. They seem to be 2 different types of rashes. There does not appear to be any type of infection, and at this point the patient will be tried on prednisone on a declining dose over the next 7 days. He does not appear to be in any respiratory distress, and they were to watch closely for any difficulty breathing. He was to follow up with his physician in 2 days to evaluate whether or not he will require a dermatologic consult or if his physician can determine what is going on with his rash. The patient was discharged home in stable condition.

Jay Corm mo

Patient name: _____

Date of service: _____

GODFREY MEDICAL ASSOCIATES
1532 Third Avenue, Suite 120 • Aldon, FL 77713 • (407) 555-4000

EXERCISE 45

Level I

OFFICE NOTE

Date:	Vital signs:	T		R	
Chief complaint:		P		BP	

HISTORY: This 56-year-old man, who lives in a CBRF, this morning was noted to have swelling of his legs. There has been no injury. Patient has Down syndrome, Alzheimer's disease, and a seizure disorder. His medications are as listed. There is no allergy to medicine. He is nonverbal and unable to give any history.

Physical examination:

Eyes are clear. TMs appear normal. There is no nasal congestion. Mouth is moist. Throat reveals no redness or swelling. The neck is supple. There is no adenopathy. Heart rhythm is regular. There is no murmur. Lungs are clear. The abdomen is obese but soft with no apparent tenderness. There is edema of both lower legs, worse on the left. There is no apparent calf tenderness or palpable cord. Lab data include hemoglobin of 14.6; white count is 5000. Chemistry panel includes alkaline phosphatase of 169; other values are within normal limits. EKG shows sinus rhythm with no acute change. Chest x-ray shows no active pulmonary disease. Venous Doppler of the left leg appears normal.

Assessment:

DIAGNOSIS: Leg swelling

Plan:

DISPOSITION: Staff will restrict the patient's salt intake and recommend he elevate his legs when sitting. If they note increased swelling, discoloration, fever, or any other problem, he is to be sent to the emergency room or follow up with his usual physician.

Stany Kravtt, MD

	Patient name:
	DOB:
	MR/Chart #:

GODFREY REGIONAL OUTPATIENT CLINIC
3122 Shannon Avenue • Aldon, FL 77712 • (407) 555-7654

EXERCISE 46

Level II

OFFICE NOTE

Chief complaint: _____

Date: _____

Vital signs: BP_____ P_____ R_____

History:

S: This 67-year-old female new patient presents with a complaint of neck discomfort, right knee discomfort, left ankle discomfort, and an abrasion on her nose after she fell out of bed this evening. She was asleep after going to bed at approximately 11:00 p.m. and was evidently having a nightmare. Her husband noted that she was screaming. She fell to the floor as she was attempting to get out of bed. She immediately woke up and was alerted to the situation and was able to stand to her feet and come to the clinic. She is mainly concerned about her neck pain.

Exam:

O: On physical exam, she is afebrile. Pulse is 90. Respirations 22. Blood pressure 169/104. Her pulse is 90. She is in no obvious distress, other than some abrasions and some bruises noted. She has a mildly stiff neck. Pupils are equal, round, and reactive to light and accommodating. Extraocular muscles are intact. Funduscopic exam is grossly normal. She has a small abrasion over her nose. There is no nasal crepitus. There is no zygomatic crepitus noted. There is no obvious tooth damage. She has no bite marks on her tongue or inside her mouth. There are no lesions in the throat. Neck is supple with no lymphadenopathy. No palpable thyroid abnormalities. She has stiffness over the posterior aspect. No specific exquisite tender points. She exhibits fairly normal range of motion in flexion, extension, side bending, and rotation. Sensation in the arms is normal. Deep tendon reflexes normal throughout. No obvious wrist, elbow, or shoulder injury. She has a large bruise on her right wrist from an IV today. She did have a colonoscopy today and was given midazolam and meperidine for sedation earlier today. Chest reveals normal lung sounds and normal heart sounds. No thoracic or lumbar tenderness to palpation. She exhibits normal thoracic and lumbar range of motion. Her gait is unaffected and normal. Hips are without crepitus and specific pain. She has had some chronic right hip pain but nothing new since her fall tonight. Lower extremities reveal a bruise over the medial aspect of the right knee. She exhibits normal range of motion with normal weightbearing, however. She has a skin abrasion and contusion of the left lower extremity just superior to the ankle. She exhibits normal range of motion of the ankle and normal weightbearing as well.

Diagnosis/assessment:

A: 1. Questionable night terror—evidently husband states she has had several episodes of this in the past. Initially, it was thought that maybe some of her symptoms were due to her sedation for her colonoscopy; however, her husband states that this has happened frequently over the last couple of years. 2. Contusion, right medial knee. 3. Skin abrasion and contusion, left lower extremity superior to the ankle. 4. Abrasion of the nose.

P: Ice to affected areas. Rest. Follow-up with her usual physician. A sleep study may need to be considered if this has been a chronic issue for her. Any further symptoms, headaches, or worsening neck pain should result in another visit to the physician.

Willem Obst MD

Patient name: _____

Date of service: _____

GODFREY MEDICAL ASSOCIATES
1532 Third Avenue, Suite 120 • Aldon, FL 77713 • (407) 555-4000

EXERCISE 47

Level II

EMERGENCY ROOM RECORD

Name:	Age:	ER physician:
	DOB:	

Allergies/type of reaction:	Usual medications/dosages:

Triage/presenting complaint:

HISTORY OF INJURY
Patient is a 65-year-old male brought in by EMS in a full code. Apparently, he was working on converting a pickup truck to a dump trunk. The dump truck box, weighing at least 2000 pounds, fell off a forklift onto him. He was curled up. There was anywhere from 8 to 12 minutes before anything was done. They got him intubated right away, put in an interosseous IV, and were

Initial assessment:

Time	T	P	R	BP	Other:					

Medication orders:

Lab work:

X-ray:

Physician's report:

He had an obvious open fracture of the right lower leg, an open fracture of the right forearm, deformity of his left forearm, and also left upper arm had a deformity with obvious fracture. CPR was continued. A needle thoracentesis was performed in the right second intercostal space midclavicular line with no release of air. However, a serous and bloody fluid was obtained from this needle.

The patient was repeated epinephrine 3 mg IV x 2 and atropine 1 mg IV with no real response. He had no pulse. He was in asystole and then also did get some mild electrical activity, but no pulse was obtained. Chest x-ray showed whiteout of the left lung, and the right thorax had multiple rib fractures in multiple locations of each rib with probable fluid in the right lung also. White count was 2.82; hemoglobin was 14.4, hematocrit 42.0. The endotracheal tube was in good position. Patient had no response to all this, and with the multiple trauma, the code was stopped at 0941 with no cardiorespiratory effort. After the patient was moved, there was also obvious damage to the posterior skull area just above the C-spine.

Diagnosis:	Physician sign/date
ASSESSMENT Cardiopulmonary arrest secondary to multiple trauma	

Discharge	Transfer	Admit	Good	Satisfactory	Other:

GODFREY REGIONAL HOSPITAL
123 Main Street • Aldon, FL 77714 • (407) 555-1234

Continued

EMERGENCY ROOM RECORD

Name:	Age:	ER physician:
	DOB:	

Allergies/type of reaction:	Usual medications/dosages:

Triage/presenting complaint: doing CPR before he arrived here. He had received 2 mg of epinephrine and 2 mg of atropine through the interosseus IV. Initially, the paramedic said he was in a PEA with no pulse, and he was not breathing on arrival here. His pupils were fixed and dilated. He had an obvious laceration head injury to the right side of his head. C-collar was in place. His chest had obvious deformity with CPR. Right side appeared to be flail chest. Breath sounds were heard bilaterally,

Initial assessment:

Time	T	P	R	BP	Other:					

Medication orders:

Lab work:

X-ray:

Physician's report:

Diagnosis:	Physician sign/date

PLAN
The family was notified. He may be a corneal donor. The coroner was also notified. There were obvious multiple crush injuries to this patient including head and chest;

Discharge	Transfer	Admit	Good	Satisfactory	Other:	

GODFREY REGIONAL HOSPITAL
123 Main Street • Aldon, FL 77714 • (407) 555-1234

Continued

EMERGENCY ROOM RECORD

Name:		Age:	ER physician:
		DOB:	

Allergies/type of reaction:	Usual medications/dosages:

Triage/presenting complaint:	however, decreased bilaterally with lots of crackles bilaterally. There were no heart sounds. Abdomen was soft. No masses were palpable. There was no response whatsoever neurologically.

Initial assessment:

Time	T	P	R	BP	Other:					

Medication orders:

Lab work:

X-ray:

Physician's report:

Diagnosis:	Physician sign/date
and on chest x-ray, his heart also appeared to have a different shape than usual. With the severe rib injuries, there probably were intraabdominal injuries also—liver and possibly spleen.	*Robert Rai MD*
Discharge Transfer Admit Good Satisfactory Other:	

GODFREY REGIONAL HOSPITAL
123 Main Street • Aldon, FL 77714 • (407) 555-1234

E X E R C I S E   4 8

Level II

EMERGENCY ROOM RECORD

Name:		Age:	ER physician:
		DOB:	

Allergies/type of reaction:	Usual medications/dosages:
States it was like "penmycin," which maybe was a penicillin or erythromycin.	Prevacid

Triage/presenting complaint:	HISTORY OF PRESENT ILLNESS: Michael presents to the ER with complaints of pain now for the past few days. He has had flu-like symptoms for some days, with achy joints and feeling feverish, has had sweats, some chills. About two weeks ago, he had cough and cold symptoms, which seemed to be getting a little bit better now. He started with fatigue and symptoms mentioned above. He vomited a few times but hasn't had any vomiting the last few days.

Initial assessment:

Time	T	P	R	BP	Other:					

Medication orders:

Lab work:	CBC shows a normal white count, and his liver enzymes are markedly elevated. We'll get an amylase on him; it is pending at this time.

X-ray:

Chest x-ray is unremarkable.

Physician's report:

REVIEW OF SYSTEMS: As noted in the HPI

PHYSICAL EXAMINATION:

VITALS: He is afebrile. BP is stable

HEENT: TMs normal; oral mucosa is pink and moist; throat is pink and moist, no exudate.

NECK: supple, no adenopathy. Negative carotid bruits.

LUNGS: clear

CARDIAC: Rate and rhythm is regular. No murmurs, clicks, or rubs.

ABDOMEN: Has good bowel sounds in all four quadrants. He has had no tenderness, no rebound, or guarding. No organomegaly or masses.

BACK: He has no spinal or CVA tenderness.

EXTREMITIES: intact. He has a trace of edema on the left lower extremity.

Diagnosis:	Physician sign/date
ASSESSMENT: Elevated liver enzymes with upper abdominal pain; probable cholelithiasis. PLAN: We'll go ahead and admit him to the hospital and get an ultrasound in the morning.	

Discharge	Transfer	Admit	Good	Satisfactory	Other:	

GODFREY REGIONAL HOSPITAL
123 Main Street • Aldon, FL 77714 • (407) 555-1234

Continued

EMERGENCY ROOM RECORD

Name:	Age:	ER physician:
	DOB:	

Allergies/type of reaction:	Usual medications/dosages:

Triage/presenting complaint:	He has been passing gas, and he has had diarrhea earlier this week. He has had no firm stool yesterday and today, but he is passing gas as mentioned. He has had no urinary symptoms, no frequency, urgency, dysuria, or hematuria. He has had no noted changes in his stools as far as blood. He has some back discomfort, which is rather generalized underneath the ribs and goes around to the abdomen. He appears not SOB, and he has not had chest pain. The

Initial assessment:

Time	T	P	R	BP	Other:					

Medication orders:

Lab work:

X-ray:

Physician's report:

Diagnosis:	Physician sign/date

| Discharge | Transfer | Admit | Good | Satisfactory | Other: | |

GODFREY REGIONAL HOSPITAL
123 Main Street • Aldon, FL 77714 • (407) 555-1234

Continued

EMERGENCY ROOM RECORD

Name:		Age:	ER physician:
		DOB:	

Allergies/type of reaction:	Usual medications/dosages:

Triage/presenting complaint: cough seems to be a little bit better at this time.
PAST MEDICAL HISTORY: He has had previous fracture of the left extremity and status-post fracture. After taking anti-inflammatories, developed some GI problems and he has been on Prevacid since then.

Initial assessment:

Time	T	P	R	BP	Other:					

Medication orders:

Lab work:

X-ray:

Physician's report:

Diagnosis:	Physician sign/date
	Robert Rai MD
Discharge Transfer Admit Good Satisfactory Other:	

GODFREY REGIONAL HOSPITAL
123 Main Street • Aldon, FL 77714 • (407) 555-1234

EXERCISE 49

Level I

OFFICE NOTE

Chief complaint: _____

Date: _____

Vital signs: BP_____ P_____ R_____

History:

S: Patient presents with complaints of chest pain. He states that he had a single-vessel bypass with internal mammary done in April three years ago. He had been doing fairly well on his medical regimen until about two months ago, when he started having some twinges of chest pain with exertion. This has been gradually worsening over the last 2 months, and now he gets chest pain when he is doing outdoor activities, activities in the heat, or indoor activities such as vacuuming. As soon as he rests, the pain goes away. Upon arrival, his pain resolved with just lying down and putting on O2. This pain has been coming and going and has not been persistent.

Exam:

O: Chest clear. Heart regular rate and rhythm without murmurs. EKG showed only some nonspecific STT-wave changes, no evidence of an acute MI. Chest x-ray also appeared to be clear.

Diagnosis/assessment:

A: Chest pain, appears to be stable worsening angina.

P: Discussed with Cardiology. After discussion, we recommended to the patient to stop his Norvasc, start him on metoprolol, 250 mg Zlx tab bid, for now, and then probably increase him to a full tablet bid, titrating up as he tolerates it, and start him on Imdur, 30 mg qd. Prescriptions were given for these. Recommended follow-up in about a week with his regular physician. Recheck sooner if he has any chest pain that comes on at rest. Recommended against any exertional activity at this time until we can find out how the medications work for him.

Maurice Doater, MD

Patient name: _____

Date of service: _____

GODFREY MEDICAL ASSOCIATES
1532 Third Avenue, Suite 120 • Aldon, FL 77713 • (407) 555-4000

EXERCISE 50

Level I

EMERGENCY ROOM RECORD

Name:		Age:	ER physician:
		DOB:	

Allergies/type of reaction:	Usual medications/dosages:

Triage/presenting complaint:	HISTORY: 77-year-old man, at about 8:30 tonight, was eating a piece of steak that hung up in his lower esophagus. Since then, he has been unable to drink water without regurgitating. He

has a long history of similar esophageal obstruction that usually resolves spontaneously. He had one prior EGD about 6 years ago. He has a past history of repair of an abdominal aortic aneurysm complicated by a BK amputation on the right because of an embolus. His medications include Persantine and Coumadin. There is no allergy to medicine.

Initial assessment:

Time	T	P	R	BP	Other:					

Medication orders:

Lab work:	Lab data include a hemoglobin of 15.2; white count is 10,800. Chemistry panel includes a glucose of 164. Other values are within normal limits. INR is 3.4.

X-ray:	Chest x-ray shows no active pulmonary disease.

Physician's report:

REVIEW OF SYSTEMS: He denies chest pain or palpitations. He has no cough or shortness of breath. He denies abdominal pain. His bowel function is regular. He has no dysuria.

EXAMINATION: Reveals an alert, pleasant, elderly gentleman. Eyes are clear. TMs appear normal. There is no nasal congestion. Mouth is moist. Throat reveals no redness or swelling. The neck is supple with no adenopathy. Heart rhythm is regular. There is no murmur. Lungs are clear. The abdomen is soft and nontender. EKG shows sinus rhythm and appears normal.

EMERGENCY ROOM COURSE: A saline lock was inserted. He was given 1 mg of glucagon intravenously. He was observed for approximately one hour and was still unable to swallow water without regurgitating.

Diagnosis:	Physician sign/date
Esophageal obstruction. DISPOSITION: Endoscopist called to perform EGD and foreign body removal.	*Robert Rai MD*

Discharge	Transfer	Admit	Good	Satisfactory	Other:

GODFREY REGIONAL HOSPITAL
123 Main Street • Aldon, FL 77714 • (407) 555-1234

EXERCISE 51

Level I

OFFICE NOTE

Chief complaint: _____

Date: _____

Vital signs: BP_____ P_____ R_____

History:

This 82-year-old woman, who is a nursing home resident, noted throat irritation after swallowing her pills this morning. For months she has noted shortness of breath in the morning. Her breathing improves over the course of the day. She has no cough or sputum production. She takes nebulized albuterol twice daily. She also has a longstanding history of bladder pressure and feeling that her bladder is not emptying. She also has arthritic pain. She had taken a brief course of Celebrex with significant relief but has now run out. There is a history of cerebral palsy with spasticity. She is known to have an abdominal aneurysm and has chronic anxiety. Her medications are as listed. There is no allergy to medicine.

Exam:

Reveals an alert, pleasant elderly woman. Eyes are clear. Mouth is moist. Throat reveals no redness or swelling. The neck is supple with no adenopathy. There is no heart murmur. Lungs are clear. The abdomen is soft and nontender. There is no bladder distension. There is no calf tenderness or ankle edema. Lab data include a hemoglobin of 12.5; white count is 6600. Urinalysis is negative. Chest x-ray shows COPD but no infiltrate or congestive heart failure.

TREATMENT COURSE: The patient was initially seen by another physician who prescribed Mylanta with Xylocaine that seemed to soothe her throat. She had no difficulty swallowing water. After voiding, a Foley catheter was inserted, and no significant residual urine was found.

Diagnosis/assessment:

1. Throat irritations
2. COPD
3. Neurogenic bladder
4. Degenerative arthritis

DISPOSITION: She is to continue her medications. Her Celebrex, 100 mg bid, was refilled. She and her daughter were told that if she continues to have difficulty swallowing, she will need a barium swallowing study. If she has increased difficulty swallowing, she is to follow up with her personal physician.

Stny Knatt MD

Patient name: _____

Date of service: _____

GODFREY MEDICAL ASSOCIATES
1532 Third Avenue, Suite 120 • Aldon, FL 77713 • (407) 555-4000

EXERCISE 52

Level II

EMERGENCY ROOM RECORD

Name:	Age:	ER physician:
	DOB:	

Allergies/type of reaction:	Usual medications/dosages:

Triage/presenting complaint:	CHIEF COMPLAINT: Collapse

SUBJECTIVE: This gentleman has a long history of bad disease. He has been known to have ischemic coronary disease, dysrhythmia, COPD, and diabetes. He has been on oxygen and multiple medications. There is a standing health care power of attorney, and advanced directives are written in his chart where he clearly states he would not want any heroic treatments, just

Initial assessment:

Time	T	P	R	BP	Other:					

Medication orders:

Lab work:

X-ray:

Physician's report:

On arrival to the emergency room, he had no palpable pulse or blood pressure. His rhythm complex showed a slow neuro complex QRS. Without a pulse, he was judged to be in pulseless CIA. He was given atropine and then epinephrine and his pulse did speed up and was palpable. He then went back into V fib and was re-shocked. He then went back into V tachycardia and was shocked. Approximately 50 minutes after the arrest with recurrent V tachycardia, V fibrillation, and with no response to treatment, efforts were called. He had dilated fixed pupils. He was judged expired at approximately 0945.

Diagnosis:	Physician sign/date
ASSESSMENT: Expired. Cause of death likely myocardial infarction and contributing factors of longstanding coronary disease, intermittent dysrhythmias, COPD, and diabetes. PLAN: Appropriate notifications.	

Discharge	Transfer	Admit	Good	Satisfactory	Other:

GODFREY REGIONAL HOSPITAL
123 Main Street • Aldon, FL 77714 • (407) 555-1234

Continued

EMERGENCY ROOM RECORD

Name:		Age:	ER physician:
		DOB:	

Allergies/type of reaction:	Usual medications/dosages:

Triage/presenting complaint:	comfort care only. Today he was out feeding chickens without his oxygen on and collapsed. There was apparently some response initially, and a couple of nitroglycerin were given before 911 was called. There were attempts to try to direct CPR over the phone. First responder came somewhere between 8 and 15 minutes afterwards and started CPR. The ambulance arrived 15 or 20 minutes afterwards, and he was transported 30 minutes en route. En route the

Initial assessment:

Time	T	P	R	BP	Other:					

Medication orders:

Lab work:

X-ray:

Physician's report:

Diagnosis:	Physician sign/date

Discharge	Transfer	Admit	Good	Satisfactory	Other:	

GODFREY REGIONAL HOSPITAL
123 Main Street • Aldon, FL 77714 • (407) 555-1234

Continued

EMERGENCY ROOM RECORD

Name:		Age:	ER physician:
		DOB:	

Allergies/type of reaction:		Usual medications/dosages:

Triage/presenting complaint:	automatic defibrillator deployed a shock three times and CPR was accomplished; a Combivent tube was placed.

Initial assessment:

Time	T	P	R	BP	Other:					

Medication orders:

Lab work:

X-ray:

Physician's report:

Diagnosis:	Physician sign/date
	Nancy Caully MD

Discharge	Transfer	Admit	Good	Satisfactory	Other:

GODFREY REGIONAL HOSPITAL
123 Main Street • Aldon, FL 77714 • (407) 555-1234

EXERCISE 53

Level II

EMERGENCY ROOM RECORD

Name:	Age:	ER physician:
	DOB:	

Allergies/type of reaction:	Usual medications/dosages:

Triage/presenting complaint:	SUBJECTIVE: This is an 88-year-old female resident of a nursing home who was brought in by ambulance today after she was walking in the hallway and fell, striking the back of her head. There has been some question of possible heart arrhythmia. She has been very bradycardic

Initial assessment:

Time	T	P	R	BP	Other:				

Medication orders:

Lab work:

X-ray:

Physician's report:

OBJECTIVE: This is a somewhat obtunded female who is moaning. Her BP is unable to be picked up. Pulse is unable to be picked up via monitors. With palpation of her femoral artery, pulse appeared to be about 20 beats per minute. She is hooked up on a cardiac monitor and this shows atrial activity, but only a rare ventricular capture. Pupils equal, round, and reactive to light. TMs are clear bilaterally. Oropharynx is clear. Neck is supple. No JVD. Heart is bradycardic. Lungs are clear to auscultation in all fields. Abdomen is soft, nontender, not distended. Extremities are free of any cyanosis, clubbing, or edema.

EMERGENCY ROOM COURSE: Patient did have an IV line established and was given IV atropine, 1 mg. This did not help her BP tremendously; therefore, with consultation with Dr. Obert, who is the internist on call and who had arrived in the ER to help resuscitate the patient, external pacing was done. She was set at a capture rate of 60 beats per minute and did well with this with a good pulse. Once she had her heart rhythm restored, she was alert. She was not complaining of any chest pain. No shortness of breath. She was unsure why she fell. EKG was done after the pacer was turned off because she was maintaining a sinus rhythm on her own. This revealed sinus bradycardia with first-degree AV block with a PR interval of 0.28 second. There was no ST-T wave elevation. There was some downward sloping of the ST segment in V5 and VS. There was evidence of a left bundle branch block. Chest x-ray was done, which was clear. Upon further examination of the patient, it did reveal a contusion to the back right side of her occiput with significant soft tissue ecchymosis, but no laceration that needed repair. This was cleansed. Neurological examination demonstrated movement in all four extremities. Toes were pointing downward bilaterally. Sensation was intact in distal extremities. A CT of her head was done, which revealed no bleed or acute findings per the radiologist's report. Troponin was 0.0. White count 13.2, hematocrit 39, Hgb 13.1, platelets 238.000. Glucose was elevated at 278, BUN 32, creatinine 1.7. This was up a little bit from her last readings. Albumin 3.1, alk phos 211, AST 46, ALT 85. This was up from

Diagnosis:	Physician sign/date
ASSESSMENT: This is an 88-year-old female with evidence of heart block now in sinus rhythm. No current evidence to suggest any acute ischemia. Neurological examination today demonstrates no focal findings.	

Discharge	Transfer	Admit	Good	Satisfactory	Other:	

GODFREY REGIONAL HOSPITAL
123 Main Street • Aldon, FL 77714 • (407) 555-1234

Continued

EMERGENCY ROOM RECORD

Name:		Age:	ER physician:
		DOB:	

Allergies/type of reaction:	Usual medications/dosages:

Triage/presenting complaint:	ever since the ambulance service got to her. Currently, the patient is moaning and unable to provide any history.

Initial assessment:

Time	T	P	R	BP	Other:					

Medication orders:

Lab work:

X-ray:

Physician's report:

normal levels of the previous tests. Sodium 135, potassium 3.7, chloride 99, bicarb 18. Patient remained stable and breathing on her own throughout her stay in the emergency room. Her heart remained in the sinus rhythm. It appeared to be a little bit tachycardic. EKG was repeated, which showed a sinus rhythm with a rate of 88 with continued first-degree AV block and left bundle branch block. Patient, who was diaphoretic and clammy when she came into the emergency room, then had normalizing of her body temperature with no further diaphoresis.

Diagnosis:	Physician sign/date
PLAN: Due to her heart block, patient was discussed with the cardiologist on call. He feels that the patient needs to be transferred down for further work-up and possible pacemaker placement; she will be transferred by ALS ambulance. She is in stable condition.	*Nancy Cauley* MD
Discharge Transfer Admit Good Satisfactory Other:	

GODFREY REGIONAL HOSPITAL
123 Main Street • Aldon, FL 77714 • (407) 555-1234

EXERCISE 54

Level I

EMERGENCY ROOM RECORD

Name:	Age:	ER physician:
	DOB:	

Allergies/type of reaction:	Usual medications/dosages:

Triage/presenting complaint:

SUBJECTIVE: This 45-year-old male was brought by ambulance to the emergency room after being involved in a motor vehicle accident. The patient was the driver; we don't know if he was seat-belted. He seems to have lost control of his car either because of falling asleep or because of alcohol, which I could smell while he was in the ER. He crossed the midline of the road and headed towards another van on the other side, and had a head-on collision. The patient's car,

Initial assessment:

Time	T	P	R	BP	Other:					

Medication orders:

Lab work:

X-ray:

Physician's report:

OBJECTIVE: On physical exam, he was awake, alert, oriented. He was in moderate distress from pain, especially when being moved; he would scream and shout. His initial vitals in the ER revealed a pulse rate 68 and blood pressure 136/95, saturation 97% on room air. HEENT: head normocephalic, atraumatic. He had some abrasions to the upper part of his forehead. There was no deformity, no swelling to the facial bones. His cranial nerves seemed to be intact. He had a C-collar around his neck. There was no bleeding from his ears or nostrils. Chest was symmetrical; there was no deformity, no tenderness. Lungs were clear to auscultation bilaterally. Heart: S1, S2, regular rate and rhythm. Abdomen: Patient had some bruises over his right upper abdomen; however, it was not tender; bowel sounds were positive. He had good femoral pulses bilaterally. There was no blood seen from the urethral meatus. The patient had a very tender left hip, especially pressing on the pelvic brim. He had a deformed left thigh. He had a deformed left leg with a long laceration to the left lower leg almost 12 cm in length involving the skin and subcutaneous tissue and muscle. I could see and feel the fibular bone through the laceration; however, no small bony fragments or broken bony fragments could be felt. Patient had his left foot externally rotated. Both feet were pink and warm. He had positive dorsalis pedis pulses bilaterally and good capillary filling of his toes. Upper extremities: He had a swollen right hand, mostly on the dorsal aspect, very tender thumb. He had good radial pulses bilaterally. He had good range of motion of shoulders, elbows, and wrist joints.

EMERGENCY ROOM COURSE: An IV line was started, and the patient was placed on 0.9 saline wide open. In the meantime, x-rays were done of the right wrist, right hand, left hip, chest, c-spine, left lower leg. Urinalysis was done. CBC, chemistry comprehensive metabolic panel and police officer requested an ETOH level that the patient did consent to.

His x-rays revealed a left comminuted intertrochanteric fracture and left distal comminuted transverse fracture of the femur. There was also the possibility of fracture of the distal phalanx of the right thumb. There was no pneumothorax, no rib fractures. C-spine: We could not get C7,

Diagnosis:	Physician sign/date
ASSESSMENT: Status motor vehicle accident with comminuted fracture of the left intertrochanteric femur, left distal femur, and frank hematuria, which could be due to bladder injury; but cannot rule out kidney injury.	

Discharge	Transfer	Admit	Good	Satisfactory	Other:

GODFREY REGIONAL HOSPITAL
123 Main Street • Aldon, FL 77714 • (407) 555-1234

Continued

EMERGENCY ROOM RECORD

Name:		**Age:**	**ER physician:**
		DOB:	

Allergies/type of reaction:	**Usual medications/dosages:**

Triage/presenting complaint: which was a pickup truck, slid into the ditch, and he had to be extricated from the vehicle. On arrival to the ER, the patient was in moderate distress from pain, especially when he was moved to the exam bed, complaining of severe pain to his left lower extremity. His left lower extremity was completely deformed; his left foot was 90 degrees rotated to the outside. The patient does not remember the accident or how it happened and he did not know any details. He

Initial assessment:

Time	T	P	R	BP	Other:					

Medication orders:

Lab work:

X-ray:

Physician's report:

so the C-collar was left on. Patient's alcohol level was 0.15. White blood cell count 8000, hemoglobin 14.1, hematocrit 41.3, and his platelets were 120. Chemistry: glucose 188, BUN 5, creatinine 1.0, sodium 137, potassium 4.4, chloride 100, bicarb 28, amylase 67, and lipase 381.

For the pain, the patient was given 4 mg intravenous morphine before going to X-ray and that seemed to relieve his pain almost down to 50%. The patient claims that he is from out of town and that he would rather be transferred to a hospital back home.

The case was discussed with the orthopedic physician on call, who accepted the transfer. The patient's left foot was rotated internally, and I placed his left lower extremity in a posterior splint. He was transferred to the emergency room of the hospital he selected by ambulance. Before transferring him, a Foley catheter was placed, which revealed frank hematuria. I re-examined the patient's abdomen; he had some bruises in the right upper quadrant; there was no tenderness or rebound tenderness.

Diagnosis:	**Physician sign/date**
PLAN: The patient was transferred by ambulance. His condition at the time of transfer was stable; his vitals were stable including blood pressure of 130/85 and pulse rate of 84/minute.	
Discharge Transfer Admit Good Satisfactory Other:	

GODFREY REGIONAL HOSPITAL
123 Main Street • Aldon, FL 77714 • (407) 555-1234

Continued

EMERGENCY ROOM RECORD

Name:		Age:	ER physician:
		DOB:	

Allergies/type of reaction:	Usual medications/dosages:

Triage/presenting complaint:	denies any headache or blurred or double vision. He denies neck pain. He denies chest pain or shortness of breath. He denies abdominal pain. Most of his pain was in his left lower extremity, especially in the left hip and mid thigh. Patient's past medical history is significant for noninsulin-dependent diabetes, asthma, and hepatitis C. The patient claims that he was up to date with his tetanus, having had it a few years ago.

Initial assessment:

Time	T	P	R	BP	Other:				

Medication orders:

Lab work:

X-ray:

Physician's report:

Diagnosis:	Physician sign/date
	Robert Rai MD

Discharge	Transfer	Admit	Good	Satisfactory	Other:

GODFREY REGIONAL HOSPITAL
123 Main Street • Aldon, FL 77714 • (407) 555-1234

EXERCISE 55

Level I

OFFICE NOTE

Chief complaint: _____

Date: _____

Vital signs: BP_____ P_____ R_____

History:

SUBJECTIVE: This 78-year-old female claims she woke up feeling short of breath and a little chest pain. She was here about 24 hours ago with dizziness, weakness, and emesis and was diagnosed with benign positional vertigo. She was prescribed Antivert that she says she is using, but it isn't helping. The patient agreed to be seen by me when she realized ambulance costs to another city wouldn't be covered.

PAST MEDICAL HISTORY: Seems to be positive for a number of emergency visits for similar complaints. She does have an artificial porcine valve and apparently has had bypass surgery.

MEDICATIONS: Vioxx, Tagament, Slow Iron, Norvasc, and the Antivert mentioned.

ALLERGIES: Apparently to Tylenol, ASA, ibuprofen, and, I believe, sulfa.

Exam:

She is afebrile. Vital signs are stable. She seems to be sleepy but is also anxious. Color is normal. She is not diaphoretic. NECK: supple. JVP is flat. Carotids are normal. CHEST: clear with good air entry bilaterally. Heart sounds are normal. She has aortic stenosis type murmur. ABDOMEN: soft and nontender, perhaps a little mild tenderness in the left upper quadrant. Pulses are normal.

LAB AND X-RAYS: ECG did not reveal any acute changes.

TREATMENT: She was originally given sublingual nitro, which she said helped. By the time the lab results came back, she had talked to the nurse and came to the conclusion that she had overreacted when she woke up, was likely just anxious, but now was feeling fine. She wants to go home.

Diagnosis/assessment:

1. Questionable anxiety

PLAN: She will go home on the usual medications.

William Oler MD

Patient name: _____

Date of service: _____

GODFREY MEDICAL ASSOCIATES
1532 Third Avenue, Suite 120 • Aldon, FL 77713 • (407) 555-4000

EXERCISE 56

Level II

EMERGENCY ROOM RECORD

Name:	Age:	ER physician:
	DOB:	

Allergies/type of reaction:	Usual medications/dosages:

Triage/presenting complaint: S: The patient is a 12-year-old child visiting this community for the first time. She was staying with her aunt. She and her aunt had been taking a nap. The aunt woke up, was puttering around the house, and then looked in on the patient when she awakened with a c/o severe headache, c/o numbness on the left side of the face, hand, and leg. The aunt became alarmed and brought her to the ER. When seen in the ER, the child was crying continuously

Initial assessment:

Time	T	P	R	BP	Other:					

Medication orders:

Lab work:

X-ray:

Physician's report:

O: On physical exam, optic fundi could initially be visualized when she was more cooperative. The optic fundi showed sharp disks and normal vascular pattern. PERRLA. EOMI with no nystagmus or weakness. There was no facial asymmetry. TMs were normal. Oropharynx showed a symmetric palate and tongue motion. There were no palpable masses in the neck. She showed symmetric ROM of upper and lower extremities. DTRs were brisk and symmetric. Romberg normal. Tandem walk normal. Finger pursuit, finger midline, heel shin were normal.

Following the initial examination, her symptoms seemed to deteriorate, and as attempts at diagnostic procedures were made, her level of objection and c/o discomfort accelerated. Over the next hour and a half, an attempt was made to locate an on-call pediatric neurologist to discuss the case. The child's vital signs remained stable throughout that time, although she continued to cry out almost continuously during that waiting period. An adult neurologist was contacted at another hospital who felt that she could not be helpful because she was not a pediatric neurologist.

Finally, a pediatric neurologist was located at another hospital. He agreed that she needed urgent transfer and evaluation under sedation if necessary. Arrangements were made with the ambulance service and she was transferred.

Total patient contact time: 11/2 hours

Diagnosis:	Physician sign/date

Discharge   Transfer   Admit   Good   Satisfactory   Other:

GODFREY REGIONAL HOSPITAL
123 Main Street • Aldon, FL 77714 • (407) 555-1234

Continued

EMERGENCY ROOM RECORD

Name:		Age:	ER physician:
		DOB:	

Allergies/type of reaction:	Usual medications/dosages:

Triage/presenting complaint: complaining that "it hurts, it hurts." She was nauseated and vomited twice. The location of the pain was not clear, but from time to time, she would describe pain in her head; other times, in her extremities, and would be inconsistent about the complaints. Dimming the lights in the room decreased her complaints. She demonstrated a waxing and waning course with lapsing into rest and calmness for several minutes, followed by an accelerating c/o pain that was

Initial assessment:

Time	T	P	R	BP	Other:					

Medication orders:

Lab work:

X-ray:

Physician's report:

Diagnosis:	Physician sign/date

Discharge   Transfer   Admit   Good   Satisfactory   Other:

GODFREY REGIONAL HOSPITAL
123 Main Street • Aldon, FL 77714 • (407) 555-1234

Continued

EMERGENCY ROOM RECORD

Name:	Age:	ER physician:
	DOB:	

Allergies/type of reaction:	Usual medications/dosages:

Triage/presenting complaint: nonspecific, followed by vomiting. She exhibited at least two and possibly three of these cycles during the ER period. Attempts to draw blood, insert an IV, and accomplish a CT scan were all met with hysterical objection and strenuous resistance.

Initial assessment:

Time	T	P	R	BP	Other:					

Medication orders:

Lab work:

X-ray:

Physician's report:

Diagnosis:	Physician sign/date
	Nancy Caully MD

Discharge   Transfer   Admit   Good   Satisfactory   Other:

GODFREY REGIONAL HOSPITAL
123 Main Street • Aldon, FL 77714 • (407) 555-1234

EXERCISE 57

Level II

EMERGENCY ROOM RECORD

Name:	Age:	ER physician:
	DOB:	

Allergies/type of reaction:	Usual medications/dosages:
none	none

Triage/presenting complaint:

S: The patient is a pleasant 47-year-old gentleman who was standing on a tire, cleaning the top of the cab of his truck. He lost his balance and landed on his right elbow. He had intense pain and was unable to flex or change position of his elbow. Given the severity of his injury and the acute pain, his wife notified the ambulance and he was brought into the ER. He had no LOC. No head injury. No shortness of breath, chest pain, GI/GU complaints. No previous trauma

Initial assessment:

Time	T	P	R	BP	Other:					

Medication orders:

Lab work:

X-ray:

X-rays reveal a fracture dislocation of the distal humerus in the elbow joint and also a fracture of the distal radius, ulna, and scaphoid.

Physician's report:

O: The patient was in acute pain, alert, oriented, and able to converse. VS: T 98, O2 sat 100% on room air, P 90s, BP 170s/80s–90s. HEENT: AT/NC, PERRL, EOMI; conjunctivae and sclera are clear. Oropharynx clear. Neck supple. Lungs clear in all fields. Heart regular rate and rhythm; no murmurs or extra sounds. Abdomen soft and benign. Lower extremities within normal limits. Right upper extremity reveals an obvious dislocation with an open fracture. He is also tender across the distal radius and ulna. Sensation of the right and left upper extremities is equal and within normal limits.

EMERGENCY ROOM COURSE: The patient was seen and evaluated, an IV was placed, and he was treated with morphine for pain—a total of 18 mg over the course of the stay. He was also treated with 30 mg of IV Toradol. He was also treated with 1 g Ancef. He was given 75 mg Demerol and 50 mg Vistaril IM for transfer to another hospital.

Diagnosis:	Physician sign/date
A: Open fracture with fracture dislocation of the distal humerus, right elbow, and fracture of the distal radius, ulna, and scaphoid right arm. P: Transfer to the accepting hospital.	

Discharge	Transfer	Admit	Good	Satisfactory	Other:

GODFREY REGIONAL HOSPITAL
123 Main Street • Aldon, FL 77714 • (407) 555-1234

Continued

EMERGENCY ROOM RECORD

Name:		Age:	ER physician:
		DOB:	

Allergies/type of reaction:	Usual medications/dosages:

Triage/presenting complaint: to the effected extremity.
FH: Noncontributory ROS: See above. PMH: He denies any previous hospitalizations or surgeries. SH: He is married. He is an over-the-road truck driver. He does use tobacco.

Initial assessment:

Time	T	P	R	BP	Other:					

Medication orders:

Lab work:

X-ray:

Physician's report:

Diagnosis:	Physician sign/date
	Robert Rai MD

Discharge   Transfer   Admit   Good   Satisfactory   Other:

GODFREY REGIONAL HOSPITAL
123 Main Street • Aldon, FL 77714 • (407) 555-1234

EXERCISE 58

Level I

EMERGENCY ROOM RECORD

Name:	Age:	ER physician:
	DOB:	

Allergies/type of reaction:	Usual medications/dosages:

Triage/presenting complaint:

S: This is a 46-year-old gentleman who was brought in by ambulance for assessment of increasing and worsening shortness of breath. He has a long history of COPD for unknown reasons. It is a debate as to whether it is from his smoking or a welding problem, but in any event, he is totally disabled because of his lungs. He is monitored by a pulmonologist and takes all the medications listed. He started having difficulty a week ago and has been getting

Initial assessment:

Time	T	P	R	BP	Other:				

Medication orders:

Lab work:

Blood gases show a pH of 7.29 with a PCO2 of 73, PO2 of 52, with O2 sats of 87% on 10 liters.

X-ray:

Physician's report:

O: Pulse 135. General: alert, responsive, oriented, quite tachypneic, has a rebreathing mask on, and appears to be in some moderate distress. Chest: Very poor air movement, and I could hear some rhonchi with rales bilaterally, but he is not wheezing. Cardiovascular: normal S1, S2 with a very rapid rate but regular rhythm.

Diagnosis:	Physician sign/date

A: COPD with acute exacerbation and impending ARDS
P: Discussed the situation with his pulmonologist. In light of the fact that he could be heading towards some mechanical assistance for breathing, we will send him to the pulmonologist's hospital for further evaluation and treatment.

Discharge	Transfer	Admit	Good	Satisfactory	Other:

GODFREY REGIONAL HOSPITAL
123 Main Street • Aldon, FL 77714 • (407) 555-1234

Continued

EMERGENCY ROOM RECORD

Name:	Age:	ER physician:
	DOB:	

Allergies/type of reaction:	Usual medications/dosages:

Triage/presenting complaint: progressively worse to the point where tonight he just was extremely winded. He was quite diaphoretic with this but didn't really have any substernal chest pain. He complained of a diffuse chest pain that he thought was from his lungs. A lot of trouble with deep breaths, however. He does have home O2, which he used, but it didn't help, so an ambulance was called. No nausea or vomiting. He does not have a history of MI. He has never had any operations. No temperature.

Initial assessment:

Time	T	P	R	BP	Other:					

Medication orders:

Lab work:

X-ray:

Physician's report:

Diagnosis:	Physician sign/date
	Robert Rai MD

Discharge   Transfer   Admit   Good   Satisfactory   Other:

GODFREY REGIONAL HOSPITAL
123 Main Street • Aldon, FL 77714 • (407) 555-1234

Level I

OFFICE NOTE

Date:	Vital signs:	T	R
Chief complaint: Back pain		P	BP

HISTORY: This is a 56-year-old gentleman who had a little bit of soreness in his back for three days, but it got worse today. It still hurts when he moves and he gets sharp pains. This was preceded by some snow shoveling several days ago. He is not really short of breath. He has no pain elsewhere. No other symptoms. He has a history of chronic back pain that is disabling. The pain he has now is more between the shoulder blades. Hyperlipidemia, diverticulosis, and kidney stones. He has arthritis in his spine and calcified aortic stenosis with, I believe, an aortic valve replacement. He has also had an L5 laminectomy in the past. He is on Lopid, Celebrex, Lipitor, Coumadin, Lopressor, and Prilosec.

Physical examination:

O: On exam, he is uncomfortable with movement. His vital signs are stable. His lungs are clear. His heart is regular with a little slight murmur and click from his valve. He has tenderness over his paraspinal muscles between his scapulae and a little bit diffusely over the spinous processes on the upper back also. More over the ligaments between the spinous process and then over them directly.

Assessment:

A: Muscular and ligamentous upper back pain

Plan:

P: Toradol, 60 mg, and Vistaril, 50 mg IM, given. He had fair relief. He was sent home with Flexeril, one tid, for muscle spasms, No. 12, and he will follow up with physical therapy if he needs to. He was stable at discharge.

William Obst MD

	Patient name:
	DOB:
	MR/Chart #:

GODFREY REGIONAL OUTPATIENT CLINIC
3122 Shannon Avenue • Aldon, FL 77712 • (407) 555-7654

EXERCISE 60

Level I

EMERGENCY ROOM RECORD

Name:	Age:	ER physician:
	DOB:	

Allergies/type of reaction:

Triage/presenting complaint: Knife wound, left thigh
S: This is a 22-year-old male who was at a party, and someone got upset and stabbed him with a pocket knife. He has a scratch along his abdomen and a wound to his left thigh. His tetanus is up to date. He has no other injuries. He may be allergic to erythromycin. No routine medications.

Initial assessment:

Time	T	P	R	BP	Other:					

Medication orders:

Lab work:

X-ray:

Physician's report:

O: He has about a 6-cm scratch midline of his abdomen that does not require any care. He has a 3.5-cm vertical laceration to the lateral aspect of his left thigh that goes through the subcutaneous fat down to the vascular layer of the thigh muscle. This is nicked, but there does not seem to be any muscle injury, and there is no active bleeding, so that does not need any repair. CMS was intact distally.

Diagnosis:	Physician sign/date
A: Laceration, left lateral thigh
P: Betadine. Local 1% plain Xylocaine for anesthesia. He had suture repair with 4 vertical mattress and 6 simple of 4-0 Ethilon and dressing applied. Wound sheet	

Discharge	Transfer	Admit	Good	Satisfactory	Other:	

GODFREY REGIONAL HOSPITAL
123 Main Street • Aldon, FL 77714 • (407) 555-1234

Continued

EMERGENCY ROOM RECORD

Name:		Age:	ER physician:
		DOB:	

Allergies/type of reaction:	Usual medications/dosages:

Triage/presenting complaint:

Initial assessment:

Time	T	P	R	BP	Other:					

Medication orders:

Lab work:

X-ray:

Physician's report:

Diagnosis:	Physician sign/date
given. Suture removal in eight days. Return for signs of infection. He was advised he would have an achy thigh muscle for a while because of the nick to the muscle fascia. He can use ibuprofen for pain. He was stable at discharge.	*Nancy Caully MD*
Discharge Transfer Admit Good Satisfactory Other:	

GODFREY REGIONAL HOSPITAL
123 Main Street • Aldon, FL 77714 • (407) 555-1234

EXERCISE 61

Level I

OFFICE NOTE

Date:	Vital signs:	T	R
Chief complaint: Leg pain		P	BP

S: The patient is a 65-year-old gentleman with insulin-dependent diabetes mellitus, coronary artery disease, history of paroxysmal atrial fibrillation, alcohol abuse with hepatic encephalopathy due to liver cirrhosis, hypertension, and chronic renal failure. He had hospitalization just earlier this month. He has been in a couple of times since then and was seen just a week ago with leg pain. He saw his physician again on Thursday, and because of increased edema, was placed on Bumex daily in addition to his other medications. He is also on some Keflex because his legs were a little inflamed. Bumex is 1 mg for three days and then half a day. Keflex is 500 mg bid. He is here because he has had this leg pain for two weeks, but it is worse since yesterday and he is not ambulating as well. He is not short of breath. He has chronic dyspnea with activity, but that is unchanged. No fever, chills, or chest discomfort.

Physical examination:

O: On exam, he is a little tachycardic. O2 sats are fine. Respirations are 16. He is afebrile. He does have a little bit of a loose cough. Lung sounds are clear. Heart is regular with his systolic murmur. Abdomen has some bruising from his insulin shots but otherwise negative. Lower extremities: He has 2+ to 3+ edema just below his knees bilaterally. Both legs are tender to touch. Even on the dorsum of the foot he has pain. His calves are sore too. He has a little bit of inflamed stasis dermatitis also. As far as his pulses, they are hard to feel because of his edema, but I think they are both palpably present. I checked his coags, and his INR is 1.21, which is better than when he was in the hospital. Blood sugar is 217. BUN is 30. Creatinine 2.0. Those were pretty stable. Sodium 134, potassium 4.6.

Assessment:

A: Increasing edema without evidence of congestive heart failure. Stasis dermatitis.

Plan:

P: Discussion. He was given metolazone 5 mg orally and he will be on 5 mg daily and will stop the Bumex for right now. He was just given #10. Demerol 75 mg IM was given. Wrote a Rx for Demerol oral, but the pharmacy was out of this, so we changed it to Dilaudid 2 mg one every 4–6 hours prn for pain, #18. He is to follow up with his physician on Tuesday. He is also to keep his feet elevated above heart level to help with the swelling, which should help with the pain. If things worsen or he has problems with his breathing, he should return. I told him he would likely end up being in the hospital for more aggressive diuresis. He was stable at discharge and he was ambulatory.

	Patient name:
	DOB:
	MR/Chart #:

GODFREY REGIONAL OUTPATIENT CLINIC
3122 Shannon Avenue • Aldon, FL 77712 • (407) 555-7654

Continued

OFFICE NOTE

| Date: | Vital signs: | T | R |
| Chief complaint: Leg pain | | P | BP |

Presently his other medications are a multivitamin, lisinopril 10 mg daily, lactulose 15 mg bid, Zantac 150 mg bid, garlic 60 mg tid, baby aspirin daily, Lasix 20 mg bid, Bumex, and Humulin 75/25. We don't have any allergies listed. Review of systems: no HEENT complaints. Respiratory: negative. Cardiac: negative. GI: negative. Otherwise, symptoms as above.

Physical examination:

Assessment:

Plan:

Stony Kreutt, MD

Patient name:

DOB:

MR/Chart #:

GODFREY REGIONAL OUTPATIENT CLINIC
3122 Shannon Avenue • Aldon, FL 77712 • (407) 555-7654

EXERCISE 62

Level I

OFFICE NOTE

Chief complaint: _____

Date: _____

Vital signs: BP_____ P_____ R_____

History:

S: The patient is a 65-year-old gentleman who presents today with some trouble swallowing since this morning. Associated with this he has a sensation that he has a hard time taking a deep breath. He had oatmeal and some toast this morning. He didn't think anything got caught, but he is having trouble swallowing and he spits things up. He has had occasional problems with dysphagia in the past, but just a few months ago he had an EGD and there was no evidence of esophageal strictures. He did have a hiatal hernia in addition to some ulcers. I just recently saw him because of edema and leg pain and had made some medication changes. The pain pills helped and his pain is less. The fluid in his legs is down with the metolazone, but he stopped the pain pills because he thought they could be contributing to his symptoms. He has insulin-dependent diabetes, hypertension, atrial fibrillation, mitral regurgitation, alcoholism with cirrhosis, COPD, previous TIA, chronic renal failure, and CHF. His medications are as [noted] previously except for he is not on Bumex, as I had stopped that a couple of days ago and put him on metolazone 5 mg daily. He has no allergies. He has had no trouble with swelling of his tongue or lips. He hasn't had a rash.

Exam:

O: On exam, he is afebrile. Vital signs look stable. His lips and tongue are not swollen. His posterior pharynx looks unremarkable. Neck feels unremarkable. Lungs are clear. Heart is unchanged. Edema is less in his legs and his legs are less tense. We did a chest x-ray and that looks unremarkable.

Diagnosis/assessment:

A: Dysphagia. I suspect he has some kind of esophageal motility problem. He was able to drink some fluid and he felt it went down.

P: Discussion. We did try a Maxi mist treatment with albuterol and also SQ epi and that really didn't affect his symptoms, so I don't think it is an allergic problem. He is to be set up for a swallowing study and stay on just a liquid diet for now. He was stable at discharge.

William Oler MD

Patient name: _____

Date of service: _____

GODFREY MEDICAL ASSOCIATES
1532 Third Avenue, Suite 120 • Aldon, FL 77713 • (407) 555-4000

EXERCISE 63

Level I

OFFICE NOTE

Date:	Vital signs:	T		R	
Chief complaint:		P		BP	

S: The patient is an 81-year-old new patient who, sometime two weeks prior to this visit, fell when deer hunting. He has fallen again and again, has recurrent right chest wall pain. He has had some dyspnea on exertion. He does, however, have chronic COPD and mild emphysema but he is restricting his breathing and has pain with each breath.

Physical examination:

O: He is afebrile. Pulse is 88. Respirations are 20 and splinted. Blood pressure is 142/76. HEENT: No signs of obvious trauma. Some memory deficit is noted. He denies any closed head injury with his initial injury. His fall last night was unexpected and caused by tripping. He had no syncopal episode, chest pain, or palpitations, and it did not appear by history to be a drop attack. Palpation of the neck revealed no crepitus but some arthritis. There was scant trapezius pain. Palpation along the right chest, however, revealed an area of exquisite tenderness without crepitus. The x-ray suggests that there is a fracture or at least a dislocation of the costochondral joint in this rib. There was no infiltrate and no effusion.

Assessment:

A: Right rib fracture, suspect 8th rib. Mild atelectasis.

Plan:

P: Treatment in the office is Toradol 30 mg IM. The patient is given a prescription for Toradol to use with meals and at bedtime routinely, but a limited prescription of five days is given. Heat and Aspercreme were discussed. The risk of atelectasis was explained in layman's terms. A forced deep inhalation was suggested.

Maurice Doater, MD

	Patient name:
	DOB:
	MR/Chart #:

GODFREY REGIONAL OUTPATIENT CLINIC
3122 Shannon Avenue • Aldon, FL 77712 • (407) 555-7654

EXERCISE 64

Level II

EMERGENCY ROOM RECORD

Name:	Age:	ER physician:
	DOB:	

Allergies/type of reaction:	Usual medications/dosages:

Triage/presenting complaint: S: This 94-year-old female was brought in by her granddaughter because of severe substernal chest discomfort that awoke her at approximately 12:15 a.m. She immediately came here because of severe chest and upper mid-back discomfort. Nursing was transferring her from the wheelchair to the ER cot when she went unresponsive and was found to be without respirations and pulseless. They immediately were able to get her on the cot, lifted her up, and

Initial assessment:

Time	T	P	R	BP	Other:					

Medication orders:

Lab work: Her laboratory results showed a CBC revealing a white count of 11,500 with 36 percent neutrophils, 54 percent lymphocytes, hemoglobin 13, and platelets 266. Her initial troponin was 0.9. Her urinalysis was unremarkable other than 2 to 4 white blood cells. Basic metabolic profile

X-ray:

Physician's report:

O: Approximately 5 minutes later, I arrived on the scene in the ER and found the patient to be in a sinus rhythm at a rate of 120 to 140 with a blood pressure of 200/100. Her pupils were approximately 3 millimeters and equal and sluggish. She did start to wake up and was rather restless and agitated. Any time her blood pressure would be taken, she would flex. There was questionable posturing noted at times. Her lung sounds were heard in both lungs after she was intubated. She was placed on the ventilator with a tidal volume of initially 900 by the medics. This was decreased to 800. She was initially hyperventilated, and her ABGs returned, showing O2 sats over 400 and a CO2 that was low at 26. The respiratory rate was decreased from 20 down to 16, and her tidal volume, as noted, was decreased down to 800. Repeat ABGs thereafter showed a PO2 of 477, PCO2 of 28, and a pH of 7.47. After she converted with the second shock, she was started on lidocaine. After a 50 cc bolus, she was started on a 30 cc drip. Life Flight was called immediately by nursing and paramedics. At approximately 1:00 a.m. she started to have more frequent PVCs. Her blood pressure was rather high, in the 220s/130. Her lidocaine drip was increased to 50 cc. 12-lead EKG was taken at that time as well, showing acute MI in the inferior, anterior, and lateral leads. She was starting to get even more restless. She was given an mg of Versed. Chest x-ray was taken and showed adequate tube placement. No obvious pulmonary edema. Lung fields actually looked rather clear. Approximately 7 minutes later, she was still rather agitated. She was given a second mg of Versed. Two IVs were started initially: one for the lidocaine drip, and a second extra IV was also started. Her temperature was noted to be 94. A Baer hugger was placed. She was then given 5 mg of Lopressor IV. Her blood pressure came down to the 150 to 140 systolic/80 diastolic. She was given 4 mg of morphine also at that same time. A Foley catheter was then also placed. NG tube was inserted. At approximately 1:40 a.m., another mg of Versed was given for a total of 3 mg up until this point. Her temperature had increased to 97.2 rectally. She continued to be rather agitated. Another 4 mg of Versed was given.

Diagnosis:	Physician sign/date
IMPRESSION: 1. Cardiorespiratory arrest with a witnessed code. 2. Ventricular fibrillation converted with 300 joules. 3. Acute anterolateral and anteroseptal and inferior myocardial infarction. 4. Mild hypokalemia.	

Discharge   **Transfer**   **Admit**   **Good**   **Satisfactory**   **Other:**

GODFREY REGIONAL HOSPITAL
123 Main Street • Aldon, FL 77714 • (407) 555-1234

Continued

EMERGENCY ROOM RECORD

| Name: | Age: | ER physician: |
| | DOB: | |

| Allergies/type of reaction: | Usual medications/dosages: |
| | |

Triage/presenting complaint: initiated ACLS protocol. They immediately put a cardiac monitor on and found her to be in ventricular fibrillation and immediately shocked her at 200 joules. A rhythm did appear on the monitor that was apparently sinus. She had a bradycardic rate and was still pulseless and spontaneously reverted back into ventricular fibrillation. She was then shocked at 300 joules, again converting into a sinus rhythm. A pulse was then palpated. Chest compressions were

Initial assessment:

| Time | T | P | R | BP | Other: | | | | | |

Medication orders:

Lab work: revealed a glucose of 130, BUN of 38, creatinine 1.3, sodium 142; and potassium was mildly low at 3.3. Chloride was 106, CO2 27, calcium 8.9, magnesium 2.9; AST and ALT were normal. LDH: 667, CK: 110.

X-ray:

Physician's report:

At approximately 1:50 a.m. Life Flight arrived. A repeat temperature showed tympanic temp of 94.2. Another 2 mg of Versed was given, and the paramedics from Life Flight also gave Zemuron to paralyze her. Just prior to this she actually looked rather alert. Her eyes were focusing on me, and she was still rather agitated. Care was then transferred to the ER physician at the receiving hospital to be taken over by the Life Flight crew. She was transferred via Life Flight to the receiving hospital for further evaluation and treatment. Further considerations and treatment had included a nitro drip, which we decided not to start after her blood pressure dropped in the 150s to 140 systolic after the Lopressor. Also, possibility of thrombolytic was considered. I consulted the receiving physicians at this time. Because of her age, it is felt that the risks outweigh the benefits for her. I also discussed with the patient's daughter and granddaughter the risks of thrombolytic therapy, and their decision at this time was to withhold thrombolytics.

Diagnosis:	Physician sign/date
PLAN: As noted above, the patient was transferred in critical condition to a receiving hospital under the care of the ER physician.	
Discharge Transfer Admit Good Satisfactory Other:	

GODFREY REGIONAL HOSPITAL
123 Main Street • Aldon, FL 77714 • (407) 555-1234

Continued

EMERGENCY ROOM RECORD

| Name: | Age: | ER physician: |
| | DOB: | |

| Allergies/type of reaction: | Usual medications/dosages: |
| | |

| Triage/presenting complaint: | started with immediate intubation by paramedics on the scene here in the hospital. CPR was continued in between shocks when she was found to be pulseless until she was shocked again. After the second shock, as noted, she was in a sinus bradycardia with a palpable pulse. |

Initial assessment:

Time	T	P	R	BP	Other:					

Medication orders:

Lab work:

X-ray:

Physician's report:

| Diagnosis: | Physician sign/date |
| | *Nancy Cauley MD* |

Discharge   Transfer   Admit   Good   Satisfactory   Other:

GODFREY REGIONAL HOSPITAL
123 Main Street • Aldon, FL 77714 • (407) 555-1234

EXERCISE 65

Level I

OFFICE NOTE

Chief complaint: _____

Date: _____

Vital signs: BP_____ P_____ R_____

History:

S: This is a 26-year-old white female who is brought in by friends after she was riding as a passenger on a snowmobile and she fell off the back end. The patient states that she was going about 80 miles an hour. Bystanders say she was only going about 40 miles per hour. They evidently hit a bump, and she went airborne and fell onto her shoulders on a smooth trail. It didn't sound like she hit anything other than the ground. She has pain from the base of her neck down to her tailbone. It seems to be worse in her low back. She does have a history of previous low back injuries. The accident occurred at approximately 2300 hours. She denies any numbness or tingling. She does not have loss of consciousness. She was wearing a helmet.

Exam:

O: On examination, the patient is awake, alert, and appropriate. She is moving all extremities well. She complains of pain mostly in the low back. We palpated in this region with the patient laying flat, and she has tenderness more in the paraspinal muscles than over the spinous processes. She has spasm and tenderness up the paraspinal muscles involving most of her lower thoracic and lumbar spine. Also a little bit in the paraspinal muscles of her cervical spine. Her head was blocked by the nurse as soon as she got here. Lateral C-spine appeared normal down through C7. Therefore, completion of cervical, lumbosacral, and thoracic spine was obtained. She did not appear to have any acute fractures. There is a question of a very slight old compression fracture in her lower thoracic spine, but this was subtle and did not appear to be acute.

Diagnosis/assessment:

A: Contusion, back after falling off a snowmobile. History of low back pain.

P: Cyclobenzaprine 10 mg qhs, Ibuprofen OTC three tablets four times a day. Tylenol in addition to this prn for pain. Recommended being up and walking at least once every hour for about five minutes and to try to avoid any heavy lifting. She is to try and maintain physical activity as much as possible. If she seems to worsen or doesn't improve over the next couple of weeks, then consider follow-up to consider physical therapy. In the meantime, she should use her pain as her guide for her activities.

Felix Warden MD

Patient name: _____

Date of service: _____

GODFREY MEDICAL ASSOCIATES
1532 Third Avenue, Suite 120 • Aldon, FL 77713 • (407) 555-4000

EXERCISE 66

Level II

EMERGENCY ROOM RECORD

Name:	Age:	ER physician:
	DOB:	

Allergies/type of reaction:	Usual medications/dosages:
Penicillin	Zoloft 50 mg qd and decongestant spray.

Triage/presenting complaint: CHIEF COMPLAINT: Collapse

An ambulance was summoned to the house after the patient was found collapsed on the floor. No CPR was done when they arrived. ECG initially showed some ventricular fibrillation. A shock was unsuccessful. Intubation was unsuccessful. He then had a Combi-tube placed. CPR was performed throughout, and he was transported to the hospital.

Initial assessment:

Time	T	P	R	BP	Other:				

Medication orders:

Lab work:

X-ray:

Physician's report:

When he arrived, CPR was being done adequately. There was fair to good ventilation of the lungs with a Combi-tube. No IV had been successfully placed. Anesthesia was present and exchanged the Combi-tube for a T-tube. There was good ventilation bilaterally, but his color remained somewhat dusky. He had rhonchi in both lungs. He was in asystole. IVs were started—initially 2 mg of epinephrine through the ET tube, and then additional epinephrine through the IV. He had 2 mg of atropine IV. Attempted external pacing with 120 milliamps output created some muscle movement of pectoralis, but there was no capture of the hearts. He remained asystolic when there was no CPR or pacing and essentially died a cardiac death.

Of note, time down with no CPR before the ambulance arrived was at least 5 minutes, probably closer to 8.

Additional history from family: He had fallen around noon today, and afterwards the family noticed he had a little bit of slurred speech. He has a history of intermittent atrial fibrillation. He is on Coumadin. His son has had coronary stents, and there is a question if he has stents. He has a history of COPD, and near the time he was being evaluated for his cardiovascular unresponsiveness, the family indicated that he had not wanted CPR.

Diagnosis:	Physician sign/date
CAUSE OF DEATH: Probable stroke. Cannot rule out myocardial infarction. Clearly sudden death. Patient with multiple risk factors. Usual physician is Dr. Smith. Message has been left for him to call back. No signs of foul play. His daughter and son who live with him were here. Several neighbors were here. Other family	

Discharge	Transfer	Admit	Good	Satisfactory	Other:	

GODFREY REGIONAL HOSPITAL
123 Main Street • Aldon, FL 77714 • (407) 555-1234

Continued

EMERGENCY ROOM RECORD

| Name: | Age: | ER physician: |
| | DOB: | |

| Allergies/type of reaction: | Usual medications/dosages: |
| | |

Triage/presenting complaint:

Initial assessment:

Time	T	P	R	BP	Other:				
Medication orders:									

Lab work:

X-ray:

Physician's report:

| Diagnosis: | Physician sign/date |
| members have been contacted. Representative from cathedral has been here. Grandson is here, as well as former daughter-in-law. We are contacting the organ donation group, but because of his age, he is an unlikely organ donor, and no autopsy was requested by us. | *Robert Rai MD* |

| Discharge | Transfer | Admit | Good | Satisfactory | Other: | |

GODFREY REGIONAL HOSPITAL
123 Main Street • Aldon, FL 77714 • (407) 555-1234

EXERCISE 67

Level I

OFFICE NOTE

Date:		Vital signs:	T	R
Chief complaint:			P	BP

Patient is 4 years old, and her parents bring her in because she sustained trauma to her back and the back of her head. She was sledding down a hill, did not wait as she was asked to, and the sled went down and started to spin around. Finally she hit a tree with her back. She also apparently hit the back of her head. She never had loss of consciousness, cried right away, and has been complaining of back pain since.

The patient is otherwise healthy. Her vaccinations are up to date.

Examination:

PHYSICAL EXAMINATION: Well nourished and developed, no acute distress. Interactive and cooperative. Vital signs are stable. She was actually quite playful also by the end of the interview. HEENT: normocephalic, atraumatic. No pallor or jaundice. Hydration is normal. Both TMs are intact without discharges. Neck supple without lymphadenopathy. Lungs: clear to auscultation. Heart: regular rate and rhythm. No murmurs or tachycardia. Back: no asymmetries, no evidence of trauma. She is a little sore on palpation of the lumbar area without any specific tenderness. Neurological exam is intact. Abdominal exam is negative. Her gait is normal.

Impression:

Status post trauma to the back without loss of consciousness. Concerned for kidney trauma.

Plan:

Will obtain a UA. If this is negative, I think that she should be treated symptomatically with acetaminophen for pain relief. If indeed her UA is negative, as expected, then she will be discharged and asked to come back if she has worsening symptoms.

Jay Corzen MD

	Patient name:
	DOB:
	MR/Chart #:

GODFREY REGIONAL OUTPATIENT CLINIC
3122 Shannon Avenue • Aldon, FL 77712 • (407) 555-7654

EXERCISE 68

Level I

EMERGENCY ROOM RECORD

Name:	Age:	ER physician:
	DOB:	

Allergies/type of reaction:	Usual medications/dosages:
Penicillin	Zoloft 50 mg qd and decongestant spray.

Triage/presenting complaint:

SUBJECTIVE: Patient is a 41-year-old gentleman who presents by ambulance today complaining of shortness of breath. He reports he was sitting watching TV when he started to feel short of breath, get tingly in his hands and feet, and just generally not feel well. He was a little bit nauseous with it. He wasn't having any chest pain or pressure with it. He did have a Cardiolite in September that was negative. Also had some pulmonary function tests indicative of

Initial assessment:

Time	T	P	R	BP	Other:					

Medication orders:

Lab work: CBC is within normal limits. Chemistry panel within normal limits. CK is 56, troponin 0. EKG shows a normal sinus rhythm with no acute changes.

X-ray:

Physician's report:

OBJECTIVE: Thin gentleman, fairly anxious appearing. Color is good. P 86, R 12, BP 109/85, O2 sat 98% on 3 liters when he arrived from the ambulance. CHEST: lungs bilaterally clear to auscultation. HEART: regular rate and rhythm without murmurs. ABDOMEN: positive bowel sounds. Soft, nontender. Nondistended. EXTREMITIES: normal strength and sensation. No cyanosis or edema.

PLAN:
1. Given that he had a normal Cardiolite fairly recently and symptoms are not terribly suggestive of heart disease, as well as all the normal labs and EKG, I think we are fairly safe in saying that this is probably not cardiac related.
2. I discussed with the patient that I am concerned that the Zoloft may be worsening some of his anxiety symptoms and may actually be causing some more manic symptoms. I have asked him to stop the Zoloft. I did give him some Xanax, 0.5 mg po q6h prn. 20 tabs given. It was discussed with him that this is not a long-term solution, but more short-term to help with the immediate anxiety symptoms.
3. I have set up for the patient to be seen at the mental health center tomorrow.

Diagnosis:	Physician sign/date

ASSESSMENT: An episode of shortness of breath; suspect some anxiety. I would also be concerned that he may be going into a more manic episode, especially given the recent starting of Zoloft. No evidence on exam or laboratory and EKG testing of heart disease.

Discharge   **Transfer**   **Admit**   **Good**   **Satisfactory**   **Other:**

GODFREY REGIONAL HOSPITAL
123 Main Street • Aldon, FL 77714 • (407) 555-1234

Continued

EMERGENCY ROOM RECORD

Name:		Age:	ER physician:
		DOB:	

Allergies/type of reaction:	Usual medications/dosages:

Triage/presenting complaint: some chronic obstructive pulmonary disease. He has had some intermittent spells of shortness of breath. He also reports he was started on Zoloft last week for some anxiety. He had been on 25 mg a day and just bumped up to 50 mg a day. He also gives a history of bipolar disorder. He is not sure when his last manic episode was, but certainly feels it has been in the last few years. Those records are in another city where he lived previously. He has not seen anyone in

Initial assessment:

Time	T	P	R	BP	Other:					

Medication orders:

Lab work:

X-ray:

Physician's report:

Diagnosis:	Physician sign/date

Discharge	Transfer	Admit	Good	Satisfactory	Other:	

GODFREY REGIONAL HOSPITAL
123 Main Street • Aldon, FL 77714 • (407) 555-1234

Continued

EMERGENCY ROOM RECORD

| Name: | Age: | ER physician: |
| | DOB: | |

| Allergies/type of reaction: | Usual medications/dosages: |
| | |

Triage/presenting complaint: Mental Health here.
PAST MEDICAL HISTORY: Otherwise negative per his report.
SOCIAL HISTORY: The patient denies any alcohol use. He smokes about a pack a day, although he says this is quite a bit cut down from his past. He is not currently working.

Initial assessment:

| Time | T | P | R | BP | Other: | | | | | |

Medication orders:

Lab work:

X-ray:

Physician's report:

| Diagnosis: | Physician sign/date |
| | *Nancy Cauly MD* |

| Discharge | Transfer | Admit | Good | Satisfactory | Other: |

GODFREY REGIONAL HOSPITAL
123 Main Street • Aldon, FL 77714 • (407) 555-1234

EXERCISE 69

Level I

OFFICE NOTE

Date:	Vital signs:	T		R	
Chief complaint:		P		BP	

73-year-old fell down at home today while carrying a box. She complains of pain on the mid lateral thigh and in the left hip area. Was brought in by ambulance secondary to difficulty ambulating. This accident happened a couple of hours before she got here. Denies any nausea or vomiting. No numbness or tingling sensation. No loss of consciousness either before the fall or afterwards.

MEDICATIONS: Actos 30 mg a day, Aciphex 20 mg a day, verapamil, doxepin, Zocor, sucralfate.

ALLERGIES: Morphine sulfate, Novocain, and Demerol.

PAST MEDICAL HISTORY: Diabetes, peptic ulcer disease, hypertension, and hypercholesterolemia.

Physical examination:

REVIEW OF SYSTEMS: Patient has a persistent cough, productive for the past several weeks. Has been treated with antibiotics but has not had relief of symptoms—is still putting out greenish sputum. Some degree of chills at home.

Alert and oriented times three, does not appear to be in acute distress. T 98.0, P 70, R 20, BP 122/67, saturating 89%. When she arrived, 97% with 2 liters oxygen. However, when oxygen was taken off later, it was 92% on room air. HEENT: PERRLA, EOMI. Anicteric sclerae. Throat clear. Ears clear. CHEST: coarse rhonchi, no wheezing, no crackles. CARDIOVASCULAR: S1, S2 normal. ABDOMEN: soft. Tenderness in the left hip joint. Straight leg raising test positive. Pain on lateral rotation of the hip; however, can elevate both legs on her own. Muscle power 5/5 all over; reflexes 21.

LAB AND X-RAY: Chest x-ray negative for any infiltrate, pleural effusion, or cardiomegaly. X-ray done of the left hip and pelvis—both negative for fracture or dislocation.

Assessment:

Upper respiratory infection/bronchitis. Negative for any fracture of the hip, most likely contusion or pulled muscle.

Plan:

Advised patient to take it easy. Was put on Percocet one tablet po qid as needed for pain control. Will also start on Zithromax Z-Pak as well for bronchitis and Robitussin-AC 1 tsp, po tid for ten days. Follow up with primary care physician in the next couple of days. Seek medical attention if she develops any severe pain or difficulty walking.

Felix Wanden M

Patient name:
DOB:
MR/Chart #:

GODFREY REGIONAL OUTPATIENT CLINIC
3122 Shannon Avenue • Aldon, FL 77712 • (407) 555-7654

EXERCISE 70

Level I

EMERGENCY ROOM RECORD

Name:		Age:	ER physician:
		DOB:	

Allergies/type of reaction:	Usual medications/dosages:

Triage/presenting complaint:	SUBJECTIVE: Patient is a 1-year-old brought in by his mom with concerns of burns to the fingertips of his middle and ring fingers on his right hand. Mom states

that she was baking cookies when he reached onto the counter and touched the hot cookie pan. He started crying right

Initial assessment:

Time	T	P	R	BP	Other:					

Medication orders:

Lab work:

X-ray:

Physician's report:

PHYSICAL EXAMINATION: Reveals on the tips of the middle and ring fingers of the right hand there is an area of whiteness. He does pull back a little bit when these are palpated very lightly; these don't appear to be vesicular but may soon become vesicles. He has surrounding erythema around this, basically just involving minimally proximal to the DIP fold on the palmar aspect of these fingers. He also has some erythema on the small finger pad, but there doesn't appear to be any vesicle here.

Diagnosis:	Physician sign/date
ASSESSMENT: 2nd degree burns to the fingertips of the middle and ring fingers of the right hand with 1st degree burns to the small fingertip of the right hand. PLAN: We did apply Silvadene ointment and a bandage. Recommend that she continue	

Discharge	Transfer	Admit	Good	Satisfactory	Other:

GODFREY REGIONAL HOSPITAL
123 Main Street • Aldon, FL 77714 • (407) 555-1234

Continued

EMERGENCY ROOM RECORD

Name:		Age:	ER physician:
		DOB:	

Allergies/type of reaction:	Usual medications/dosages:

Triage/presenting complaint:	away. Mom took his fingers and ran them under cool and cold water. Then after that, she brought him up to the emergency department.

Initial assessment:

Time	T	P	R	BP	Other:					

Medication orders:

Lab work:

X-ray:

Physician's report:

Diagnosis:	Physician sign/date
keeping these covered. Continue with an antibiotic ointment cream. Watch for any signs of infection and return to the clinic should he have any signs of infection.	*Nancy Crawley* MD
Discharge Transfer Admit Good Satisfactory Other:	

GODFREY REGIONAL HOSPITAL
123 Main Street • Aldon, FL 77714 • (407) 555-1234

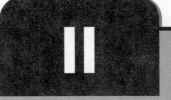

SURGERY

INTEGUMENTARY EXERCISES

EXERCISE 1

Level I

OPERATIVE REPORT

Patient information:	
Patient name: DOB: MR#:	Date: Surgeon: Anesthetist:

Preoperative diagnosis:

CA nose

Postoperative diagnosis:

CA nose

Procedure(s) performed:

OPERATIONS: Excision nasal lesion and coverage with pedicle flap

This patient is kindly referred for a lesion involving the right alar surface. It is 1 cm in diameter, has a typical rolled edge with central ulceration. Given the size along with the patient's current medications and anticoagulant status, the surgery was done in the operating room with monitors. IV sedation was given due to the fact that the area was fairly significant and a flap was needed for coverage.

Anesthesia:

Assistant surgeon:

Description of procedure:

After the skin was carefully prepped and draped, the lesion was carefully outlined. It indeed measured 1.3 cm in diameter. It looks as if I am well around the margin. The base was gently electrocoagulated. The suture was marked with a superior margin, having a suture located in it. A pedicle flap was then elevated along the nasal labial area and this in turn was rotated into its anatomic position. This was sutured in place with 5-0 chromic and 6-0 Prolene sutures. Excellent coverage was noted. Dressing was placed over the nose. The standard precautions are noted for discharge. A careful recheck will be made over the next couple of weeks. After the wound was sutured, the wound was carefully dressed with Xeroform and a standard 4 × 4 dressing. There were no complications.

Rachel Perez MD

GODFREY REGIONAL HOSPITAL
123 Main Street • Aldon, FL 77714 • (407) 555-1234

EXERCISE 2

Level I

OPERATIVE REPORT

Patient information:

Patient name: Date:
DOB: Surgeon:
MR#:   Anesthetist:

Preoperative diagnosis:

Extensive basal cell carcinoma in the left retroauricular area

Postoperative diagnosis:

Same

Procedure(s) performed:

OPERATION: 1. Wide excision basal cell carcinoma of the left auricular area
2. Harvesting skin graft of the left thigh and then skin graft application to the area of excisional therapy left auricular area
The patient had been seen in referral from his family doctor. He had local extensive basal cell carcinoma. Because of its size, 4 × 5 cm, it was clear that primary repair could not be accomplished, so I advised that possible skin graft would be necessary. I advised them to go home and talk it over, and if they wished to go through with the procedure, I would be delighted to do that. So, after they talked it over, the wife called me and they gave their consent to proceed. The procedure was done under local.

Anesthesia:

Assistant surgeon:

Description of procedure:

He was brought to surgery. The area in the left retroauricular area was shaved. The area in question, lesion with ulcerations, etc., was marked out. Then, starting on the left thigh, the appropriate area was chosen, cleaned with Betadine, and draped. 2% Xylocaine was then infiltrated, and appropriate split-thickness skin graft of appropriate thickness was harvested using the disposable Dynatome. This was saved in ice, wrapped in a sponge soaked in ice. Then the lesion behind the left ear was now addressed. This was infiltrated again with 2% Xylocaine. Once anesthesia took, the lesion was excised completely and submitted to Pathology for clearance. No marginal involvement was identified. Hemostasis was achieved. Then the graft harvested previously was now fashioned by nicking it in several places to allow for adequate drainage, and then sutured to the skin margins. In the lowermost aspect the graft was inadequate, so the wound defect was closed for now with 2-0 nylon with total closure of the wound with the graft. Operation terminated. Appropriate dressings were applied to the donor site on the left thigh as well as the op site in the left retroauricular area.

Patient was discharged to follow up on Friday just to check the status of the wound. Nursing was then advised to make sure patient doesn't pull off the dressings, or we are back to square one.

Stacy Knott, MD

GODFREY REGIONAL HOSPITAL
123 Main Street • Aldon, FL 77714 • (407) 555-1234

EXERCISE 3

Level I

OPERATIVE REPORT

Patient information:	
Patient name: DOB: MR#:	Date: Surgeon: Anesthetist:

Preoperative diagnosis:

Left leg squamous cell carcinoma

Postoperative diagnosis:

Left leg squamous cell carcinoma

Procedure(s) performed:

Excision of left leg CA with full-thickness skin graft and complex repair of the left thigh.

Anesthesia:

Assistant surgeon:

Description of procedure:

Under local anesthesia with Xylocaine 1% (used about 20 cc) and IV sedation by anesthesiologist, the left leg was prepped with Betadine, sterile towel draped, and incised. The lesion was in the distal leg at the anterior side and it is about 2 cm. I infiltrated the skin at this area and I did circular incision around the lesion, staying about 8 mm from the edge of it. Cut through the skin and subcutaneous tissue and sent the specimen to the pathologist. They told me the margin was free of tumor. Hemostasis was done with cautery.

We were then supposed to do a split-thickness skin graft from the left thigh, but the dermatome was not available, so I had to do it full-thickness skin graft. I cut the skin in the left upper thigh area anteriorly with Xylocaine 1% and used about 12 cc. Then I did an elliptical incision about 3 inches × 1 inch, cut the skin and subcutaneous tissue, took the lesion off, and then mobilized the skin flap on both sides of the thigh, superiorly and inferiorly. Hemostasis was done with cautery. Closed the edges together with chromic.

3-0 without tension, and the subcutaneous tissue and the skin was approximated with nylon 3-0 and a mattress suture. I applied sterile dressing, then cleaned the skin graft from the subcutaneous fat, and applied it over the left leg and sutured it in interrupted layers with nylon 4-0. I applied Vaseline gauze and a cotton ball on the top of it. I tied the suture on top of it and applied sterile dressing. I put an Ace bandage over the dressing of the graft. The patient tolerated the procedure well.

GODFREY REGIONAL HOSPITAL
123 Main Street • Aldon, FL 77714 • (407) 555-1234

Rachel Perez MD

EXERCISE 4

Level II

OPERATIVE REPORT

Patient information:

Patient name: Date:
DOB: Surgeon:
MR#:   Anesthetist:

Preoperative diagnosis:

Mass right breast

Postoperative diagnosis:

Same

Procedure(s) performed:

Ultrasound-guided needle localization of right breast lesion. Excision biopsy of lesion of right breast following ultrasound localization. Frozen-section exam, all revealing benign fibroadenoma of the right breast.

Anesthesia:

Assistant surgeon:

Description of procedure:

The patient was admitted this morning for surgery. She had recently been evaluated and found to have a right breast lump. Ultrasound suggested a solid mass, and excision was recommended. We obtained an informed consent and she was admitted this morning for the same. I explained to her that the procedure was to be done with needle localization so that the exact lump palpated was the one that was removed. On admission this morning, an IV line was started in the ED. She was then taken to the x-ray suite where under ultrasound guidance the lump was localized with the needle. She was then brought up for surgery. Preoperatively, she received 1 gram of Ancef IV. Surgery was to be done with local plus IV sedation monitored anesthesia. In surgery, she was appropriately positioned. The right breast area was cleaned with DuraPrep and draped, and the entry point was at the 3-4 o'clock position. The incision site was then infiltrated with my usual anesthetic mix. Once this took, a small incision was then made just abutting to the entry point of needle. Entering the breast substance, hemostasis was achieved. The needle was localized and then followed to its termination. Prior to termination, the area in question was identified; a generous excision margin was now achieved and encompassed the needle and the node in question. All of this was taken in one piece and submitted for radiologic evaluation. This confirmed that the area in question had been removed. Subsequently, frozen section was then done, which showed benign fibroadenoma. At this junction the operation was terminated, and hemostasis was achieved. The breast was then reconstructed in layers: subcu with 2-0 chromic, skin with 3-0 nylon. Appropriate dressings were applied. I will be visiting with the patient's mother, and patient was advised as to our findings and the successful outcome with benign results. Upon discharge, she will see me in the office a week from today. Sponge and instrument counts were correct on two occasions.

Adr Westy MD

GODFREY REGIONAL HOSPITAL
123 Main Street • Aldon, FL 77714 • (407) 555-1234

EXERCISE 5

Level II

OPERATIVE REPORT

Patient information:	
Patient name: DOB: MR#:	Date: Surgeon: Anesthetist:

Preoperative diagnosis:

Thickened endometrium by way of ultrasound

Postoperative diagnosis:

1. Same with path pending suggestive of either an endometrial polyp or a small submucous fibroid
2. Lesions to the right infraclavicular area, right cheek, and right parascapular area

Procedure(s) performed:

OPERATION:
1. Excision of lesions to the right clavicular area, right preauricular area, and right parascapular area
2. Cystoscopy and D&C

FINDINGS: Six 2-mm raised lesions to the right infraclavicular area. Approximately 5-mm lesion to the right preauricular area. Approximately 1.2-cm lesion to the right parascapular area. The general bimanual exam was negative.

Anesthesia:

Assistant surgeon:

Description of procedure:

In lithotomy position under general anesthesia, the patient is appropriately prepped and draped. The bimanual exam is done, which reveals the uterus to be retroverted, retroflexed. There appear to be no adnexal masses. Subsequently, a weighted vaginal speculum is introduced into the vagina. The anterior lip of the cervix is picked up with a tenaculum. The uterus sounded to a depth of approximately 9 cm. The uterus, as mentioned, is noted to be retroverted. The hysteroscope is introduced into the endometrial canal and advanced. There is noted to be somewhat of a polypoid lesion on the mid anterior uterine wall just past the cervix. The rest of the intrauterine cavity appears to be negative. Subsequently, the cervix is then further dilated with Hegar's dilator sufficient enough to admit the uterine curette, the uterine cavity is curetted with a sharp curette, and the mass to the anterior portion of the uterus is removed with a curettage and sent to Pathology. The uterine cavity is checked for other masses and none are noted. The hysteroscope is reintroduced. There appear to be no further lesions noted in the uterine cavity. The tissue was then sent to Pathology. Tenaculum and speculum are removed.

Attention is carried to the lesions to the infraclavicular area, right preauricular area, and the right parascapular area. These areas are all cleaned with Betadine and subsequently curetted off and cauterized with electrocautery. Hemostasis is to be noted quite adequate.

The patient tolerated the procedure well and left operating room in good condition. Estimated blood loss is minimal.

Rachel Perez MD

GODFREY REGIONAL HOSPITAL
123 Main Street • Aldon, FL 77714 • (407) 555-1234

EXERCISE 6

Level I

OPERATIVE REPORT

Patient information:	
Patient name: DOB: MR#:	Date: Surgeon: Anesthetist:

Preoperative diagnosis:

INDICATION:
The patient is a 7-year-old white male who reportedly fell off bleachers and suffered lacerations to his face along the inferior aspect of the lip on the right side, and also small lacerations over the lip itself and intraorally along the mucosa and just at the sulcus inferiorly near the mandible. The patient's family denies any loss of consciousness of the child, and he was brought immediately to the emergency room.

Postoperative diagnosis:

Procedure(s) performed:

Debridement irrigation, closure of facial and intraoral lacerations

Anesthesia:

Assistant surgeon:

Description of procedure:

In the operating room the patient underwent general anesthesia with endotracheal intubation. The face and mouth were then prepped and draped in the usual sterile fashion. The necrotic tissue from the edges of the wound were sharply debrided with a 15 blade scalpel and tenotomy scissors. Hemostasis was achieved with bipolar cautery. The intraoral lesions measured 1 cm along the mucosa near the commissure of the lip and 2.5 cm at the sulcus inferiorly. These lacerations were irrigated, bleeding was cauterized, necrotic tissue was debrided sharply, and it was closed with a running 4-0 Vicryl suture using locking stitches. The small laceration along the mucosa was closed with interrupted 4-0 Vicryl sutures.

The external lacerations measured 2.5 cm below the right side of the lower lip. This was debrided sharply and hemostasis was achieved with bipolar cautery. The laceration was closed in layers using 4-0 Vicryl for the deep layer to reapproximate the orbicularis oris muscle and 5-0 Vicryl for the subdermal layer; 5-0 plain gut was used to close the skin. A small portion of the laceration extended across the vermilion border and the majority of it was on the skin. A small 3-mm laceration oriented vertically on the lower lip was also closed with interrupted plain gut suture. And a small 3-mm laceration on his chin was closed also with interrupted plain gut.

The patient tolerated the procedure well. At the end of the procedure a plain x-ray of the face was taken to rule out any fractures. The patient was successfully extubated in the operating room and then taken to the PACU for recovery.

GODFREY REGIONAL HOSPITAL   *Maurice Doater, MD*
123 Main Street • Aldon, FL 77714 • (407) 555-1234

EXERCISE 7

Level I

OPERATIVE REPORT

Patient information:	
Patient name: DOB: MR#:	Date: Surgeon: Anesthetist:

Preoperative diagnosis:

Mass right breast

Postoperative diagnosis:

Infiltrating ductal carcinoma

Procedure(s) performed:

Excisional biopsy of right breast with frozen section, followed by lumpectomy and axillary node dissection

Anesthesia:

Assistant surgeon:

Description of procedure:

The patient was placed in the operating room on the operating table in the supine position. After induction of general anesthesia, the right breast and axilla were prepped with DuraPrep and draped in the usual manner. The patient had a palpable lump in the upper right breast, correlating with the normal mammogram and sonogram. A transverse incision of about 5 cm was made. This was deepened through subcutaneous tissue. Bleeders were cauterized. The palpable mass was felt and excision was carried around this lesion down to the deeper layer. The lesion was about 2 inches above the areola. The specimen was removed and x-rayed, and this confirmed that the lesion was removed. This was then sent to Pathology for frozen section. The results were infiltrating ductal carcinoma less than 1 cm in diameter with adequate margin, the closest margin being 6 mm from the tumor. While we were waiting for the frozen section, the incision was closed. The decision was made to proceed with lumpectomy and axillary node dissection; this had been agreed to by the patient earlier.

The skin was then marked, and an elliptical incision was made at least 2 cm from each edge of the incision. An elliptical incision was made, and the incision was carried down to the pectoralis fascia. The previous biopsy site was not entered. The specimen was completely removed. The wound was irrigated and packed with wet saline gauze. We then proceeded with the axillary node dissection, which was made through a separate axillary incision about 6 cm in length. This was deepened through subcutaneous tissue. The axilla was entered. The axillary vein was identified. Palpable nodes were noted. A few were enlarged and suspicious, about 1–2 cm in diameter. The long thoracic nerve and thoracodorsal nerve were seen and preserved. The veins in the lymphatics were hemoclipped and divided, and the axilla was cleared between the two nerves, and the thoracodorsal vessels were preserved. There was no evidence of any lymph nodes adherent to the nerves

GODFREY REGIONAL HOSPITAL
123 Main Street • Aldon, FL 77714 • (407) 555-1234

Continued

OPERATIVE REPORT

Patient information:	
Patient name: DOB: MR#:	Date: Surgeon: Anesthetist:

Preoperative diagnosis:

Postoperative diagnosis:

Procedure(s) performed:

Anesthesia:

Assistant surgeon:

Description of procedure:

or the axillary vein, and the apex of the axilla was clear. The dissection was completed and submitted for pathology. The wound was irrigated. A Jackson-Pratt was placed in the wound in the axilla through a separate stab wound and was secured with 2-0 silk. After irrigation, the incisions were closed with interrupted 2-0 Vicryl. Then another layer of running 3-0 Vicryl on the dermis and the skin with subcuticular 4-0 Dexon was used. Neosporin and dressings were applied. The breast was covered with an Ace bandage on the chest for compression. Blood loss was about 100 cc.

Adm Westg MD

GODFREY REGIONAL HOSPITAL
123 Main Street • Aldon, FL 77714 • (407) 555-1234

EXERCISE 8

Level II

OPERATIVE REPORT

Patient information:

Patient name:	Date:
DOB:	Surgeon:
MR#:	Anesthetist:

Preoperative diagnosis:

Right lower eyelid, right upper arm, right forearm, upper back skin lesions, and left hand wound

Postoperative diagnosis:

Right lower eyelid, right upper arm, right forearm, upper back skin lesions, and left hand wound

Procedure(s) performed:

OPERATIVE PROCEDURE:
Excision of right lower eyelid, right upper arm, right forearm, upper back skin lesions, and debridement of left hand wound
INDICATIONS FOR PROCEDURE:
The patient is a 68-year-old white female who is on chronic steroids and has all the stigmata of chronic steroid use. She is

Anesthesia:

Assistant surgeon:

Description of procedure:

The patient was brought to the operating room and placed supine on the operating room table. The patient's right forearm, upper arm, left hand, and face were prepped and draped in the usual sterile fashion.

After adequate IV sedation, the skin lesions on the right lower eyelid, right upper arm, and right forearm were anesthetized with 1% lidocaine with epinephrine. The wound over the left hand was anesthetized with 1% lidocaine plain. After adequate local anesthesia was achieved, the skin lesion from the right lower eyelid was excised using curved iris scissors. The wound edges were closed with simple stitches using 6-0 fast-absorbing catgut sutures.

Next, the lesions on the upper arm and forearm were excised using a 15 blade scalpel, which was used to form a fusiform incision around the lesions, providing a 3-mm border. The lesion was then sent to Pathology for permanent sections. The wound edges were undermined and then closed with 3-0 nylon sutures using horizontal mattress stitches.

These wounds were then cleaned, covered with antibiotic ointment and gauze on the arm; and the lesion on the right lower eyelid was covered with bacitracin ophthalmic ointment.

The lesion on the left hand, dorsal surface, was debrided sharply with a 15 blade scalpel. All necrotic tissue was removed

GODFREY REGIONAL HOSPITAL
123 Main Street • Aldon, FL 77714 • (407) 555-1234

Continued

OPERATIVE REPORT

Patient information:	
Patient name:	Date:
DOB:	Surgeon:
MR#:	Anesthetist:

Preoperative diagnosis:

Postoperative diagnosis:

Procedure(s) performed:

also a kidney transplant patient on immunosuppression. She has a history of multiple skin cancers and now presents with four lesions that are suspicious for skin cancers. She wishes to have these excised. The patient also suffered a traumatic injury to the dorsum of her left hand within the last week; the wound has some necrotic tissue within it and needs debridement.

Anesthesia:

Assistant surgeon:

Description of procedure:

sharply. The wound was then irrigated, hemostasis was achieved with electrocautery, and the wound was then covered with Silvadene and a sterile gauze dressing.

At the end of the procedure, the patient was sat up on the operating room table. The lesion on the patient's upper back below her neck was prepped and draped in the usual sterile fashion. It was then anesthetized with 1% lidocaine with epinephrine. The lesion was then excised using a fusiform incision, and this lesion, too, was sent to Pathology for analysis. The wound edges were then undermined and closed with interrupted 3-0 nylon sutures using horizontal mattress stitches. The patient tolerated the procedure well. Her wounds were cleaned, covered with antibiotic ointment and gauze, and she was then taken to PACU for recovery in stable condition.

Maurice Doater, MD

GODFREY REGIONAL HOSPITAL
123 Main Street • Aldon, FL 77714 • (407) 555-1234

EXERCISE 9

Level II

OPERATIVE REPORT

Patient information:	
Patient name: DOB: MR#:	Date: Surgeon: Anesthetist:

Preoperative diagnosis:

Gynecomastia, right breast

Postoperative diagnosis:

Same

Procedure(s) performed:

OPERATION: Excision gynecomastia right breast with frozen section

INDICATIONS: Patient was admitted for the operation. In the distant past we had excised the gynecomastia of the left breast. No cause could be found for this. He saw me a few weeks ago, having developed another gynecomastia in the right breast and he wanted it removed, so he was brought in this morning for surgery. On admission, he received 1 gram of Ancef on call to surgery. He was then brought to surgery. The procedure was to be done under local with monitored anesthesia.

Anesthesia:

Assistant surgeon:

Description of procedure:

In surgery with an IV line in place, he received IV anesthetics for sedation. Then the right breast, right chest wall was cleaned with DuraPrep and draped and the operation started. The right breast was markedly enlarged, consistent with gynecomastia, and benign. My incision was going to be a circumareolar incision. The area of my planned incision was then marked out with a marking pen, infiltrated with my usual anesthetic mix for an appropriate distance until adequate analgesia/anesthesia was obtained. The incision was then made. The areolar complex was immobilized and elevated. Then the margins of the breast around the areola were now dissected circumferentially until all breast tissue was marked out. It was then dissected out from the pectoralis muscle until all of the tissue was removed. The breast was then removed in toto and submitted for frozen section exam that confirmed that this was a benign gynecomastia. The empty space resulting was now cleaned. Hemostasis was achieved using the cautery as needed. A small Penrose drain was then inserted prior to closure. The breast was then closed in layers: subcu 2-0 chromic, skin with 3-0 nylon and appropriate pressure dressings were applied. The patient is to see me again on Friday. At that time I will decide whether it would be appropriate to remove the drain or not.

I talked with the patient in the recovery room post recovery, and advised him as to findings and as to when I will be seeing him. He will be discharged on pain meds and I will see him on Friday.

GODFREY REGIONAL HOSPITAL
123 Main Street • Aldon, FL 77714 • (407) 555-1234

EXERCISE 10

Level I

OPERATIVE REPORT

Patient information:	
Patient name: DOB: MR#:	Date: Surgeon: Anesthetist:

Preoperative diagnosis:

Chronic ulcer, left hallux toe, secondary to neuropathy

Postoperative diagnosis:

Same

Procedure(s) performed:

Debridement of ulceration with bone biopsy

Anesthesia:

Assistant surgeon:

Description of procedure:

The patient was prepped and draped in the usual aseptic manner. Attention was directed to the ulcer on the plantar aspect of the left hallux toe. Two converging semi-elliptical incisions were made about the ulcer. The ulcer edges were incised in toto. The incision was carried proximally along the course of the tunnel, which did course proximal and medial. It was noted that there was inflamed, swollen, infected, and necrotic tissue, which included the tendon sheath but not the flexor hallucis longus tendon. The tendon did appear white and glistening.

The incision was made in capsule, and there was a serosanguineous type fluid that drained from the wound/incision. Bone debridement was made for biopsy. Culture was made. The wound was flushed with copious amounts of sterile saline using Pulse Vac. The wound was inspected, and it was noted that all devitalized tissue had been removed. The wound was closed with 3-0 Polysorb simple interrupted sutures, and a 1/4-inch Penrose drain was inserted into the wound.

The incision was not closed in normal fashion, but I used about half the sutures that I would normally use so as to allow for drainage. I applied Xeroform gauze plus a sterile gauze bandage for compression and hemostasis.

The patient tolerated the procedure and anesthesia well and was transported to the recovery room with vital signs stable and in good condition.

GODFREY REGIONAL HOSPITAL
123 Main Street • Aldon, FL 77714 • (407) 555-1234

EXERCISE 11

Level II

OPERATIVE REPORT

Patient information:

Patient name:	Date:
DOB:	Surgeon:
MR#:	Anesthetist:

Preoperative diagnosis:

Right middle finger nail bed injury with subungual hematoma

Postoperative diagnosis:

Right middle finger nail bed injury with subungual hematoma with right middle nail bed laceration and necrotic nail bed with bone exposure

Procedure(s) performed:

PROCEDURE: Right middle finger nail plate removal, evacuation of subungual hematoma, debridement of necrotic nail bed, repair of nail bed laceration, suture removal

INDICATION FOR SURGERY: The patient is a 56-year-old white male who suffered a blunt trauma injury to his right middle finger approximately one week ago. He presented yesterday with this injury that had been repaired at an outside hospital emergency room. He now presents for evacuation of a subungual hematoma and repair of nail bed injuries.

Anesthesia:

Assistant surgeon:

Description of procedure:

The patient underwent a digital block of his right middle finger prior to coming into the operating room. There he underwent sedation, and his right hand and forearm were prepped and draped in the usual sterile fashion. A tourniquet was placed over his upper arm. At the beginning of the procedure, the hand was elevated and pressure was held for exsanguination. The tourniquet was inflated to 250 mm Hg pressure. Two sutures were removed from the nail plate and the skin using a blunt mosquito forceps. The nail plate was dissected off of the remaining nail bed and the nail plate was then removed. The underlying nail bed had a laceration across the mid portion and was necrotic at the distal portion along the radial side of the finger. The necrotic tissue was sharply debrided with a 15 blade scalpel. Upon completion of the nail bed debridement, there was exposed bone under the wound. The patient has a fracture of this distal phalanx, which was noted on preoperative x-ray. The wound was thoroughly irrigated with saline solution. The nail bed laceration in this open wound was then closed using 4-0 Vicryl suture. After repair of the nail bed and closure of this open wound, the nail bed and finger were assessed for bleeding by deflating the tourniquet. There was good hemostasis over the operative field. Preoperatively, it was noted that the patient's fingertip, which had been lacerated in the injury, was repaired but appeared dusky. A 25-gauge needle was poked into this flap of skin at the distal pulp of the finger and there was poor blood return. This suggests that there may be partial necrosis and loss of the skin in this part of the finger. The wound was then covered with antibiotic ointment, Xeroform gauze, clean gauze, and paper tape. It was then placed into a splint. The patient was then successfully taken to the PACU for recovery in stable condition.

GODFREY REGIONAL HOSPITAL
123 Main Street • Aldon, FL 77714 • (407) 555-1234

EXERCISE 12

Level I

OPERATIVE REPORT

Patient information:

Patient name: Date:
DOB: Surgeon:
MR#:   Anesthetist:

Preoperative diagnosis:

Thin melanoma left arm

Postoperative diagnosis:

Thin melanoma left arm

Procedure(s) performed:

TITLE OF PROCEDURE:
Re-excision of melanoma left arm with 1-cm margins
FINDINGS:
There was no gross tumor left

Anesthesia:

Assistant surgeon:

Description of procedure:

TECHNICAL PROCEDURES USED:
After placement on the table in the supine position with the appropriate area overlying the triceps of the left arm exposed, the left arm was prepped and draped in the usual fashion. A measuring device was utilized to mark off 1-cm margins around the previous excision. An ellipse was then removed, being certain to obtain at least 1-cm margins around the previous area of excision. This was oriented transversely. Dissection was carried straight down through the skin incision down to the fascia, and all underlying connective tissue was removed with the specimen down to the fascial level. Hemostasis was obtained using electrocautery. The wound was then closed using interrupted 4-0 Ethilon sutures, followed by a sterile dressing. The patient tolerated the procedure with no complications.

GODFREY REGIONAL HOSPITAL
123 Main Street • Aldon, FL 77714 • (407) 555-1234

EXERCISE 13

Level I

OPERATIVE REPORT

Patient information:	
Patient name: DOB: MR#:	Date: Surgeon: Anesthetist:

Preoperative diagnosis:

Possible basal cell carcinoma of the right upper lid

Postoperative diagnosis:

Pending surgical pathology

Procedure(s) performed:

Anesthesia:

Lid block using 2% lidocaine with epinephrine

Assistant surgeon:

Description of procedure:

After written informed consent was obtained, the patient was brought to the operating room where she was prepped and draped in the usual sterile fashion. The area of the right upper lid neoplasm was marked in a wedge shape, and the lid block consisting of 2 ccs of 2% lidocaine with epinephrine was given to the right upper lid.

Next a wedge resection was performed using Westcott scissors. Next the bleeding vessels were cauterized. Three 4-0 Vicryl sutures were used to close the tarsus so that they opposed each other. Then 2 6-0 silk sutures were passed through the anterior and posterior lid margin to oppose the lid margins together. 6-0 Vicryl sutures were used to close the orbicularis oculi layer superior to the tarsus.

Then interrupted 6-0 nylon sutures were used to close the skin incision, taking care to tag the silk sutures around the nylon sutures. At the end of the case, the wedge defect had been closed and the lid margins were nicely opposed to each other without any notching of the lid margin.

Bacitracin ointment was applied to the wound and a patch was placed. The patient was taken to the recovery room in excellent condition.

COMPLICATIONS: None

Adm Westg MD

GODFREY REGIONAL HOSPITAL
123 Main Street • Aldon, FL 77714 • (407) 555-1234

EXERCISE 14

Level I

OPERATIVE REPORT

Patient information:

Patient name: Date:
DOB: Surgeon:
MR#:   Anesthetist:

Preoperative diagnosis:

Right gynecomastia, skin tag

Postoperative diagnosis:

Same

Procedure(s) performed:

OPERATIVE PROCEDURE: Right subcutaneous mastectomy; excision of skin tag, right groin
INDICATIONS: The patient is a 75-year-old gentleman who has had enlargement and tenderness in the right breast for about six months. His sonogram and mammogram show changes consistent with gynecomastia.
OPERATIVE FINDINGS: Beneath the right areola there was a 4 × 3 cm condensation of fibrous breast tissue. There was no clinical evidence of malignancy. The pathologic examination is pending at this time.

Anesthesia:

Assistant surgeon:

Description of procedure:

TEXT OF NOTE:
The patient was brought to the operating room and identified by myself as Andrew Smith for the purpose of the above stated procedure. Intravenous sedation was administered. The right breast was sterilely prepped and draped. Under a satisfactory level of sedation, I inscribed a circumareolar incision oriented in the lower outer quadrant. The dermis and subcutaneous breast tissue were infiltrated with 1% lidocaine with epinephrine. The incision was made with the 15 blade. The areola was elevated off of the breast tissue using the scalpel and electrocautery. The lesion was circumferentially excised with the electrocautery and removed. Some minor bleeding points were cauterized. The wound was irrigated with antibiotic solution and sponged dry. Satisfactory hemostasis was observed. The wound was closed with interrupted 3-0 Monocryl and running 4-0 subcuticular Monocryl. Mastisol, Steri-strips, and an Opsite dressing were applied.

The right groin was exposed and prepped with Betadine. The dermis at the base of the skin tag was infiltrated with lidocaine with epinephrine and the skin tag was removed by shave excision. The base was cauterized. A bandage dressing was applied. The final instrument, sponge, and needle counts were correct. Estimated blood loss was minimal. The patient tolerated the procedure well and was returned to the recovery room in satisfactory condition.

Adm Westg MD

GODFREY REGIONAL HOSPITAL
123 Main Street • Aldon, FL 77714 • (407) 555-1234

EXERCISE 15

Level I

OPERATIVE REPORT

Patient information:	
Patient name:	Date:
DOB:	Surgeon:
MR#:	Anesthetist:

Preoperative diagnosis:

1. Traumatic amputation, tip left 3rd toe
2. Open fracture, distal phalanx, left second toe

Postoperative diagnosis:

Same

Procedure(s) performed:

Irrigation and debridement of wounds with revision of amputation, left third toe

Anesthesia:

Assistant surgeon:

Description of procedure:

The patient was placed supine on the operating room table and a satisfactory general anesthetic was given. The patient was given preoperative Kefzol intravenously in the emergency room. No pneumatic tourniquet was used. The left foot, ankle, and lower leg were prepped sterilely with DuraPrep and the left foot was draped in the usual sterile fashion. 2.5 liters of normal saline antibiotic solution were then used to irrigate out the second and third toes to very healthy and clean tissue. Any debris was removed before and during the irrigation. A spike of bone was protruding from the amputation site of the third toe. This was cleared to soft tissue when resected back beneath the tissue. The toe was not shortened further to provide a closure of the amputation site. Rather, the amputation site was discussed with the patient in the emergency room, and will remain open to allow for granulation. The tip of the second toe was not completely amputated and was actually a flap or open Bookman type of laceration with underlying fracture of the distal phalanx. This was tacked closed loosely with a single simple suture of 3-0 Ethilon. The wounds were irrigated again with 0.5 liters of normal saline antibiotic solution. Neosporin ointment was copiously applied as well as dry sterile dressings and sterile Kerlix wrap.

The patient tolerated the procedure well. There were no complications. He was awakened in the operating room and transported to the recovery room in stable condition.

GODFREY REGIONAL HOSPITAL
123 Main Street • Aldon, FL 77714 • (407) 555-1234

EXERCISE 16

Level II

OPERATIVE REPORT

Patient information:

Patient name:　　　　　　　　　　　Date:
DOB:　　　　　　　　　　　　　　　Surgeon:
MR#:　　　　　　　　　　　　　　　Anesthetist:

Preoperative diagnosis:

Cutaneous wound fistula with probable suture abscesses

Postoperative diagnosis:

Cutaneous wound fistula with probable suture abscesses

Procedure(s) performed:

Right subcostal wound exploration; removal of suture abscess; scar revision

INDICATIONS: The patient is a 70-year-old Native American gentleman who underwent an emergency cholecystectomy via a right subcostal incision late last year in Texas. The patient has had problems with the incision itself for many months since then, and suture material has been removed from the wound on several occasions by both the patient and his primary care provider, a PA-C. The area has never healed and there have been two persistent fistulas now for many months, which have resisted topical therapy.

Anesthesia:

General endotracheal anesthesia by CRNA

Assistant surgeon:

Description of procedure:

The patient was identified and taken to the operating suite where he received a gram of intravenous Ancef. A general endotracheal anesthetic was then induced and the patient positioned appropriately for abdominal surgery. The abdomen was then prepped and draped in the usual sterile fashion.

The medial portion of the previous incision was opened to include the two cutaneous fistulae. The suture was immediately apparent. This was grasped and divided at the deepest level. The granulomatous reaction in the adjacent fascia was then debrided sharply. Hemostasis was achieved with electrocautery. The wound edges at the skin level were then freshened using a sharp blade. Hemostasis was achieved with electrocautery. The wound was then irrigated with Bacitracin solution.

With hemostasis assured, closure was performed in a single layer using titanium skin clips. Sterile bandage and dressing were then placed.

The patient's anesthetic was then reversed. He was uneventfully extubated and taken from the operative suite to the postanesthetic care unit in stable cardiovascular condition.

GODFREY REGIONAL HOSPITAL
123 Main Street • Aldon, FL 77714 • (407) 555-1234

Continued

OPERATIVE REPORT

Patient information:

Patient name: Date:
DOB: Surgeon:
MR#:   Anesthetist:

Preoperative diagnosis:

Postoperative diagnosis:

Procedure(s) performed:

The patient was referred for surgical evaluation at which time he was advised that a wound exploration, removal of the offending suture material, and scar revision would be the most appropriate treatment. He was given a description of this procedure and various other alternatives and ultimately agreed to proceed. He was given a description of the potential perioperative complications including persistence or recurrence of the fistulous problem. The patient gave his full informed consent.
EBL: Less than 20 cc

Anesthesia:

Assistant surgeon:

Description of procedure:

FINDINGS: The findings at the time of surgery include the presence of a typical suture abscess present with the suture of the anterior fascial closure of this right Kocher incision. The suture had not degraded; it appeared to be a braided-type material. This was removed with no disruption of the fascial closure and the wound closed in a single layer with titanium skin clips. There was no sign of any active infection. The skin of the wound had a probable yeast superficial infection.
COMPLICATIONS: None

Adm Westg MD

GODFREY REGIONAL HOSPITAL
123 Main Street • Aldon, FL 77714 • (407) 555-1234

EXERCISE 17

Level II

OPERATIVE REPORT

Patient information:

Patient name:	Date:
DOB:	Surgeon:
MR#:	Anesthetist:

Preoperative diagnosis:

Bloody nipple discharge, right nipple, 8 o'clock radius

Postoperative diagnosis:

Same

Procedure(s) performed:

Duct exploration and excision
SPECIMEN: Breast tissue, frozen section benign papilloma and fibrocystic changes
CONDITION: Stable
PROGNOSIS: Excellent
INDICATIONS: The patient presented with bloody nipple discharge, Hemoccult-positive on testing in the office. I had asked her not to express this, and we scheduled her for nipple duct exploration.

Anesthesia:

Assistant surgeon:

Description of procedure:

She was brought to the operating room and placed in the supine position. After appropriate anesthesia was achieved, she was prepped and draped over the right breast. Curvilinear incision was made in the areolar border through a field of injected lidocaine with epinephrine. I elevated an areolar flap until the ductal tissues were encountered and an enlarged blue-black looking duct was encountered. It was circumferentially dissected; actually, it was opened and I was able to pass a lacrimal duct cannula into the duct, and held that in place with a hemostat. I then took the duct down off of the back of the nipple. I then further excised ductal tissue off the back of the nipple as a separate specimen. I then elevated flaps circumferentially and excised the underlying breast tissue in that quadrant. It was oriented with sutures for the pathologist. I then sent it to Pathology for sectioning. Excision was done with the Bovie; controlled bleeding was done with the Bovie. The patient tolerated the procedure without apparent difficulty. The wound was marked with clips circumferentially. I then closed the subcutaneous tissues with 3-0 Vicryl and the skin with 5-0 Prolene, followed by a sterile dressing.

With the patient still under sedation I went to Pathology, reviewed the specimen with the pathologist and the frozen section, which just came back benign. There was a papilloma present. There were fibrocystic changes present. We then released the patient from the OR. She is in stable condition.

Adm Westg MD

GODFREY REGIONAL HOSPITAL
123 Main Street • Aldon, FL 77714 • (407) 555-1234

EXERCISE 18

Level II

OPERATIVE REPORT

Patient information:	
Patient name:	Date:
DOB:	Surgeon:
MR#:	Anesthetist:

Preoperative diagnosis:

Skin lesion over right flank and back, possible melanoma in situ

Postoperative diagnosis:

Skin lesion over right flank and back, possible melanoma in situ

Procedure(s) performed:

Excision of right flank and back skin lesions with complex closure

INDICATION FOR SURGERY:
The patient is a 47-year-old white female with shave biopsies of lesions over her right flank and back. The specimens were not clearly labeled and it is unclear which of these areas was truly a melanoma in situ. The other lesion is consistent with some atypia. Because of the uncertainty of the diagnosis for melanoma in the location, both lesions are being excised with the presumptive diagnosis of melanoma in situ.

Anesthesia:

Assistant surgeon:

Description of procedure:

The patient was placed in a left decubitus position. The areas were prepped and draped in the usual sterile fashion. The skin and subcutaneous tissue around these lesions were anesthetized with 1% lidocaine with epinephrine. A total of 22 cc of local anesthetic was used. Fusiform incisions were made around these lesions, allowing for a 0.5 cm border. The border was marked around the biopsy scar. The scar over the right flank measured 1.5 cm and the scar over the back measured 0.8 cm. After the fusiform incisions were made, further dissection was carried out with the scalpel. Separate instruments were used for both locations. When the specimen was removed, it was sent to Pathology for permanent sections.

Using skin hooks, the wound edges were retracted, and electrocautery was used to extensively undermine the wound edges to allow for tension-free closure. Once the wound edges were thoroughly mobilized in the subcutaneous plane, bleeding was controlled with electrocautery. The wound was then thoroughly irrigated with saline solution. The right flank wound was then closed with 3-0 Vicryl for the deep layer and running 3-0 nylon for the skin. The lesion over the back was also extensively mobilized by retracting the wound edges with skin hooks and using electrocautery to undermine the skin flaps. The bleeding was controlled with electrocautery, and the deep layer was closed with 3-0 Vicryl suture and the skin was closed with running 2-0 nylon suture.

The patient tolerated the operation well, and the wounds were cleaned and covered with antibiotic ointment and pressure dressings. The patient was then taken to the postanesthesia care unit for recovery in stable condition.

GODFREY REGIONAL HOSPITAL *Maurice Doater, MD*
123 Main Street • Aldon, FL 77714 • (407) 555-1234

EXERCISE 19

Level I

OPERATIVE REPORT

Patient information:	
Patient name: DOB: MR#:	Date: Surgeon: Anesthetist:

Preoperative diagnosis:

Morpheaform basal cell carcinoma of the nose

Postoperative diagnosis:

Morpheaform basal cell carcinoma of the nose

Procedure(s) performed:

Excision of basal cell carcinoma of the nose (2 cm × 1¼ cm). Full-thickness skin graft reconstruction of the nose from left preauricular donor site.
ESTIMATED BLOOD LOSS: Less than 10 cc

Anesthesia:

IV sedation/attended local

Assistant surgeon:

Description of procedure:

OPERATIVE NOTE: The patient was brought to the operating room and placed on the operating room table in a supine position. IV sedation was administered, and using 1% lidocaine with 1:100,000 parts epinephrine. The nose and left preauricular regions were injected. The face was prepped and draped in sterile fashion. Using a marking pen, the area of visualized tumor with margins was marked along the dorsum and nasal tip region. Using 15-blade scalpel, an incision was made along the marked areas, measuring approximately 1¼ cm, and full-thickness skin graft was removed, labeled, and sent to Pathology for frozen and permanent sections. Frozen section showed residual tumor on the lateral 6 to 9 o'clock margins and additional section removed was clear on frozen section. Deep margins were clear. Meticulous hemostasis was obtained with bipolar and Bovie cautery. Left preauricular incision was made and an elliptical full-thickness skin tag taken from this region. It was cut to size and sutured in place with interrupted 6-0 nylon sutures to the nasal tip defect. The preauricular incision was undermined and then closed with running interlocking 5-0 nylon sutures. Bacitracin ointment was placed to both wounds, followed by Telfa dressing over the left preauricular area, and a Telfa pressure dressing over the left nasal tip skin graft site.

The patient was fully awakened from IV sedation and brought to the recovery room in stable condition, having tolerated the procedure well.

Adm Westg MD

GODFREY REGIONAL HOSPITAL
123 Main Street • Aldon, FL 77714 • (407) 555-1234

Continued

OPERATIVE REPORT

Patient information:

Patient name: Date:
DOB: Surgeon:
MR#:   Anesthetist:

Preoperative diagnosis:

Postoperative diagnosis:

Procedure(s) performed:

CLINICAL NOTE: The patient is a 60-year-old white female who has had recurrent basal cell carcinoma of the nose removed on two previous occasions. The last occasion was found to be consistent with morpheaform basal cell carcinoma with positive residual tumor present. She is being brought to the operating room for wide local excision with frozen sections and reconstruction using full-thickness skin graft.

Anesthesia:

Assistant surgeon:

Description of procedure:

GODFREY REGIONAL HOSPITAL
123 Main Street • Aldon, FL 77714 • (407) 555-1234

EXERCISE 20

Level II

OPERATIVE REPORT

Patient information:	
Patient name: DOB: MR#:	Date: Surgeon: Anesthetist:

Preoperative diagnosis:

Traumatic scalp wound with bone exposure

Postoperative diagnosis:

Traumatic scalp wound with bone exposure

Procedure(s) performed:

Debridement and irrigation of traumatic scalp wound with flap coverage

INDICATION FOR SURGERY: The patient is a 76-year-old white male who initially fell from a seawall. He suffered a traumatic injury to his scalp with bone exposure, excessive bleeding, and had a foreign body within the scalp tissue. He did not seek medical attention initially and approximately three days later presented to the emergency room with an infected wound. There he underwent initial debridement and irrigation of his wound along with antibiotic therapy. He now presents for elective closure of his scalp following debridement and irrigation.

Anesthesia:

Assistant surgeon:

Description of procedure:

The patient was brought to the operating room and placed in supine position on the operating room table. After adequate general anesthesia and endotracheal intubation, the patient was prepped and draped in the usual sterile fashion. Using 1% lidocaine with epinephrine 1:100,000, a total of 20 cc of local anesthesia was used to infiltrate the scalp tissue around the wound. The wound measured approximately 12 cm × 6 cm in greatest dimensions. There was approximately 3.5 cm of exposed bone at the center of the wound. Currently, there is no purulence, crepitus or fluctuance or erythema associated with this wound, and there is no foreign body within it. However, there is still some necrotic material in the scalp wound. After adequate infiltration and anesthesia of area, skin hooks were used to retract the wound edges, and debridement was performed to tissue and fascia. Fibrinous material and other necrotic tissue was debrided with a curet. After the skin edges, subcutaneous tissue, muscle, and fascia were all thoroughly debrided and cleaned, the scalp was extensively undermined circumferentially. The wound was pulled together; however, it was not able to cover the area of bone exposure, thus a flap was constructed by incising the scalp over the left temporal area to allow for a rotation of the scalp flap into the central portion of the wound to cover the exposed bone. After the flap had been incised, it was mobilized with blunt and sharp dissection. Hemostasis was achieved with electrocautery. After the flap had been adequately immobilized, the wound was

GODFREY REGIONAL HOSPITAL
123 Main Street • Aldon, FL 77714 • (407) 555-1234

Continued

OPERATIVE REPORT

Patient information:	
Patient name:	Date:
DOB:	Surgeon:
MR#:	Anesthetist:

Preoperative diagnosis:

Postoperative diagnosis:

Procedure(s) performed:

Anesthesia:

Assistant surgeon:

Description of procedure:

thoroughly irrigated with three liters of normal saline solution mixed in with 50,000 units of Bacitracin.

After the wound and the flap had been thoroughly cleansed with irrigation, hemostasis was rechecked with electrocautery. After adequate hemostasis was achieved, the wound edges were reapproximated with interrupted 0 Vicryl sutures. In addition, 2-0 Vicryl was used to close the remaining areas. After closure of the deep layer, the rotation flap covered all of the exposed bone and the wound edges were not under tension. The skin was then closed with interrupted 2-0 nylon using simple stitches. The posterior and lateral aspects of the incisions were closed with running 3-0 nylon sutures.

The patient tolerated the procedure well. The wound was cleaned and covered with Bacitracin ointment, 4 × 4s, fluffs, and Kerlix rolls. The patient in the operating room was successfully extubated and taken to PACU for recovery. He went to PACU in stable condition.

Adm Westg MD

GODFREY REGIONAL HOSPITAL
123 Main Street • Aldon, FL 77714 • (407) 555-1234

EXERCISE 21

Level II

OPERATIVE REPORT

Patient information:	
Patient name: DOB: MR#:	Date: Surgeon: Anesthetist:

Preoperative diagnosis:

1. Intraoral tumor
2. Right nasal ala skin lesion

Postoperative diagnosis:

1. Intraoral tumor
2. Right nasal ala basal cell carcinoma measuring 0.9 cm

Procedure(s) performed:

OPERATIVE PROCEDURE:
Excision of intraoral tumor, excision of right nasal ala basal cell carcinoma with bilobed flap reconstruction

INDICATIONS FOR SURGERY:
The patient is a 70-year-old white female who presents with an intraoral lesion that has been slowly growing for the past several months, as well as a lesion on her nose over the right alar dome. She now presents for elective excision and treatment of these lesions.

Anesthesia:

Assistant surgeon:

Description of procedure:

The patient was brought to the operating room and placed supine on the operating room table. After adequate general anesthesia and endotracheal intubation, the patient was prepped and draped in the usual sterile fashion. Using 1% lidocaine with epinephrine, the skin and subcutaneous tissue around the lesion of the right alar dome were anesthetized. After adequate local anesthesia and epinephrine effect, a shave biopsy was performed of this basal cell carcinoma that measured 0.9 cm in size. The specimen was sent to Pathology and came back positive for basal cell carcinoma, all margins involved. The patient then had a 3-mm margin excised and sent to Pathology with sutures orienting the pathologist. Frozen section of this excision was negative for any tumor at the margins. A bilobed flap was outlined along the right nasal sidewall. Using skin hooks, the bilobed flap was undermined widely in the submuscular plane. Once this myocutaneous flap was adequately mobilized, the remaining wound edges were also mobilized to allow for closure without tension. The flap was then in-set using 5-0 Vicryl sutures for the deep layer and a combination of 5-0 and 6-0 nylon sutures for the skin. Please note that during flap transfer, the skin, subcutaneous tissue, and nasal muscle were transferred together with the flap.

Using separate instruments, separate syringe and needles, the intraoral lesion was anesthetized with 1% lidocaine with epinephrine for the epinephrine effect. After adequate time had elapsed, the lesion was excised with a #15 blade scalpel. The cheek was retracted with a small intraoral retractor, and the specimen was sent to Pathology for permanent sections. Hemostasis was achieved with electrocautery. The mucosa was then closed with running and locking 2-0 chromic sutures. At the end of the procedure, the patient was successfully extubated in the operating room. Her face had been cleaned and the suture line was covered with Bacitracin ointment.

At the end of the procedure, the patient was taken to PACU for recovery in stable condition.

Maurice Doster, MD

GODFREY REGIONAL HOSPITAL
123 Main Street • Aldon, FL 77714 • (407) 555-1234

EXERCISE 22

Level I

OPERATIVE REPORT

Patient information:	
Patient name:	Date:
DOB:	Surgeon:
MR#:	Anesthetist:

Preoperative diagnosis:

Recurrent squamous cell carcinoma of the oral cavity

Postoperative diagnosis:

Recurrent squamous cell carcinoma of the oral cavity

Procedure(s) performed:

Laser ablation of recurrent squamous cell carcinoma of the left anterior floor of mouth/mandibular alveolar mucosa/and left anterior tongue
ESTIMATED BLOOD LOSS: Less than 5 cc

Anesthesia:

General

Assistant surgeon:

Description of procedure:

OPERATIVE NOTE: The patient was brought in the operating room and placed on the operating room table in a supine position. General anesthesia was administered endotracheally with a special laser tube. The left anterior tongue/floor of mouth and alveolar area of tumor were seen and examined circumferentially. With margins this was marked with Bovie cautery prior to injecting with 1% lidocaine with 1:100,000 epinephrine. Using a hand-held laser set at 15 watts, super pulse power was applied around the circumference of the lesion, and dysplasia was circumscribed with the laser. The central tumor and dysplastic tissue were then ablated and vaporized with the laser. Specimens were sent from the left anterior tongue/anterior and posterior alveolar mucosal margins and left floor of mouth deep margins from the patient after ablation of the tumor. All these returned back negative for residual squamous cell carcinoma except the posterior alveolar margin that showed one small foci of carcinoma. This area was further ablated with the laser to destroy any residual tumor. There was adequate hemostasis obtained. There was meticulous hemostasis throughout the procedure. The patient was then awakened from general anesthesia, extubated, and brought to the recovery room in stable condition, having tolerated the procedure well.

Maurice Doater, MD

GODFREY REGIONAL HOSPITAL
123 Main Street • Aldon, FL 77714 • (407) 555-1234

Continued

OPERATIVE REPORT

Patient information:	
Patient name:	Date:
DOB:	Surgeon:
MR#:	Anesthetist:

Preoperative diagnosis:

Postoperative diagnosis:

Procedure(s) performed:

CLINICAL NOTE: The patient is an 82-year-old white female who several years ago underwent wide local resection of left anterior and lateral tongue and floor of mouth, squamous cell carcinoma. She had full-course radiation therapy postoperatively. She has been doing well, when on routine follow-up visit was found to have recurrent squamous cell carcinoma that was biopsied in the office and confirmed the above. She is being brought to the operating room for resection/ablation.

Anesthesia:

Assistant surgeon:

Description of procedure:

GODFREY REGIONAL HOSPITAL
123 Main Street • Aldon, FL 77714 • (407) 555-1234

EXERCISE 23

Level II

OPERATIVE REPORT

Patient information:	
Patient name: DOB: MR#:	Date: Surgeon: Anesthetist:

Preoperative diagnosis:

SUBJECTIVE:
The patient is a 5-year-old boy brought to the OR today for light sedation and treatment of molluscum contagiosum by cryotherapy. The patient has a history of molluscum, and two attempts at treatment in the clinic have taken place. The patient has not tolerated these procedures well at all and has required people to try to hold him down. In discussion with the family, they elected to use some light sedation for treatment of all the lesions at one time.

Postoperative diagnosis:

Procedure(s) performed:

Cryotherapy, attempts at curetting molluscum contagiosum skin lesions. The patient was brought to the operating area by his father. The patient was given light MEC for sedation. Once fully sedated, the lesions were exposed. Curettage was attempted but the lesions were not easily removed. Cryotherapy was then used to treat each of the lesions through two freeze/thaw cycles. Total time probably 5 minutes. Sedation was removed and the patient was awakened. He tolerated it all very well.

Anesthesia:

Assistant surgeon:

Description of procedure:

ASSESSMENT:
Cryotherapy of molluscum contagiosum. Scars of the lesions were discussed with the father. They are encouraged to use some Bacitracin on the lesions. They are encouraged to return with any signs of infection. Father was given a Rx for Atarax 25 mg up to qid as needed for itch. I also encouraged them to use ibuprofen or Tylenol as needed for pain. They are to return to the clinic for recheck in one week.

NOTE:
The patient was admitted through Outpatient Day Surgery.

Adm Westg, MD

GODFREY REGIONAL HOSPITAL
123 Main Street • Aldon, FL 77714 • (407) 555-1234

EXERCISE 24

Level I

EMERGENCY ROOM RECORD

Name:		Age:	ER physician:
		DOB:	

Allergies/type of reaction:	Usual medications/dosages:
Codein	

Triage/presenting complaint:	CC: Fall/injury, pain Patient fell and hit head on coffee table PAST MEDICAL HISTORY: DJD, HTN

Initial assessment:	ROS: Negative nausea, vomited, headache Tripped, no loss of consciousness, no headache Integumentary: Negative for rashes Constitutional: Negative for fever All other systems have been reviewed and are negative

Time	T	P	R	BP	Other:					

Medication orders:
Fosamax 70 mg once a week, Norvasc 2.5 mg daily

Lab work:

X-ray:

Physician's report:

EXAM:
General: White 71-year-old male, well nourished and in acute distress
HEENT: 1-cm laceration to occipital scalp. Eyes, pupils equal, round and reactive to light, extraocular motion intact
Respiratory: Respirations unlabored with symmetric chest expansion. Lungs sound equal and clear bilaterally.
CV: Regular rate and rhythm
Abdomen: Soft, non-tender to palpation without guarding
Skin: Normal, except for 1-cm laceration on the occipital scalp

PROCEDURE:
The area was prepped and draped and the wound was clensed thoroughtly with betadine. Wound was irrigated with copious amounts of NS. Skin closure was accomplished with 2 staples.

Diagnosis:	Physician sign/date
IMPRESSION: 1-cm scalp laceration Patient received discharge instructions and was related from the ED.	*Robert Rai MD*

Discharge	Transfer	Admit	Good	Satisfactory	Other:

GODFREY REGIONAL HOSPITAL
123 Main Street • Aldon, FL 77714 • (407) 555-1234

EXERCISE 25

Level I

EMERGENCY ROOM RECORD

Name:		Age:	ER physician:
		DOB:	

Allergies/type of reaction:	Usual medications/dosages:

Triage/presenting complaint:

CC: 44-year-old with simple laceration

Initial assessment:

REVIEW OF SYSTEMS: Patient denies fever

HISTORY: 44-year-old presented to the ED who sustained a laceration immediately prior to arriving to the ED. Patient sustained laceration after being cut by a sharp edge of a can. Laceration is located on the eyebrow.

Time	T	P	R	BP	Other:					

Medication orders:

Lab work:

X-ray:

Physician's report:

EXAM:
General: WD, well nourished and in NAD. Vital signs normal.
Respiratory: Respirations unlabored with symmetric chest expansion.
　　　　　Lungs sound equal and clear bilaterally.
CV: Regular rate and rhythm.
Skin: Laceration, 2 cm, left eyebrow, extending through the dermis and into the subcutaneous tissue. Wound was closed with the placement of Steri-strips to the area.

Diagnosis:	Physician sign/date
The patient was discharged from the ED with treatment instructions.	*Robert Rai MD*

Discharge	Transfer	Admit	Good	Satisfactory	Other:

GODFREY REGIONAL HOSPITAL
123 Main Street • Aldon, FL 77714 • (407) 555-1234

MUSCULOSKELETAL EXERCISES

EXERCISE 1

Level II

OPERATIVE REPORT

Patient information:

Patient name: Date:
DOB: Surgeon:
MR#:   Anesthetist:

Preoperative diagnosis:

Severe retracted rotator cuff tear (acute), chronic impingement, acromioclavicular arthritis, right shoulder

Postoperative diagnosis:

Severe retracted rotator cuff tear, chronic impingement, acromioclavicular arthritis, right shoulder

Procedure(s) performed:

Neer anterior acromioplasty and coracoacromial ligament release, acromioclavicular joint debridement with excision of distal tip of clavicle, repair of chronic avulsion and rotator cuff tendon with transosseous sutures, and interrupted and inverted suture repair of right shoulder.

Anesthesia:

Assistant surgeon:

Description of procedure:

After informed consent and complete discussion of the alternatives and complications with no guarantees, implied or given, the patient was taken to the operating room. After an adequate level of an intravenous sedation had been obtained, the patient's lower neck, shoulder, and upper extremity were surgically scrubbed with Betadine soap, prepped with Betadine solution, and draped in the usual sterile fashion utilizing the double Vi-drape technique. Next, the incision was marked along the anterolateral aspect of the shoulder in a longitudinal fashion. 0.1% epinephrine was utilized for hemostasis. Under 3Z\x wide field loupe magnification, an incision was made and the dissection was carried down through the subcutaneous fat and fascia. Hemostasis was obtained with Bovie coagulation. The fascia was divided in a longitudinal fashion overlying the AC joint and anterior aspect of the acromion. The dissection was carried down subperiosteal and anterior to the AC joint and anterolateral acromion. The elongated and beak type III acromion was identified. The anterior acromioplasty was carried out to transform this to a type I acromion. Following this, marked adhesions were noted anteriorly, laterally, and posteriorly. Severe impingement was noted under the undersurface of the AC joint. The AC joint was exposed and the osteotome was utilized to remove the tip of the distal clavicle. This allowed marked improvement in the space in the area beneath the distal clavicle. Wax was placed on the cancellous bone face. Next, attention was turned to the rotator cuff.

The rotator cuff was severely retracted and was noted to be torn from the area adjacent to the subscapularis, well posteriorly into the teres minor. The cuff was freshened at the area of the tear. The cuff was approximately two inches in width. The tear was carefully advanced and mattress sutures of 0 Ethibond were utilized X6 for the repair. A trough was made in the area of avulsion and soft tissue was removed down

GODFREY REGIONAL HOSPITAL
123 Main Street • Aldon, FL 77714 • (407) 555-1234

Continued

OPERATIVE REPORT

Patient information:	

Patient name: Date:
DOB: Surgeon:
MR#:   Anesthetist:

Preoperative diagnosis:

Postoperative diagnosis:

Procedure(s) performed:

Anesthesia:

Assistant surgeon:

Description of procedure:

to bleeding cancellous bone. A margin of cuff was present on the greater tuberosity area, and this was subsequently utilized for interrupted inverted suture repair with 0 Ethibond, following the passage of the transosseous sutures tied along the lateral aspect of the cortex with the arm abducted. Excellent repair was noted with the transosseous sutures and interrupted inverted sutures of 0 Ethibond. There was no tension on the repair with the arm in the neutral position. The rotator cuff, upon evaluation, revealed thinning under the undersurface. Some horizontal portions of the anterior cuff were debrided. There were obvious degenerative changes within the cuff tissue. Marked bursal inflammation and thickening of the subacromial bursa was noted. Partial bursectomy was performed. Thorough irrigation was carried out with triple antibiotic solution throughout the procedure. 0.5% Marcaine was instilled in the glenohumeral joint, as well as in the subacromial area, for analgesia. The reconstruction of the deltoid was carried out with transosseous and interrupted inverted sutures of 0 Ethibond. The subcutaneous layers were approximated with 3-0 Vicryl in an interrupted and inverted fashion. The skins were reapproximated with subcutaneous 4-0 Prolene.

Sterile dressings were applied to the shoulder, and the patient was immediately placed in a sling and slough. The patient received cephalosporin antibiotics thirty minutes prior to the procedure prophylactically. Irrigation was carried out throughout the procedure with triple antibiotic solution.

The patient tolerated the operative procedure and anesthesia satisfactorily. No breaks in sterile technique occured. No complications occured.

In regard to physical therapy, the patient was instructed preoperatively and expected postoperatively to undergo rotator cuff tear rehabilitation protocol, and the patient voiced understanding of the importance of this to maximize healing potential. This was discussed with the patient at length and in detail. The patient voiced understanding of the above and wished to proceed.

GODFREY REGIONAL HOSPITAL
123 Main Street • Aldon, FL 77714 • (407) 555-1234

EXERCISE 2

Level II

OPERATIVE REPORT

Patient information:

Patient name:	Date:
DOB:	Surgeon:
MR#:	Anesthetist:

Preoperative diagnosis:

Lateral patellar facet syndrome, left knee

Postoperative diagnosis:

Same

Procedure(s) performed:

Arthroscopy, left knee with open lateral retinacular release

Anesthesia:

Assistant surgeon:

Description of procedure:

The patient was placed supine on the operating room table and a satisfactory general anesthetic was given. Preoperative intravenous cephalosporin antibiotic was given. Pneumatic tourniquet was placed high about the left thigh. No leg holder was used. The left knee was shaved in the proposed incisional location. The leg was prepped sterilely with DuraPrep from the tourniquet to the foot, and the left knee was draped in the usual sterile fashion. Tourniquet was inflated to 350 mm of mercury. Arthroscope cannula was introduced via an anteromedial portal at the joint line, followed by the arthroscope. Inflow to the knee from the arthroscopy pump to the cannula at a setting of 15 mm of mercury. The knee was distended with normal saline in this fashion. Outflow from the cannula to suction. A flow of irrigation was maintained for purposes of visualization and removal of debris. There was no pathology or loose body in the medial gutter. The cartilaginous surfaces of the medial femoral condyle and medial tibial plateau were intact without evidence of fibrillation or breakdown. The medial meniscus showed no evidence of intrasubstance tear or peripheral detachment. The intercondylar notch showed no evidence of pathology. The visualized portions of the anterior and posterior cruciate ligaments were intact without evidence of stretching or tearing of their fibers or hemorrhage on their surfaces. The cartilaginous surfaces of the lateral femoral condyle and lateral tibial plateau were intact without evidence of fibrillation or breakdown. The lateral meniscus showed no evidence of intrasubstance tear or peripheral detachment except for the usual detachment in the region of the popliteus tendon, which was not elongated. The lateral gutter showed no evidence of pathology or loose body. There was no pathology or loose body in the suprapatellar area. The medial plica showed no evidence of pathology or damage. The cartilaginous surface of the patella, as well as the intracondylar notch, showed no evidence of fibrillation, breakdown, or pathology. There was a tight lateral

GODFREY REGIONAL HOSPITAL
123 Main Street • Aldon, FL 77714 • (407) 555-1234

Continued

OPERATIVE REPORT

Patient information:

Patient name: Date:
DOB: Surgeon:
MR#:   Anesthetist:

Preoperative diagnosis:

Postoperative diagnosis:

Procedure(s) performed:

Anesthesia:

Assistant surgeon:

Description of procedure:

retinaculum noted through a range of motion of the knee. A longitudinal skin incision was made laterally adjacent to the patella. The incision was carried through subcutaneous tissue. Hemostasis was achieved as necessary. Full-thickness skin flaps were raised. A nick was made in the lateral patellar retinaculum and a lateral patella release was performed in its entirety. This freed up the lateral aspect of the patella as visualized arthroscopically, which allowed better lift-off and enhanced medial glide of the patella. The knee was copiously irrigated with normal saline antibiotic solution from the arthroscopy pump during the procedure. As much fluid as possible was suctioned from the knee at the conclusion of the procedure. The arthroscope portal was closed with a single simple suture of 3-0 Ethilon. The lateral release incision was closed with interrupted vertical mattress sutures of 3-0 Ethilon. A total of 30 ccs of a combination of 0.5% Marcaine with epinephrine plus 5 mgs of morphine was injected into the knee. Dry sterile dressings were applied, followed by sterile circumferential cast padding. Tourniquet was deflated. All drapes were removed, including the tourniquet. Ace bandage was applied about the knee area.

The patient tolerated the procedure well. There were no complications. He was awakened in the operating room and transported to the recovery room in stable condition.

Patrick Chris MD

GODFREY REGIONAL HOSPITAL
123 Main Street • Aldon, FL 77714 • (407) 555-1234

EXERCISE 3

Level II

OPERATIVE REPORT

Patient information:	
Patient name: DOB: MR#:	Date: Surgeon: Anesthetist:

Preoperative diagnosis:

Complex open wounds to the left ring and small fingers with open fractures of these fingers; simple laceration to the long finger

Postoperative diagnosis:

1. 1 cm dorsal laceration, left long finger
2. 3 cm complex laceration, left ring finger
3. Extensor tendon laceration, left ring finger
4. Intra-articular fracture of proximal phalanx of the left ring finger
5. Intra-articular fracture of the middle phalanx of the left ring finger
6. Complex laceration, approximately 2 cm, left small finger
7. Extensor tendon laceration, left small finger
8. Osteochondral fracture of the proximal phalanx of left small finger

Procedure(s) performed:

1. Debridement and irrigation of open left ring finger proximal phalanx fracture, ring finger middle phalanx fracture, small finger proximal phalanx fracture
2. Open reduction and internal fixation of proximal phalanx fracture of the ring finger and middle phalanx fracture of the ring finger
3. Excision of osteochondral fragment of small finger
4. Extensor tendon repair of the ring finger
5. Extensor tendon repair of the small finger
6. Laceration repair of long, ring, and small fingers
7. Intraoperative use of fluoroscopy
8. Short-arm splinting

Anesthesia:

Assistant surgeon:

Description of procedure:

The patient was taken to the operating room where, after general anesthesia was administered, the left upper extremity was prepped and draped in a sterile fashion. Copious amounts of antibiotic irrigation were used to irrigate all the open fractures. There was a complex intra-articular injury to the PIP joint of the ring finger, and a smaller injury with some small osteochondral fragments at the proximal interphalangeal joint of the small finger. Any loose bony fragments and debris were debrided. Once this was completed, along with debriding the skin edges, attention was turned to the fractures.

The small finger PIP joint had some very small osteochondral fragments that were unable to be affixed in any fashion and these were excised. The majority of the joint here was intact. The ring finger had a complex intra-articular injury with fractures involving the joint surfaces of the proximal and middle phalanges. These were affixed using the mini-frag set 1.5-mm screws and K-wires. Care was taken to seat the K-wire used on the proximal phalanx articular surface beneath the articular surface. Once fixation here was achieved, I was pleased with the articular congruity and the range of motion able to be achieved. The extensor tendons were then repaired. The small finger extensor tendon had a laceration that was somewhat complex, but a good repair was able to be achieved. 4-0 Ethibond mattress and figure-of-eight sutures were used here. The finger was able to be flexed down to 90 degrees without undue tension. The ring finger had a more complex injury to the extensor tendon with some missing tissue, especially along the radial aspect. Despite this, adequate repair was able to be achieved. The central slip was repaired back down to bone through bony drill holes, and the remainder of the tendon was repaired with horizontal mattress

GODFREY REGIONAL HOSPITAL
123 Main Street • Aldon, FL 77714 • (407) 555-1234

Continued

OPERATIVE REPORT

Patient information:	
Patient name: DOB: MR#:	Date: Surgeon: Anesthetist:

Preoperative diagnosis:

Postoperative diagnosis:

Procedure(s) performed:

Anesthesia:

Assistant surgeon:

Description of procedure:

and figure-of-eight 4-0 Ethibond sutures. The finger here was able to be flexed to about 30 degrees before some tension was noted. At this point the wound was irrigated out again and the complex lacerations were closed with 4-0 nylon sutures. Sterile bulky hand dressing and short-arm splint were applied. Fluoroscopy was used throughout the case, and fixation of the fractures and permanent pictures were saved on this. The patient was awakened and taken to the recovery room in stable condition. There were no complications. On admission to the recovery room, his fingers were pink with good color and capillary refill.

[signature]

GODFREY REGIONAL HOSPITAL
123 Main Street • Aldon, FL 77714 • (407) 555-1234

EXERCISE 4

Level II

OPERATIVE REPORT

Patient information:	
Patient name: DOB: MR#:	Date: Surgeon: Anesthetist:

Preoperative diagnosis:

Loose ulnar collateral ligament of metacarpophalangeal joint, right thumb

Postoperative diagnosis:

Same

Procedure(s) performed:

Excision of bone fragment with repair of ulnar collateral ligament, metacarpophalangeal joint right thumb; application of short-arm thumb spica cast

Anesthesia:

Assistant surgeon:

Description of procedure:

The patient was placed supine on the operating room table and a satisfactory general anesthetic was given. Preoperative intravenous cephalosporin antibiotic was given. Pneumatic tourniquet was placed about the right arm. The right hand, wrist, forearm, and elbow to the tourniquet level were prepped with DuraPrep, and the right hand was draped in the usual sterile fashion. Tourniquet was inflated to 250 mm of mercury. Skin incision was made at the ulnar base of the thumb overlying the metacarpophalangeal joint. The incision was carried through subcutaneous tissue. Hemostasis was achieved as necessary. Full-thickness skin flaps were raised. The conjoined tendon was elevated, and the small displaced bony fragment off the ulnar base of the proximal phalanx was noted to not be healed. It was easily moveable adjacent to the proximal phalanx of the thumb. It was very difficult to rotate this piece into appropriate position and the decision was made to simply remove this small fragment and to repair the ulnar ligament. The wound was irrigated with normal saline antibiotic solution. A 2-0 Prolene suture was weaved into the ulnar collateral ligament and conjoined tendon and placed via a Keith needle drilled from the normal ligament attachment site across the proximal phalanx out its radial side and radial aspect of the thumb. Each end of the Prolene suture was placed in two different drill holes. Attention was turned to the ulnar collateral ligament and the Prolene was then tied over a plastic button at the radial aspect of the thumb over dressings to protect the skin. A good tight repair was obtained, and there was no laxity to stress testing of the ulnar collateral ligament. The wound was

GODFREY REGIONAL HOSPITAL
123 Main Street • Aldon, FL 77714 • (407) 555-1234

Continued

OPERATIVE REPORT

Patient information:	
Patient name:	Date:
DOB:	Surgeon:
MR#:	Anesthetist:

Preoperative diagnosis:

Postoperative diagnosis:

Procedure(s) performed:

Anesthesia:

Assistant surgeon:

Description of procedure:

irrigated with normal saline antibiotic solution. The skin was reapproximated with interrupted vertical mattress sutures of 3-0 Ethilon. Dry sterile dressings were applied, followed by sterile circumferential cast padding. Tourniquet was deflated. All drapes were removed, including the tourniquet. A well-padded short-arm thumb spica cast was then applied. The patient tolerated the procedure well. There were no complications. She was awakened in the operating room and was transported to the recovery room in stable condition.

Patrick Chung mD

GODFREY REGIONAL HOSPITAL
123 Main Street • Aldon, FL 77714 • (407) 555-1234

EXERCISE 5

Level II

OPERATIVE REPORT

Patient information:		
Patient name: DOB: MR#:		Date: Surgeon: Anesthetist:

Preoperative diagnosis:

1. Torn calcaneal fibular ligament, left
2. Attenuated anterior talofibular ligament, left

Postoperative diagnosis:

Same

Procedure(s) performed:

1. Primary repair of calcaneal fibular ligament
2. Primary repair of anterior talofibular ligament left

Anesthesia:

Local with MAC

Assistant surgeon:

Description of procedure:

HEMOSTASIS: Pneumatic ankle tourniquet on the left

ESTIMATED BLOOD LOSS: Less than 1 cc
Under mild sedation, the patient was brought into the operating room and placed on the operating table in a supine position. A pneumatic ankle tourniquet was then placed about the patient's ankle. Following IV sedation, local anesthesia was obtained about the left ankle. The foot was then scrubbed, prepped, and draped in the usual aseptic manner. An Esmarch bandage was then utilized to exsanguinate the patient's left foot and a pneumatic ankle tourniquet was then inflated. Attention was then directed to the lateral aspect of the left foot where a 5-cm curvilinear incision was made, beginning at the anterior distal end of the fibula and curving distal to the plantar aspect of the fibula overlying the calcaneal fibular ligament. Dissection was continued using sharp and blunt dissection down to the level of the ankle capsule where identification of the torn calcaneal fibular ligament was then made. A curvilinear capsulotomy was performed over the dorsal aspect of the anterior talofibular ligament and the calcaneal fibular ligament. Attention was directed to the distal aspect of the fibula where, utilizing a #64 blade, the periosteum was then released from the fibula and the overlying bone was then scraped utilizing a rongeur. Utilizing double 0 Panacryl, a total of 7 sutures were then placed within the distal aspect of the anterior talofibular ligament and calcaneal fibular ligament and attached to the distal aspect of the fibula beneath the periosteum. The overlying periosteum was then further imbricated into the superior portion of the inferior extensor retinaculum. At this time, an anterior drawer sign was no longer positive. The area was flushed with copious amounts of sterile normal saline solution, and the subcuticular tissues were reapproximated and coapted utilizing 4-0 Vicryl, and the skin was

GODFREY REGIONAL HOSPITAL
123 Main Street • Aldon, FL 77714 • (407) 555-1234

Continued

OPERATIVE REPORT

Patient information:	
Patient name: DOB: MR#:	Date: Surgeon: Anesthetist:

Preoperative diagnosis:

Postoperative diagnosis:

Procedure(s) performed:

Anesthesia:

Assistant surgeon:

Description of procedure:

reapproximated and coapted utilizing 5-0 Vicryl subcuticular suture technique. Upon completion of the procedure, a total of 1 cc of Decadron phosphate was infiltrated about the incision site. A postoperative block consisting of 0.5% Marcaine plain was also injected. The incision was dressed with Mastisol and Steri-strips and covered with a sterile compressive dressing consisting of 4 × 4s and Kling, and the pneumatic ankle tourniquet was then deflated and a prompt hyperresponse was noted to all digits of the left foot. A mono-valved B-K cast was then applied.

The patient tolerated the procedure and anesthesia well. She was transferred to recovery with vital signs stable and vascular status intact to all of the left foot. Following a period of postoperative monitoring, patient will be discharged home with written and oral postoperative instructions. Patient has instructions to stay nonweight bearing times a period of weeks and will reappoint in my office within a period of one week for follow-up.

GODFREY REGIONAL HOSPITAL
123 Main Street • Aldon, FL 77714 • (407) 555-1234

EXERCISE 6

Level I

OPERATIVE REPORT

Patient information:

Patient name: Date:
DOB: Surgeon:
MR#:   Anesthetist:

Preoperative diagnosis:

Chondromalacia patella, left knee, and possible medial meniscal tear, left knee

Postoperative diagnosis:

Chondromalacia patella and diffuse grade IV; chondromalacia medial femoral condyle from 0 to 80° and synovitis of the notch

Procedure(s) performed:

Left knee arthroscopy, synovectomy of the notch, chondroplasty patella and medial femoral condyle

Anesthesia:

Assistant surgeon:

Description of procedure:

After suitable general anesthesia had been achieved, the patient's left knee was prepped and draped in the usual manner. Prior to prepping, thigh tourniquet was applied, and after draping, inflated to 300 mm of mercury. Arthroscope was inserted through an anterior medial portal. The patient was noted to have marked synovitis of the notch. Thickened synovial tissue was excised with the shaver, and synovial bleeders were cauterized using the radiofrequency probe. Lateral compartment revealed intact articular surfaces and a stable intact lateral meniscus. Examination of the medial compartment revealed a lot of flakes of loose articular cartilage floating free inside the knee. Medial meniscus was intact and stable with probing. There was noted to be diffuse grade IV changes, 80% of the medial femoral condyle from 0–80°. Articular cartilage flaps were smoothed with the shaver. Examination of the patellofemoral joint revealed diffuse grade IV changes, but minimal articular cartilage flaps except at the inferior pole of the patella where there was a substantial cluster of articular cartilage flaps. These were smoothed with the shaver. Synovial bleeders were cauterized with the radiofrequency probe after excision of a thickened medial plica. Knee joint was then thoroughly irrigated, and the arthroscope was removed. Stab wounds were closed with 4-0 nylon. Dressing was then applied. Tourniquet was released. Following tourniquet release, good circulation was noted to return to the foot.

Patient tolerated the procedure well and returned to the recovery room in stable condition.

[signature]

GODFREY REGIONAL HOSPITAL
123 Main Street • Aldon, FL 77714 • (407) 555-1234

EXERCISE 7

Level I

OPERATIVE REPORT

Patient information:	
Patient name: DOB: MR#:	Date: Surgeon: Anesthetist:

Preoperative diagnosis:

Chondromalacia patella, lateral patellar tilt and lateral retinacular tightness

Postoperative diagnosis:

Same

Procedure(s) performed:

Right knee arthroscopy and chondroplasty of patella; right knee arthroscopy lateral release

Anesthesia:

Assistant surgeon:

Description of procedure:

After suitable general anesthesia had been achieved, the patient's right knee was prepped and draped in the usual manner. Prior to prepping, a thigh tourniquet was applied, and after draping, inflated to 300 mm of mercury. Inflow cannula was inserted to the suprapatellar pouch on the medial side. The arthroscope was inserted through an anterior lateral portal. The medial compartment was examined first. There was noted to be intact stable medial meniscus and intact articular surfaces. Examination of the notch revealed intact and stable ACL and PCL. Examination of the lateral compartment revealed intact articular surfaces and intact and stable lateral meniscus. Examination of the patellofemoral joint revealed localized chondromalacia at the lateral aspect of the inferior pole of the patella. This was smoothed with a shaver and further smoothing was done using an Oratec probe. The patient was noted to have a small medial synovial plica and this was trimmed with the shaver as well. Using an arthroscopic cautery, arthroscopic lateral release was done from the superior pole of the patella to the joint line. Following this, the knee joint was thoroughly irrigated and the arthroscope removed. Patellar tracking was then reassessed and the patella lateral retinaculum tightness had been corrected. Knee joint was thoroughly irrigated again and no bleeding was noted. Dressing was applied. Tourniquet was released. Following tourniquet release, good circulation was noted to return to the foot.

The patient tolerated the procedure well and returned to the recovery room in stable condition.

[signature]

GODFREY REGIONAL HOSPITAL
123 Main Street • Aldon, FL 77714 • (407) 555-1234

E X E R C I S E   8

Level I

OPERATIVE REPORT

Patient information:

Patient name: Date:
DOB: Surgeon:
MR#:   Anesthetist:

Preoperative diagnosis:

Postoperative diagnosis:

Procedure(s) performed:

Diagnostic and surgical arthroscopy of the right shoulder with findings of small rotator cuff tear with significant impingement, as well as torn labrum. For this she underwent surgical and diagnostic arthroscopy of the right shoulder with anterior acromioplasty, resection of the coracoacromial ligament, and trimming of the under and outer surfaces of the rotator cuff, as well as the torn labrum, and through a mini-arthrotomy a repair of the rotator cuff.

Anesthesia:

Assistant surgeon:

Description of procedure:

The patient initially was placed under general anesthesia and placed in a left lateral decubitus position. The right arm was suspended with the aid of an arm holder and the right shoulder was prepped and draped in the usual sterile fashion. A 30-degree scope was introduced through a posterior portal in the glenohumeral joint. This looked reasonably normal. However, there was diffuse degenerative fraying of the labrum, as well as the under surface of the rotator cuff, and both these were trimmed with a 4-mm shaver introduced through the anterior portal. The bicipital tendon was intact. The scope was then removed and introduced into the subacromial area, and a 5-mm shaver was introduced through a lateral portal. Initiation was carried out, relieving a fairly significant subacromial impingement, as well as removing the coracoacromial ligament. Following initial decompression and light trimming of the rotator cuff, the scope was removed and introduced through a lateral portal. The motorized shaver was introduced through a posterior portal. Additional bone was removed to ensure that a straight line could be projected from posterior to anterior. Following inspection, the rotator cuff showed a significant wear, but there was only one area involving the rotator cuff tear. This was non-displaced. Consequently, we made a mini-arthrotomy, placed a single Mitek ligament suture, and in a horizontal mattress fashion, tied this down into the sulcus just lateral to the humeral head. This was repaired under no tension. Following irrigation with Ancef-impregnated irrigant, the split in the deltoid measured about 2 cm. It was repaired with running 2-0 clear Vicryl suture. The subdermal tissue was approximated with interrupted 3-0 clear Vicryl, and the skin was closed with running 3-0 vertical mattress nylon, as were the stab wounds.

GODFREY REGIONAL HOSPITAL
123 Main Street • Aldon, FL 77714 • (407) 555-1234

Continued

OPERATIVE REPORT

Patient information:	
Patient name:	Date:
DOB:	Surgeon:
MR#:	Anesthetist:

Preoperative diagnosis:

Postoperative diagnosis:

Procedure(s) performed:

Anesthesia:

Assistant surgeon:

Description of procedure:

A pain pump catheter was placed. This was hooked up to the pain pump. Light dressing was applied.

The patient was taken to the recovery room in a shoulder immobilizer. She tolerated the procedure well.

[signature] MD

GODFREY REGIONAL HOSPITAL
123 Main Street • Aldon, FL 77714 • (407) 555-1234

EXERCISE 9

Level II

OPERATIVE REPORT

Patient information:	
Patient name: DOB: MR#:	Date: Surgeon: Anesthetist:

Preoperative diagnosis:

Hallux limitus

Postoperative diagnosis:

Hallux limitus

Procedure(s) performed:

1. Distal L osteotomy with pin fixation
2. Cheilectomy

Anesthesia:

Assistant surgeon:

Description of procedure:

Patient was brought back to the operating room, properly identified, and placed on the OR table in the supine position. Following IV sedation, the foot was anesthetized with 10 cc of 50/50 mixture of 2% lidocaine plain and 0.5% Marcaine plain in a Mayo H block fashion around the right first ray. The foot was then prepped and draped in the usual sterile aseptic technique.

Utilizing an Esmarch dressing, the foot was exsanguinated, and the previously well-padded ankle tourniquet was inflated to 250 mm of mercury. Attention was then directed to the first dorsal aspect of the first metatarsal-phalangeal joint where a 10-cm curvilinear incision was made. The incision site was deepened down to the joint capsule and care was taken to protect the neurovascular structures. The joint capsule was noted and a linear capsulotomy was performed. The joint capsule was then freed from the metatarsal head dorsally and medially. Next, utilizing a sagittal saw, the medial eminence of the first metatarsal was introduced in the surgical field and resected from the surgical site in total. Next, the dorsal eminence was introduced into the surgical field, and utilizing the sagittal saw, the dorsal eminence was resected from the surgical site in toto. Next, attention was directed to the lateral aspect of the first metatarsal into the first interspace where the intermetatarsal ligament, the abductor tendon, and the sesamoid ligaments were freed from their attachments. Attention was then directed back to the medial aspect of the first metatarsal head where a 0.045 K-wire was introduced, running from medial to lateral with light plantar flexion as a guide. Next utilizing a sagittal saw, the distal L osteotomy cut was performed with the plantar cut first and the dorsal cut second. Next, the K wire guide was removed from the surgical site in toto and the metatarsal head was put into proper position. Next utilizing the

GODFREY REGIONAL HOSPITAL
123 Main Street • Aldon, FL 77714 • (407) 555-1234

Continued

OPERATIVE REPORT

Patient information:	
Patient name:	Date:
DOB:	Surgeon:
MR#:	Anesthetist:

Preoperative diagnosis:

Postoperative diagnosis:

Procedure(s) performed:

Anesthesia:

Assistant surgeon:

Description of procedure:

sagittal saw, a 3-mm wedge of bone was resected from the dorsal arm of the osteotomy cut and removed from the surgical site en toto. Next, the distal metatarsal osteotomy was positioned in its proper position, slightly laterally and impacted on the metatarsal. Next, a 0.045 K wire was used to secure the osteotomy in place. The wire was then bent and cut. Attention was then directed to the redundant bone on the metatarsal. Utilizing the sagittal saw, the redundant bone was removed from the surgical site en toto. Next the joint itself was inspected and noted to have large yellow cartilaginous deficits and two large red, denuded areas of bone. The denuded bone and the yellow cartilaginous deficits were drilled with 0.045 K wire to promote blood flow to the cartilaginous caps. Next, the surgical site was copiously irrigated with normal saline. The joint capsule was reapproximated with 3-0 Vicryl. The skin tissue was then reapproximated with 4-0 Proline. The foot was then dressed with adaptic fluffs and Kling and Coban.

The patient tolerated the procedure well and anesthesia well and left the OR with vital signs stable and vascular status intact.

Patrick Chang md

GODFREY REGIONAL HOSPITAL
123 Main Street • Aldon, FL 77714 • (407) 555-1234

Level II

OPERATIVE REPORT

Patient information:	
Patient name: DOB: MR#:	Date: Surgeon: Anesthetist:

Preoperative diagnosis:

Dupuytren contractures, both hands

Postoperative diagnosis:

Dupuytren contractures, both hands

Procedure(s) performed:

OPERATION SUMMARY: Release Dupuytren contractures, both hands

OPERATIVE FINDINGS: Dupuytren contractures, both hands

TISSUE REMOVED: Dupuytren contractures

Anesthesia:

Assistant surgeon:

Description of procedure:

Under adequate regional anesthetic, patient was prepped and draped in a sterile manner, and the left hand was released first. Incision was made over the palm. The 4th and 5th fingers were the ones that were tight, and these were carefully released, dissecting down, removing the thickened fascia scar layer of Dupuytren. This was completed while carefully preserving all neurovascular structures, both of the fingers were released so they would extend nicely without any tension and were quite free. Once release was completed and meticulous hemostasis was obtained, the incision was closed with Proline sutures. Dressings were applied. Attention was then turned to the opposite, that is, the right hand. On this hand the thumb was quite tight and this had to be released. Incision was made over the contracture and it was carefully dissected off and removed completely. This freed the thumb completely and it moved well and easily. Following this, then the 5th finger was released as well. However, there was ankylosis of the joint, that is the proximal interphalangeal joint, and this could not be freed. The contracture portion was freed so that the MP joint would move well, but with the ankylosed joint this could not be released. Upon release of these while carefully protecting all neurovascular structures and with meticulous hemostasis being obtained, these incisions as well were closed with Proline sutures. Dressings were applied and the patient was discharged to recovery in a stable condition. Patient tolerated this procedure well. Estimated blood loss, 25 cc. Sponge and needle count report is correct.

POSTOPERATIVE PLAN: He will follow up Saturday for dressing changes and next week for reexamination and dressing change.

[signature]

GODFREY REGIONAL HOSPITAL
123 Main Street • Aldon, FL 77714 • (407) 555-1234

EXERCISE 11

Level I

OPERATIVE REPORT

Patient information:	
Patient name: DOB: MR#:	Date: Surgeon: Anesthetist:

Preoperative diagnosis:

Chronic dislocation and subluxation, anterior left shoulder

Postoperative diagnosis:

Same

Procedure(s) performed:

Anterior capsulorrhaphy, left shoulder

Anesthesia:

Assistant surgeon:

Description of procedure:

The patient was placed supine on the operating room table on the beach chair attachment and a satisfactory general anesthetic was given. The patient was placed in the modified beach chair position. Preoperative intravenous cephalosporin antibiotic was given. The left shoulder was widely prepped sterilely with DuraPrep times two.

A skin incision was made along the course of the cephalic vein, commencing at the coracoid process and extending distally.

The incision was carried through subcutaneous tissue. Hemostasis was achieved as necessary. Full-thickness skin flaps were raised. The cephalic vein was identified and freed and retracted medially. The deltopectoral interval was bluntly opened down to the clavipectoral fascia. This fascia was then incised and reflected. The lateral edge of the conjoint tendon was freed up, and via retractors, the deltoid muscle and conjoint tendons were separated. Fascia was cleared off the anterior portion of the glenohumeral joint and subscapularis muscle. The subscapularis muscle was then split perpendicularly to its fibers to encounter the joint capsule. The joint capsule was freed up. The articular surfaces of the glenoid and humeral head were intact without evidence of fibrillation breakdown or cartilaginous cracking. The anterior labrum was noted to be well situated on the anterior glenoid. The shoulder joint was irrigated with normal saline antibiotic solution. An anterior capsulorrhaphy was then performed in a north-south type fashion with 0 Ethibond sutures. The

GODFREY REGIONAL HOSPITAL
123 Main Street • Aldon, FL 77714 • (407) 555-1234

Continued

OPERATIVE REPORT

Patient information:	
Patient name: DOB: MR#:	Date: Surgeon: Anesthetist:

Preoperative diagnosis:

Postoperative diagnosis:

Procedure(s) performed:

Anesthesia:

Assistant surgeon:

Description of procedure:

subscapularis was reapproximated to its normal length with interrupted figure-of-eight suture of 0 Ethibond. The wound was again irrigated with normal saline antibiotic solution. The subcutaneous tissue was closed with interrupted inverted sutures of 2-0 Vicryl, followed by closure of the skin with staples. Dry sterile dressings were applied, which were held in place during removal of the drapes. Dressings were taped into place. A shoulder immobilizer was applied.

The patient tolerated the procedure well. There were no complications. She was awakened in the operating room and transported to the recovery room in stable condition.

Patrick Chris MD

GODFREY REGIONAL HOSPITAL
123 Main Street • Aldon, FL 77714 • (407) 555-1234

EXERCISE 12

Level II

OPERATIVE REPORT

Patient information:

Patient name: Date:
DOB: Surgeon:
MR#:   Anesthetist:

Preoperative diagnosis:

1) Osteomyelitis, right 2nd distal phalanx.
2) Non-healing ulceration, right 2nd digit.

Postoperative diagnosis:

1) Osteomyelitis, right 2nd distal phalanx.
2) Non-healing ulceration, right 2nd digit.

Procedure(s) performed:

1) Amputation of the distal phalanx.
2) Removal of the nail plate and nail bed of the right distal phalanx.

Anesthesia:

Assistant surgeon:

Description of procedure:

The patient was brought back to the operating room, properly identified, and placed on the OR table in a supine position. Following IV sedation, the right 2nd digit was anesthetized with 3 cc of 50/50 mixture of 1% lidocaine plain and 0.5% Marcaine plain. The foot was then prepped and draped in the usual sterile, aseptic manner.

Attention then was directed to the distal aspect of the right 2nd digit where a fishmouth incision was placed at the distal top over the ulceration. The incision site was deepened down to the distal phalanx, which was noted to be open down through the cortical bone, and the bone was very soft. The soft tissue was freed from the distal phalanx plantarly, medially, and laterally. The dorsal attachment was noted to be void of coverage; the dorsal aspect of the phalanx was exposed and a void of soft tissue coverage under the nail plate. The nail plate was loose and the bone was exposed underneath the nail plate. The phalanx was removed from the surgical site in toto. The intermediate phalanx was inspected and noted to be healthy and had no breakdown. The nail plate was not attached except to the proximal nail fold. The nail plate was noted to be nonviable and void of nail bed secondary to the underlying bone exposure. The nail was then removed from the surgical site in toto. The area was then flushed with copious amounts of saline with Ancef in the solution. The redundant tissue was removed from the surgical site, closed with 4-0 Prolene. The foot was then dressed with adaptic 3x3 and Kling.

The patient tolerated the procedure well and left the OR with vital signs stable and vascular status intact to all digits.

Patrick Chug MD

GODFREY REGIONAL HOSPITAL
123 Main Street • Aldon, FL 77714 • (407) 555-1234

EXERCISE 13

Level I

OPERATIVE REPORT

Patient information:	
Patient name:	Date:
DOB:	Surgeon:
MR#:	Anesthetist:

Preoperative diagnosis:

Dupuytren's contracture of right ring finger extending secondary into palm

Postoperative diagnosis:

Dupuytren's contracture of right ring finger extending secondary into palm

Procedure(s) performed:

Excision of Dupuytren's contracture

Anesthesia:

Assistant surgeon:

Description of procedure:

The patient was brought to the operating room and placed in the supine position. After adequate block, the area was prepped and draped in the sterile fashion. We made a straight incision down the 5th finger from just proximal to the DIP crease and then crossing over at about the MP joint to catch the band that went up into the 4th palmar area. We did sharp dissection on both sides of the skin to clear the skin edges up. We then identified the Dupuytren's. We followed both neurovascular bundles down, dissecting them free as we went, and then we were able to remove the Dupuytren's contracture once we had the neurovascular bundles protected. We were able to straighten the finger out with a little bit of release of the contracture, and then we released the tourniquet and obtained hemostasis. The finger pinked up quite nicely and quickly. We then did a couple Z-plasties and then repaired the skin with 4-0 nylon. The wound was dressed with an adaptic, followed by sheet wadding and plaster for a short-arm splint in extension. Patient was taken to the recovery room in good condition.

[signature] Patrick Chung MD

GODFREY REGIONAL HOSPITAL
123 Main Street • Aldon, FL 77714 • (407) 555-1234

EXERCISE 14

Level I

OPERATIVE REPORT

Patient information:

Patient name: Date:
DOB: Surgeon:
MR#:   Anesthetist:

Preoperative diagnosis:

Saw injury to right small finger

Postoperative diagnosis:

1. Open proximal phalanx fracture
2. Traumatic arthrotomy of the proximal interphalangeal joint
3. Ulnar-sided digital neurovascular laceration
4. Complex laceration of the entire fifth digit

Procedure(s) performed:

1. Debridement and irrigation of open proximal phalanx fracture
2. Debridement and irrigation of open proximal interphalangeal joint
3. Debridement, irrigation, and primary repair of complex laceration (approximately 5 cm)
4. Digital nerve repair
5. Pinning of proximal phalanx fracture
6. Short-arm splint application
7. Fluoroscopy

Anesthesia:

Assistant surgeon:

Description of procedure:

The patient was taken to the operating room where, after general anesthesia was administered, the right upper extremity was prepped and draped in a sterile fashion. The skin edges were debrided as needed. The joint was debrided of any foreign bodies. Minimal foreign material was actually seen. The fracture was curetted and irrigated out copiously as well. Copious amounts of antibiotic irrigation were used for lavage. Once this was completed, the wound was extended for about 1 cm proximally and distally to help identify the neurovascular bundle. This was identified. The digital artery had a segmental loss and it was coagulated. The digital nerve was injured over about a 2-cm segment. However, the nerve was felt to be repairable. The fracture site was somewhat unstable and, therefore, a single pin was placed from the radial aspect distally to proximally under fluoroscopic guidance. The fracture was stable after this, and excellent alignment was obtained as visualized on multiple planes with fluoroscopy. The digital nerve was repaired with 4 epineural sutures using 8-0 nylon. The PIP joint had to be flexed to about 15 degrees to allow for repair without significant tension. Once this was completed, the wound was once again irrigated out copiously with antibiotic irrigation solution. The complex laceration was closed with multiple simple and vertical mattress nylon sutures.

Xeroform and bulky hand dressing and a short-arm dorsal blocking splint were applied. Of note, the tourniquet was deflated prior to the end of the procedure, and the finger had good capillary refill and good color. Hemostasis was obtained as needed during the procedure with electrocautery. The patient was taken to the recovery room in stable condition. There were no complications.

GODFREY REGIONAL HOSPITAL
123 Main Street • Aldon, FL 77714 • (407) 555-1234

EXERCISE 15

Level II

OPERATIVE REPORT

Patient information:	
Patient name:	Date:
DOB:	Surgeon:
MR#:	Anesthetist:

Preoperative diagnosis:

1. Chronic ulcer, left foot
2. Dislocated second digit, left foot
3. Plantar flexed, second metatarsal, left foot

Postoperative diagnosis:

1. Chronic ulcer, left foot
2. Dislocated second digit, left foot
3. Plantar flexed, second metatarsal, left foot

Procedure(s) performed:

1. Amputation, second digit, left foot
2. Plantar condylectomy, second metatarsal, left foot
3. Application of Apligraf skin graft, second MPJ, left foot

Anesthesia:

Assistant surgeon:

Description of procedure:

COMPLICATIONS: None
PATHOLOGY:
1. Skin for ulcer for biopsy, left foot
2. Second digit, left foot

Under local and IV sedation the patient was prepped and draped in the usual aseptic manner. Martin's bandage was applied at the level of the left malleolus. Attention was directed to the dorsum of the left forefoot where a linear incision was made. The incision was continued circumferentially about the second digit on the left foot. The incision was deepened with care taken to clamp and ligate all superficial bleeders as they were encountered, and all neurovascular and tendinous structures were carefully identified and retracted. All soft tissue from the second digit was released away from the metatarsal where it was articulated near the dorsal neck, and the second digit was removed. Next a plastic condylectomy was performed on the second metatarsal on the left foot. All bony tissue was rasped smooth. The wound was flushed with copious amounts of sterile saline and closed in layers with subcutaneous reapproximation with 3-0 Polysorb simple interrupted sutures followed by skin reapproximation with 4-0 nylon simple interrupted sutures.

GODFREY REGIONAL HOSPITAL
123 Main Street • Aldon, FL 77714 • (407) 555-1234

Continued

OPERATIVE REPORT

Patient information:	
Patient name:	Date:
DOB:	Surgeon:
MR#:	Anesthetist:

Preoperative diagnosis:

Postoperative diagnosis:

Procedure(s) performed:

Anesthesia:

Assistant surgeon:

Description of procedure:

Next, attention was directed to the plantar aspect of the left foot, and the ulcer at the second MPJ was circumscribed and removed in toto. There was a subdermal bursa that was removed. The wound was flushed again. The tourniquet was let down, and it was noted that there was good bleeding tissue through the ulcer site. Next, the Apligraf skin graft was prepared and cut to size and stitched in place with 4-0 nylon simple interrupted sutures. I applied sterile Vaseline gauze over the incision line, followed by a sterile gauze bandage for compression and hemostasis. The patient tolerated the procedure and anesthesia well and was transported to the recovery room with vital signs stable and in good condition.

GODFREY REGIONAL HOSPITAL
123 Main Street • Aldon, FL 77714 • (407) 555-1234

EXERCISE 16

Level II

OPERATIVE REPORT

Patient information:	
Patient name: DOB: MR#:	Date: Surgeon: Anesthetist:

Preoperative diagnosis:

Subluxation with contracted toe; 2nd metatarsophalangeal joint, right and left feet

Postoperative diagnosis:

Same

Procedure(s) performed:

Extensor tendon lengthening with capsulotomy, 2nd metatarsophalangeal joint, right and left feet

Anesthesia:

Assistant surgeon:

Description of procedure:

V-lock cuffs were placed above both ankles for hemostasis and the patient was prepped and draped in the usual aseptic manner. With IV sedation, 2% Xylocaine hydrochloride plain was used to infiltrate the operative area on the right forefoot. A series of triangle-shaped skin incisions were made dorsally over the 2nd metatarsophalangeal joint and over the previous skin incision that was hypertrophic and adhesed. The skin and subcutaneous tissues were undermined and carefully retracted. The incision was then deepened to the level of the extensor digitorum longus tendon, which was identified and retracted from the wound. This tendon was found to be quite thickened and fibrotic from previous surgery. The tendon was then lengthened in a Z-plasty fashion. Incision was further deepened to the level of the capsule over the 2nd metatarsophalangeal joint, and the capsule was incised both dorsally and medially, as well as laterally, and a 2nd toe was then plantar flexed. Upon loading of the right foot, the 2nd toe was found to be much more normally positioned and in line with the adjacent toes. There appeared to be good soft tissue release dorsally over the metatarsophalangeal joint, and a subluxation was significantly reduced. While maintaining the 2nd toe in a straight and somewhat plantar flexed position, the capsular structures were then repaired with interrupted sutures of 3-0 Vicryl. Extensor tendon was then repaired with 3-0 Vicryl, and subcutaneous tissue over the tendon was repaired with a continuous strand of 3-0 Vicryl. Skin margins were then approximated with interrupted horizontal mattress sutures of 4-0 nylon. The right foot was loaded, finding the 2nd toe remaining in a normal position with significant reduction of the preoperative deformity and the dorsal skin incision free of suture tension and tightness. Celestone Solu span 5 cc was then deposited in the operative area. Adaptic was applied to the skin incision and a mild compression dressing was then placed around the right foot, maintaining the 2nd toe in a straight and slightly plantar flexed position.

GODFREY REGIONAL HOSPITAL
123 Main Street • Aldon, FL 77714 • (407) 555-1234

Continued

OPERATIVE REPORT

Patient information:	
Patient name:	Date:
DOB:	Surgeon:
MR#:	Anesthetist:

Preoperative diagnosis:

Postoperative diagnosis:

Procedure(s) performed:

Anesthesia:

Assistant surgeon:

Description of procedure:

The tourniquet was released, and returned blood flow was found to be normal. Attention was then directed to the left foot where 2% Xylocaine hydrochloride plain was used to infiltrate the operative area. The same procedure as described upon the right foot was then performed in the identical fashion to the 2nd metatarsophalangeal joint on the left foot, including extensor digitorum longus tendon lengthening and capsulotomy and closure accomplished in the same manner as described. With completion of the left foot, Celestone Solu span 5 cc was then deposited in the operative area. Adaptic was applied to the skin incision and a mild compression dressing was then placed around the left foot, maintaining the 2nd toe in a straight and slightly plantar flexed position. The tourniquet was released and returned blood flow was found to be normal.

The immediate postoperative condition of the patient was excellent and she was returned to her room.

Patrick Chug md

GODFREY REGIONAL HOSPITAL
123 Main Street • Aldon, FL 77714 • (407) 555-1234

EXERCISE 17

Level II

OPERATIVE REPORT

Patient information:	
Patient name: DOB: MR#:	Date: Surgeon: Anesthetist:

Preoperative diagnosis:

Suspicion of torn rotator cuff, left shoulder

Postoperative diagnosis:

Torn rotator cuff, left shoulder

Procedure(s) performed:

Diagnostic arthroscopy, left shoulder with arthroscopic subacromial decompression; open repair of torn rotator cuff; placement of infusion catheter

Anesthesia:

Assistant surgeon:

Description of procedure:

The patient was placed supine on the operating room table on the beach chair attachment and a satisfactory general anesthetic was given. Preoperative intravenous cephalosporin antibiotic was given. Bilateral pneumatic compression sleeves were on the calves and were operative throughout the procedure. The patient was placed in the modified beach chair position. The left shoulder was widely prepped sterilely with DuraPrep times two including the lateral neck, anterolateral, posterior torso, axilla, arm, and down to the hand. The left shoulder was draped in the usual sterile fashion.

Arthroscope cannula was introduced via a standard posterior portal into the glenohumeral joint. Inflow to the joint was via the arthroscopy pump. Normal saline was delivered in this fashion. Outflow was from the cannula to suction. A flow of irrigation was maintained for purposes of visualization and removal of debris.

Arthroscope was placed. The biceps tendon was intact without evidence of stretching or tearing of its fibers or hemorrhage on its surface. Its attachment to the glenoid was intact. The anterior and posterior labrum structures were intact without evidence of thinning or detachment. The articular surfaces of the humeral head and glenoid were intact without evidence of fibrillation or cartilaginous cracking or tears. No subchondral bone was exposed. The anterior, posterior, and inferior recesses were of normal size with no evidence of loose body. The anterior ligamentous structures were intact without evidence of pathology. The rotator cuff showed some fraying at its water-shed area. It was followed out to its attachment site and showed some detachment and retraction. Decision was made to perform an arthroscopy acromioplasty.

GODFREY REGIONAL HOSPITAL
123 Main Street • Aldon, FL 77714 • (407) 555-1234

Continued

OPERATIVE REPORT

Patient information:

Patient name: Date:
DOB: Surgeon:
MR#:   Anesthetist:

Preoperative diagnosis:

Postoperative diagnosis:

Procedure(s) performed:

Anesthesia:

Assistant surgeon:

Description of procedure:

The arthroscope was replaced through the same posterior portal into the subacromial space. A separate standard lateral portal was then made. A rotary shaver was used to perform a bursectomy, with debris produced removed via suction attached to a rotary shaver. A rotary burr was then used to perform an anterior inferior acromioplasty, with debris produced removed via suction attached to the burr. The undersurface of the distal clavicle was not prominent and did not require resection.

Because of the location of the tear and the extreme difficulty it would cause to try to repair this arthroscopically, the decision was made to perform this open.

Skin incision was made along the skin lines, roughly halfway between the acromioclavicular joint and the lateral tip of the acromion. The incision was carried through subcutaneous tissue. Hemostasis was achieved as necessary. Full-thickness skin flaps were raised. The deltoid fascia was incised perpendicularly to its fibers. The rotator cuff was identified and the detachment was identified. Two Ultra Fix suture anchors were then placed at appropriate locations and weaved into the edge of the rotator cuff tendon. The tendon was then brought to its normal attachment site without tension. The elbow was at the patient's side. A strong repair was obtained.

The wound was copiously irrigated with normal saline antibiotic solution. An 18-gauge spinal needle was placed percutaneously through the deltoid muscle into the subacromial space, followed by placement through the needle of an epidural type catheter. The tip of the catheter remained in the subacromial space as the needle was withdrawn. The catheter was taped to the patient's skin with sterile tape. The

GODFREY REGIONAL HOSPITAL
123 Main Street • Aldon, FL 77714 • (407) 555-1234

Continued

OPERATIVE REPORT

Patient information:	
Patient name: DOB: MR#:	Date: Surgeon: Anesthetist:

Preoperative diagnosis:

Postoperative diagnosis:

Procedure(s) performed:

Anesthesia:

Assistant surgeon:

Description of procedure:

acromioplasty was noted to be quite sufficient as the tip of the index finger could easily be placed between the rotator cuff and remaining acromion. The deltoid fascia was reapproximated with interrupted figure-of-8 sutures of 0 Ethibond. The subcutaneous tissue was copiously irrigated with normal saline antibiotic solution. The subcutaneous tissue was closed with interrupted inverted sutures of 2-0 Vicryl, followed by closure of the skin with staples. The subcutaneous tissue, prior to closure, was infiltrated with 0.5% Marcaine with epinephrine. This was also injected into the subacromial space. The portals were closed with staples. The end of the epidural type catheter was connected to an infusion pump filled with 100 ccs of 2% lidocaine without epinephrine at delivery rate of 2 ccs per hour.

Dry sterile dressings were applied to the incision and catheter sites and held in place during the removal of the drapes. Dressings were taped into place. Shoulder immobilizer was applied.

The patient tolerated the procedure well. There were no complications. She was awakened in the operating room and transported to the PACU in satisfactory condition.

Patrick Cherry MD

GODFREY REGIONAL HOSPITAL
123 Main Street • Aldon, FL 77714 • (407) 555-1234

EXERCISE 18

Level II

OPERATIVE REPORT

Patient information:	
Patient name: DOB: MR#:	Date: Surgeon: Anesthetist:

Preoperative diagnosis:

1. Right lateral epicondylitis
2. Possible loose body, right elbow

INDICATIONS FOR PROCEDURE: A 56-year-old gentleman with a history of bilateral radial head fractures, nondisplaced treated non-operatively, and persistent pain in his right elbow. Resulting symptoms of lateral epicondylitis had been treated with physical therapy, injections, splinting, and anti-inflammatory medications. He continues to have discomfort. After

Postoperative diagnosis:

Right lateral epicondylitis

Procedure(s) performed:

Right lateral tennis elbow release with elbow arthrotomy and exploration

Anesthesia:

Assistant surgeon:

Description of procedure:

COMPLICATIONS: None

The patient was taken to the operating room and placed supine on the operating room table. General anesthesia was obtained. The right arm was prepped and draped in the usual sterile fashion. A standard lateral incision was made directly over the lateral epicondyle. Subcutaneous tissue was dissected down to the deep fascia. The deep fascia was identified and the interval between the ECU and extensor carpi radialis longus was identified and split. As this was separated, we identified the extensor carpi radialis brevis. It was subsequently released from its origin onto the lateral humeral epicondyle, and there was significant scar tissue beneath this. This was subsequently rongeured off, and we inspected the radial capitello joint, found no evidence of any loose bodies with good smooth articular cartilage. We then closed the capsule up with 3-0 Ticron. It was then irrigated out copiously. The tourniquet was let down. Hemostasis was obtained with electrocautery. The superficial extensors were then sutured together with 2-0 Vicryl, the subcutaneous tissue with 2-0 Vicryl, and the skin was sutured with 4-0 nylon in a running fashion.

The patient tolerated the procedure well, was extubated in the operating room, transferred from the operating table to his bed, and taken to the postanesthesia recovery room in stable condition.

Patrick Chung, MD

GODFREY REGIONAL HOSPITAL
123 Main Street • Aldon, FL 77714 • (407) 555-1234

Continued

OPERATIVE REPORT

Patient information:	
Patient name: DOB: MR#:	Date: Surgeon: Anesthetist:

Preoperative diagnosis:

discussion of the options, risks, and benefits of surgery including bleeding, infection, nerve damage, continued pain and discomfort, all questions were answered and consents were signed. The patient was taken to the operating room.

Postoperative diagnosis:

Procedure(s) performed:

Anesthesia:

Assistant surgeon:

Description of procedure:

GODFREY REGIONAL HOSPITAL
123 Main Street • Aldon, FL 77714 • (407) 555-1234

EXERCISE 19

Level II

OPERATIVE REPORT

Patient information:	
Patient name:	Date:
DOB:	Surgeon:
MR#:	Anesthetist:

Preoperative diagnosis:

Medial meniscal tear, left knee

Postoperative diagnosis:

Complex posterior horn tear, medial meniscus, left knee; complete ACL tear (previous partial tear) and synovitis of the notch and medial compartment

Procedure(s) performed:

Left knee arthroscopy and partial arthroscopic medial meniscectomy

Anesthesia:

Assistant surgeon:

Description of procedure:

After suitable general anesthesia had been achieved, the patient's left knee was prepped and draped in the usual manner. Prior to prepping, thigh tourniquet was applied, and after draping, inflated to 300 mm of mercury. No inflow cannula was used. Arthroscope was inserted through an anterior medial porthole. The lateral compartment was examined first. There was noted to be stable intact lateral meniscus. Examination of the notch revealed what appeared to be an old partial ACL tear, which had been recently completed to a complete ACL tear. There was torn ACL tissue that was being impinged and was excised. There was noted to be marked synovitis of the notch. Using the radiofrequency probe, synovial bleeders were cauterized. Examination of the medial compartment revealed synovitis along the medial gutter. Using the cautery, this was cauterized. There was noted to be a complex tear of the posterior horn of the medial meniscus with a lot of large meniscal flaps. Using combination punch and shaver, the meniscus that was unstable was excised, excising pretty much the entire posterior horn. Remainder of the meniscus was contoured, and the articular surfaces medially looked in good shape. Articular surface laterally looked in good shape. The patellofemoral joint was examined, and there was noted to be some diffuse mild grade II changes on the patella with minimal articular cartilage flaps. The trochlea also showed some very mild superficial wear with no flaps. The knee joint was then thoroughly irrigated and the arthroscope removed. Stab wounds were closed with 4-0 nylon. The patient's knee was then instilled with 80 mg of Kenalog and 20 cc of 0.5% Marcaine. Dressing was then applied. Tourniquet was released. Following tourniquet release, good circulation was noted to return to the foot.

The patient tolerated the procedure well and returned to the recovery room in stable condition.   *Patrick Chung, MD*

GODFREY REGIONAL HOSPITAL
123 Main Street • Aldon, FL 77714 • (407) 555-1234

EXERCISE 20

Level II

OPERATIVE REPORT

Patient information:

Patient name:
DOB:
MR#:

Date:
Surgeon:
Anesthetist:

Preoperative diagnosis:

1) Subluxation, 2nd metatarsophalangeal joint, right foot

2) Hammer toe deformity, 2nd toe, right foot

Postoperative diagnosis:

Same

Procedure(s) performed:

1) Osteoplasty, 2nd metatarsal head, right foot

2) Arthroplasty proximal interphalangeal joint, 2nd toe, right foot

Anesthesia:

Assistant surgeon:

Description of procedure:

A V-lock cuff was placed above the right ankle for hemostasis, and the patient was prepped and draped in usual aseptic manner. With IV sedation, 2% Xylocaine hydrochloride plain was used to infiltrate the operative area on the right forefoot. A dorsolongitudinal skin incision, approximately 4 cm in length, was made extending from mid shaft of the 2nd metatarsal proximally to the base of the proximal phalanx of the 2nd toe distally. The skin and subcutaneous tissues were underscored and retracted. The incision was then deepened medial to the extensor digital and longus tendon and carried down to the level of the metatarsal head. The capsular and ligamentous structures then separated from the 2nd metatarsal head and the 2nd toe plantar flexed, thereby bringing the 2nd metatarsal head into view. Utilizing a power saw and beginning at the surgical neck of the metatarsal head, a cut was made perpendicular to the shaft approximately one half the width of the metatarsal head and then beveled at a 45-degree angle to include the plantar condyles. The severed bone was then dissected out by sharp dissection, and all rough edges were rasped smooth. The wound was then copiously flushed with normal saline solution. The right foot was loaded, finding good release of subluxation occurring at the level of the 2nd metatarsophalangeal joint but with considerable contractures still occurring at the proximal phalangeal joint of the 2nd toe. Therefore, two longitudinal ellipsing skin incisions were made directly over the head of the proximal phalanx of the 2nd toe. The created skin wedge was then sharply dissected. The skin and subcutaneous tissues were underscored and retracted. A transverse incision was then made through the capsule and extensor tendon complex at the proximal interphalangeal joint. The medial and lateral collateral ligaments were incised and the head of the proximal phalanx was delivered. Utilizing a power saw, the head of the proximal phalanx was then resected, and all bony edges were rasped smooth. The wound was then copiously

GODFREY REGIONAL HOSPITAL
123 Main Street • Aldon, FL 77714 • (407) 555-1234

Continued

OPERATIVE REPORT

Patient information:

Patient name: Date:
DOB: Surgeon:
MR#:   Anesthetist:

Preoperative diagnosis:

Postoperative diagnosis:

Procedure(s) performed:

Anesthesia:

Assistant surgeon:

Description of procedure:

flushed with normal saline solution. The right foot was loaded, finding a much more normally positioned 2nd toe with full reduction of the preoperative deformity. At the level of the 2nd metatarsophalangeal joint, the ligamentous and capsular structures were repaired with interrupted sutures of 2-0 Vicryl. Superficial tissues were then closed with 3-0 Vicryl, and the skin margins were approximated with interrupted horizontal mattress sutures of 4-0 nylon. Attention was then directed to the 2nd toe where the extensor tendon and collateral ligaments were repaired with interrupted sutures of 3-0 Vicryl. Skin margins were then approximated with interrupted horizontal mattress sutures of 4-0 nylon. Before bandaging, the right foot was again loaded, finding a normally positioned 2nd toe. Celestone Solu span 1 cc was then deposited in the operative sites. Adaptic was applied to both skin incisions and a mild compression dressing was then placed around the right foot, maintaining the 2nd toe in a straight and slightly plantar flexed position. The tourniquet was released and return blood flow was found to be normal.

The immediate postoperative condition of the patient was excellent, and she was returned to her room.

[signature]

GODFREY REGIONAL HOSPITAL
123 Main Street • Aldon, FL 77714 • (407) 555-1234

EXERCISE 21

Level I

OPERATIVE REPORT

Patient information:	
Patient name: DOB: MR#:	Date: Surgeon: Anesthetist:

Preoperative diagnosis:

Hallux abducto valgus deformity, right foot

Postoperative diagnosis:

Same

Procedure(s) performed:

Bunionectomy with distal 1st metatarsal osteotomy including K-wire fixation, right foot

Anesthesia:

Assistant surgeon:

Description of procedure:

A V-lock cuff was placed above the right ankle for hemostasis and the patient was prepped and draped in the usual aseptic manner. With IV sedation, 2% Xylocaine hydrochloride plain was used to infiltrate the operative area on the right forefoot. A longitudinal skin incision, approximately 6 cm in length, was made in the dorsomedial aspect, extending from mid shaft of the 1st metatarsal proximally to the base of the proximal phalanx of the great toe distally. The skin and subcutaneous tissues were underscored and retracted. A curvilinear incision was then made through the capsular structure over the 1st metatarsophalangeal joint, with the resultant capsular flap being dissected free of the 1st metatarsal head. The prominent hyperostosis along the medial and dorsal aspect of the 1st metatarsal head was then removed and all bony edges were rasped smooth. Likewise, the corresponding hyperostosis along the medial aspect of the base of the proximal phalanx was removed and rasped smooth. A drill hole from medial to lateral was then made through the center of the 1st metatarsal bed, thus forming the apex of the osteotomy. Beginning at the apex, at a 60-degree angle, a cut was made in the bone from medial to lateral superiorly. A similar cut was made inferiorly, thus resulting in a separated fragment of bone. The osteotomy fragment was then displaced laterally and firmly impacted back upon the 1st metatarsal shaft, thereby aligning the articular surfaces. The bony lip resulting from the displacement was removed and rasped smooth. The osteotomy was then further

GODFREY REGIONAL HOSPITAL
123 Main Street • Aldon, FL 77714 • (407) 555-1234

Continued

OPERATIVE REPORT

Patient information:	
Patient name:	Date:
DOB:	Surgeon:
MR#:	Anesthetist:

Preoperative diagnosis:

Postoperative diagnosis:

Procedure(s) performed:

Anesthesia:

Assistant surgeon:

Description of procedure:

secured utilizing a single K-wire measuring .045 and inserted obliquely through the osteotomy from dorsal medial to lateral plantar. The right foot was loaded, finding a stable osteotomy with a normally positioned great toe and normal range of motion. The wound was then copiously flushed with normal saline solution. Capsular structures, including superficial tissues, were then closed with interrupted sutures of 2-0 Vicryl. Skin margins were then approximated with interrupted horizontal mattress sutures of 4-0 nylon. The protruding K-wire was then bent and clipped. Celestone Solu span 1 cc was then deposited in the operative area. Betadine ointment was placed around a single protruding K-wire, followed by Adaptic to the skin incision, and a mild compression bandage was then placed around the right foot maintaining the great toe in a straightened position. The cuff was released and return blood flow was found to be normal.

The immediate post-op condition of the patient was satisfactory and she was returned to her room.

Patrick Chung, MD

GODFREY REGIONAL HOSPITAL
123 Main Street • Aldon, FL 77714 • (407) 555-1234

EXERCISE 22

Level I

OPERATIVE REPORT

Patient information:	
Patient name: DOB: MR#:	Date: Surgeon: Anesthetist:

Preoperative diagnosis:

Impingement, right shoulder, with tear, rotator cuff

Postoperative diagnosis:

Impingement, right shoulder, with undersurface fraying, rotator cuff and inflammation, right glenohumeral joint

Procedure(s) performed:

Arthroscopy, right shoulder with Depo-Medrol injection, right glenohumeral joint, arthroscopic subacromial decompression, placement of infusion catheter

Anesthesia:

Assistant surgeon:

Description of procedure:

The patient was placed supine on the operating room table and a satisfactory general anesthetic was given. Preoperative intravenous cephalosporin antibiotic was given. Bilateral pneumatic compression sleeves were on the calves and were operative throughout the procedure. The patient was placed in the modified beach chair position. The left shoulder was widely prepped sterilely with DuraPrep times two including the lateral neck, anterior, lateral, posterior torso, axilla, and arm down to the hand. The right shoulder was draped in the usual sterile fashion. The scope cannula was introduced via a standard posterior portal and into the glenohumeral joint, followed by the arthroscope. Inflow to the shoulder through the cannula from the arthroscopy pump at a setting of 70 mm Hg. The shoulder was distended with normal saline in this fashion. Outflow from the cannula to suction. A flow of irrigation was maintained for purposes of visualization and removal of debris.

The biceps tendon was intact without evidence of stretching or tearing of its fibers or hemorrhage on its surface. Its attachment to the superior glenoid was intact. The anterior and posterior labral structures were intact without evidence of degeneration or displacement or separation from the glenoid. The articular surfaces of the humeral head and glenoid were intact without evidence of fibrillation, cartilaginous cracking, or breakdown. The anterior ligamentous structures were intact without evidence of stretching or tearing or hemorrhage on their surface. The anterior, posterior, and inferior recesses were of normal size and showed no evidence of intrasubstance pathology or loose body. The rotator cuff was scrutinized and showed some fibrillation at the watershed area but showed no evidence of tearing. There was quite a bit of synovitis involving the glenohumeral joint as a whole. The rotator cuff was visualized through the attachment site and showed no evidence of

GODFREY REGIONAL HOSPITAL
123 Main Street • Aldon, FL 77714 • (407) 555-1234

Continued

OPERATIVE REPORT

Patient information:	
Patient name: DOB: MR#:	Date: Surgeon: Anesthetist:

Preoperative diagnosis:

Postoperative diagnosis:

Procedure(s) performed:

Anesthesia:

Assistant surgeon:

Description of procedure:

intrasubstance tear or detachment. A total of 80 mg Depo-Medrol with some Marcaine was then injected through the arthroscope cannula into the glenohumeral joint.

The arthroscope was withdrawn and redirected into the subacromial space. A standard lateral portal was made, followed by a rotary shaver with attached suction. The bursal tissue was excised as well as tissue on the undersurface of the acromion. There was obvious impingement in the subacromial space through range of motion of the shoulder.

A rotary burr with attached suction was used to perform a generous anterior inferior acromioplasty to the level of the acromioclavicular joint. The undersurface of the distal clavicle was slightly prominent and this required resection as well. Debris produced was removed via suction attached to the rotary burr. After the acromioplasty, the shoulder was placed through a range of motion and there was no further evidence of impingement.

An 18-gauge spinal needle was placed percutaneously through the deltoid muscle into the subacromial space, followed by placement through the needle of an epidural type catheter. The catheter remained in the subacromial space as the needle was withdrawn. The catheter was taped to the patient using sterile tape. A total of 30 cc of a combination of 0.5% Marcaine with epinephrine plus 5 mg morphine sulfate was injected into the subacromial space via the arthroscope cannula. The cannula was removed. Each portal was closed with a single simple suture of 3-0 Ethilon. The end of the epidural type catheter was connected to an infusion pump filled with 100 cc of 2% lidocaine without

GODFREY REGIONAL HOSPITAL
123 Main Street • Aldon, FL 77714 • (407) 555-1234

Continued

OPERATIVE REPORT

Patient information:

Patient name: Date:
DOB: Surgeon:
MR#:   Anesthetist:

Preoperative diagnosis:

Postoperative diagnosis:

Procedure(s) performed:

Anesthesia:

Assistant surgeon:

Description of procedure:

epinephrine at a delivery rate of 2 cc per hour. Dry sterile dressings were applied to the incision and catheter sites and held in place during removal of the drapes. Dressings were taped into place. Sling was applied.

The patient tolerated the procedure well. There were no complications. She was awakened in the operating room and transported to the recovery room in stable condition.

Patrick Chung MD

GODFREY REGIONAL HOSPITAL
123 Main Street • Aldon, FL 77714 • (407) 555-1234

EXERCISE 23

Level II

OPERATIVE REPORT

Patient information:	
Patient name: DOB: MR#:	Date: Surgeon: Anesthetist:

Preoperative diagnosis:

1. Extremely comminuted, displaced, unstable, interarticular fracture of the distal radius, left wrist
2. Pre-existing longstanding navicular non-union with radioscaphoid and capitolunate degenerative arthritis, left wrist

Postoperative diagnosis:

1. Extremely comminuted, displaced, unstable, interarticular fracture of the distal radial left wrist
2. Pre-existing longstanding navicular non-union with radioscaphoid and capitolunate degenerative arthritis, left wrist

Procedure(s) performed:

Closed reduction and external fixation

Anesthesia:

Assistant surgeon:

Description of procedure:

The patient is under general anesthesia and LMA. He is positioned supine. The left upper extremity is placed on a hand table. A tourniquet is applied around the left arm. The patient received two grams of Ancef IV, 15 minutes prior to inflating the tourniquet. The fracture is examined under fluoroscopic imaging. With traction on the wrist, the fracture reduces very nicely on both views. The comminution of the articular surface is extremely severe. Placing the wrist in neutral dorsiflexion and volar flexion allows anatomic reduction of the articular surface of the distal radius on both views. The fracture is very unstable. There is an obvious non-union of a navicular fracture with radioscaphoid and capitolunate degenerative arthritis. The radial styloid is pointed in shape.

Prep and drape of the left upper extremity in the usual manner. The left upper extremity is exsanguinated with an Esmarch and the tourniquet inflated to 300 mm of mercury. Total tourniquet time was 60 minutes.

A 3-cm long skin incision is made on the dorsal radial aspect of the second metacarpal shaft. Deep dissection is done with scissors. The subcutaneous veins are identified and protected. A pre-drilling technique is used to insert a 3-mm self-tapping pin in the second metacarpal shaft. The first 3-mm pin is placed into the base of the second metacarpal. The second pin is placed perfectly parallel to the first pin using the appropriate guide. The soft tissues are irrigated with normal saline, removing all bone debris. The skin is partially closed around the pins, avoiding any tension of the skin around the pins. The closure of the skin is done using 4-0 nylon.

Another 3-cm long skin incision is made on the dorsal radial aspect of the forearm, in line with the dorsal radial incision on the hand. The

GODFREY REGIONAL HOSPITAL
123 Main Street • Aldon, FL 77714 • (407) 555-1234

Continued

OPERATIVE REPORT

Patient information:

Patient name:	Date:
DOB:	Surgeon:
MR#:	Anesthetist:

Preoperative diagnosis:

Postoperative diagnosis:

Procedure(s) performed:

Anesthesia:

Assistant surgeon:

Description of procedure:

incision is made 6–7 cm proximal to the radial styloid. Deep dissection is done with scissors. The superficial branch of the radial nerve is identified and protected. The radius shaft is exposed. A pre-drilling technique is used to insert perfectly parallel 3-mm self-tapping pins. The soft tissues are irrigated with normal saline, removing all bone debris, and the skin is partially closed using 4-0 nylon, avoiding any tension of the skin around the pins.

The external fixator clamps and rod are connected to the hat pins. The reduction is repeated using the same technique described previously. The wrist is placed in neutral position of dorsiflexion/volar flexion and in neutral deviation. After tightening the external fixator, the fracture is checked under fluoroscopic imaging. Alignment of the articular surface is excellent on both views. There is no shortening. Radial inclination and the tilt of the articular surface are restored. However, there is persistent instability of the fracture.

A bulky, non-adhesive dressing is applied around the hat pins. An ulnar gutter fiberglass splint is applied. Care is taken to carefully mold the splint over the wrist area. Alignment is re-examined after the cast has hardened, unchanged.

Surgery was well tolerated and the patient left the operating room for recovery in stable condition.

Patrick Chung, MD

GODFREY REGIONAL HOSPITAL
123 Main Street • Aldon, FL 77714 • (407) 555-1234

EXERCISE 24

Level I

OPERATIVE REPORT

Patient information:

Patient name: Date:
DOB: Surgeon:
MR#:   Anesthetist:

Preoperative diagnosis:

Posttraumatic arthritis, right wrist

Postoperative diagnosis:

Same

Procedure(s) performed:

Right wrist arthrodesis with application short-arm cast

Anesthesia:

Assistant surgeon:

Description of procedure:

The patient was placed supine on the operating room table and a satisfactory general anesthetic was given. Preoperative intravenous cephalosporin antibiotic was given. Pneumatic tourniquet was placed high on the left arm. The left hand, wrist, and forearm to proximal to the elbow were prepped sterilely with DuraPrep, and the left hand and wrist were draped in the usual sterile fashion. The dorsum of the wrist was shaved as needed prior to prepping and draping in the proposed incisional location. Tourniquet was inflated to 250 mm Hg.

Longitudinal skin incision was made on the dorsum of the hand and wrist from the area of the distal radius to the level of the mid shaft of the third metacarpal. The incision was carried through subcutaneous tissue. Hemostasis was achieved as necessary. Full-thickness skin flaps were raised. The extensor pollicis longus tendon was released from its sheath and was retracted during the procedure. The dorsal hump of the distal radius was then removed with rongeurs. Soft tissue was removed from the dorsal bones, including the lunate capitate and base of the third metacarpal. A burr was used to decorticate the posterior aspects of these bones as well as the joint surfaces between the radius and lunate, lunate and capitate, and capitate and third metacarpal. The wound was copiously irrigated with normal saline antibiotic solution. A nine-hole 3.5-mm dynamic compression plate was then bent in appropriate fashion to allow 10–20 degrees of extension at the

GODFREY REGIONAL HOSPITAL
123 Main Street • Aldon, FL 77714 • (407) 555-1234

Continued

OPERATIVE REPORT

Patient information:

Patient name:
DOB:
MR#:

Date:
Surgeon:
Anesthetist:

Preoperative diagnosis:

Postoperative diagnosis:

Procedure(s) performed:

Anesthesia:

Assistant surgeon:

Description of procedure:

wrist after arthrodesis. The prepared surfaces of the bone in between the radial lunate, lunocapitate, and capitate third metacarpal were filled with Collagraft. The plate was applied and attached to the radius and third metacarpal in compression type fashion. The overall alignment of the wrist was quite good. The plate was placed beneath the extensor pollicis longus tendon that was not damaged during the procedure.

The wound was copiously irrigated again with normal saline antibiotic solution. All fingers showed full range of motion passively after the procedure. The skin was closed full thickness with staples. Dry sterile dressings were applied, followed by sterile circumferential cast padding. Tourniquet was deflated. All drapes were removed including the tourniquet. Cast padding was applied to the elbow and a short-arm fiberglass cast was applied, not limiting flexion or extension to any joint of any finger. The patient tolerated the procedure well. There were no complications. She was awakened in the operating room and transported to the recovery room in stable condition.

GODFREY REGIONAL HOSPITAL
123 Main Street • Aldon, FL 77714 • (407) 555-1234

EXERCISE 25

Level I

OPERATIVE REPORT

Patient information:	
Patient name:	Date:
DOB:	Surgeon:
MR#:	Anesthetist:

Preoperative diagnosis:

Right knee medial and lateral meniscal tear

Postoperative diagnosis:

Right knee medial and lateral meniscal tear

Procedure(s) performed:

Right knee diagnostic arthroscopy, partial lateral meniscectomy, and partial medial posterior horn meniscectomy

Anesthesia:

Spinal

Assistant surgeon:

Description of procedure:

ESTIMATED BLOOD LOSS: Minimal

TOTAL TOURNIQUET TIME: Zero

IV FLUID: 1500 cc of crystalloid

INDICATIONS AND/OR FINDINGS: The patient tolerated the procedure well and transferred back to recovery room with noted stable vital signs.

OPERATIVE TECHNIQUE:
The patient was brought to the operating room and transferred onto the operating table. Spinal anesthesia was then induced. Once an adequate level of anesthetic was achieved, the right lower extremity was prepped and draped in the usual sterile fashion. Antibiotic was given preoperatively for prophylaxis. Anterior lateral portal was established for outflow. Inferior lateral portal was established for inflow and camera portal site. Diagnostic arthroscopy began first in the suprapatellar pouch proceeding toward the medial lateral compartment, in viewing the arthritis in the patella femoral surface, as well as defibrillation of the articular surface. There is also no evidence of loose body noted. The medial compartment was then entered as the knee was placed in a valgus position. We noted that there is a small tear in the posterior medial horn of the medial meniscus. This was subsequently evaluated under a probe as we established a working port on the inferior medial port. A small trimmer was used to trim back the medial horn to a stable edge. Of note, we did appreciate some arthritis on the medial compartment.

GODFREY REGIONAL HOSPITAL
123 Main Street • Aldon, FL 77714 • (407) 555-1234

Continued

OPERATIVE REPORT

Patient information:

Patient name:
DOB:
MR#:

Date:
Surgeon:
Anesthetist:

Preoperative diagnosis:

Postoperative diagnosis:

Procedure(s) performed:

Anesthesia:

Assistant surgeon:

Description of procedure:

The articular surface appears to be minimally denuded. The intercondylar notch was evaluated. The anterior cruciate ligament appears to be intact. Some moderate amount of fibrotic tissue was debrided, and synovitis was noted in the soft tissue and fibrous tissue region in this area.

Adequate debridement with an arthroscopic incisor was performed for better visualization as we removed the infrapatellar fat pad. The leg was taken to a lateral figure-of-four position to open up and get better visualization into the lateral joint line. Upon entering into the lateral compartment, we noted an extensive amount of defibrillation of the articular surface, as well as denution in both the lateral femoral condyle and the lateral tibia plateau down to its articular surface of pink denuded bone. There is also noticeable meniscal tear on the anterior horn, tracking back to the posterior lateral horn of the lateral meniscus. This was subsequently trimmed using multiple arthroscopic incisors, as well as the arthroscopic trimmer. We trimmed the lateral meniscus back to a stable rim. The knee was taken to full range of motion and noted to be quite smooth. There was no evidence of mechanical catching or locking any further. The knee was irrigated out profusely. Intraoperative x-ray was obtained using the arthroscopic camera. The portal site was then subsequently removed and closed in the routine fashion. Sensorcaine was used to inject the portal sites for postoperative pain management. Compressive dressing was then applied.

The patient was then awakened and transferred back to recovery room with noted stable vital signs.

Patrick Chung MD

GODFREY REGIONAL HOSPITAL
123 Main Street • Aldon, FL 77714 • (407) 555-1234

EXERCISE 26

Level I

OPERATIVE REPORT

Patient information:

Patient name:
DOB:
MR#:

Date:
Surgeon:
Anesthetist:

Preoperative diagnosis:

Left chronic ankle instability

Postoperative diagnosis:

Left chronic ankle instability

Procedure(s) performed:

Left modified Brostrom procedure

Anesthesia:

Assistant surgeon:

Description of procedure:

The patient was brought to the operating suite and placed in the supine position, and a general anesthetic was given without difficulties. The left lower extremity was prepped and draped in the usual sterile fashion, and tourniquet on the left thigh was inflated to 300 mm of mercury. After exsanguination of the ligament with an Esmarch bandage, the patient's ankle was tested for stability. There was marked increased laxity on talar tilt and anterior drawer testing.

A J-shaped incision was made along the lateral aspect of the distal fibula and brought down carefully to the extensor retinaculum, which was retracted distally as well. The peroneal tendons were identified and then retracted posteriorly, and this allowed us to detach the stretched and thickened ATF and CF ligaments safely from the distal fibula. The joint was visualized. There was no articular cartilage damage in the later part of the talar dome. There was some synovitis present, and this was removed using a rongeur. A rongeur was also used to make a trough in the end of the distal fibula at the ATF and CF ligament attachments. The ligament was then pulled into the bony trough in an effort to tighten the ligament structures. This was done with 2-0 Panacryl through drill holes in the fibula. The retinaculum of the extensor tendons was then sutured to the periosteum of the distal fibula using 0 Vicryl sutures, and then a usual layered closure was done with 4-0 Monocryl sutures for the subcuticular tissue. 20 cc of 0.5% Marcaine plain was injected around the ankle joint, and then a well-padded, short-leg cast with the ankle in neutral was applied. The tourniquet was let down; the cap refill in toes appeared quite nice.

The patient was brought to the recovery room in stable condition.

GODFREY REGIONAL HOSPITAL
123 Main Street • Aldon, FL 77714 • (407) 555-1234

EXERCISE 27

Level II

OPERATIVE REPORT

Patient information:

Patient name:	Date:
DOB:	Surgeon:
MR#:	Anesthetist:

Preoperative diagnosis:

Internal derangement of the right knee with complex tear of the posterior horn of medial meniscus and associated extensive medial femoral condylar osteochondral defect with chondromalacia and early degenerative osteoarthrosis

Postoperative diagnosis:

Same

Procedure(s) performed:

Right knee arthroscopy, arthroscopic partial medial meniscectomy, and arthroscopic abrasion arthroplasty of medial femoral condylar osteochondral defect

Anesthesia:

Spinal

Assistant surgeon:

Description of procedure:

The patient was brought to the operating room and placed under spinal anesthesia without episode. He was then turned to the supine position. Tourniquet was applied high on the proximal aspect of the right thigh. The right lower extremity was then thoroughly prepped and draped in the usual sterile fashion, with the right lower extremity draped as a sterile field from the tourniquet level distally. Venous blood was exsanguinated with a sterile Ace bandage and the tourniquet inflated to 300 mm of mercury pressure. A short anteromedial portal incision was created with a #11 blade, measuring approximately 1 cm in length. The arthroscope and sharp obturator were then advanced through the skin and the capsule and into the joint. The obturator was removed. Upon removal of the obturator, moderate sized interarticular effusion was evacuated through the arthroscope and fluids submitted to the laboratory for synovial fluid studies. The arthroscope and camera were then advanced into the joint. A second superolateral stab wound was created for admission of a large trocar and inflow cannula and the sterile tubing connected to an arthroscopic pump. Arthroscopic examination of the knee was carried out sequentially. Arthroscopic examination was accompanied by several Polaroid films documenting findings throughout the procedure. Arthroscopic examination confirmed the preoperative MRI findings of a complex multiplanar tear involving the posterior horn of the medial meniscus. This tear was too extensive and fragmented for repair.

In addition to the expected tear of the medial meniscus, a substantial defect of the weightbearing surface of the medial femoral condyle was demonstrated; again, this was accompanied by cracking and fragmentation of the margins of the articular cartilage in the area of the lesion.

GODFREY REGIONAL HOSPITAL
123 Main Street • Aldon, FL 77714 • (407) 555-1234

Continued

OPERATIVE REPORT

Patient information:

Patient name: Date:
DOB: Surgeon:
MR#:   Anesthetist:

Preoperative diagnosis:

Postoperative diagnosis:

Procedure(s) performed:

Anesthesia:

Assistant surgeon:

Description of procedure:

A second stab wound was created for admission of the arthroscopic surgical equipment, and utilizing a 5-0 shaver, as well as a 4-0 shaver, arthroscopic debridement of the torn portion of the medial meniscus was carried out. This was supplemented with hand instruments to attain a clean margin at the level of resection of the posterior horn tear. Following debridement and rejection of the complex medial meniscus tear of the posterior margin, arthroscopic abrasion arthroplasty of the osteochondral defect over the medial femoral condyle was carried out until a smooth margin was created. The base of the lesion was then drilled multiply, utilizing a small smooth Steinmann pin to reach the osteochondral area for hopeful production of fibrocartilage patching of the defect. Copious and repetitive irrigation of the joint was carried out to evacuate arthroscopic debris of meniscal fragments, as well as the osteochondral lesion. This was continued until the irrigation was returning clear. At this point the joint was evacuated, and the arthroscopic instrumentation was withdrawn. The arthroscopic incisions were closed with interrupted sutures of 4-0 nylon. The joint was injected with a solution of 0.5% Marcaine with epinephrine. Sterile Adaptic gauze, sterile 4 × 4s, and sterile soft roll were applied with an Ace bandage, and on release of tourniquet, good distal circulation was noted with good distal pulses at the posterior tibial and dorsalis pedis levels.

The patient subsequently was removed from the operating room and returned to the medical-surgical unit in good condition, having tolerated the procedure without apparent incident. All needle and sponge counts were correct at the termination of the procedure.

GODFREY REGIONAL HOSPITAL
123 Main Street • Aldon, FL 77714 • (407) 555-1234

EXERCISE 28

Level I

OPERATIVE REPORT

Patient information:	
Patient name: DOB: MR#:	Date: Surgeon: Anesthetist:

Preoperative diagnosis:

Osteochondral flap, right patella

INDICATIONS: 14-year-old white male who has had persistent mechanical symptoms as well as effusion in the right knee. MRI was consistent with osteochondral flap of the patella. Alternatives, risks, and possible complications were carefully discussed with him and his family. Operative intervention was desired. Consent was obtained.

Postoperative diagnosis:

Osteochondral flap, right patella

Procedure(s) performed:

Diagnostic arthroscopy, right; debridement osteochondral flap, right knee; drilling, right patella

Anesthesia:

General

Assistant surgeon:

Description of procedure:

EBL: Minimal

TOURNIQUET TIME: 25 minutes at 300 mm Hg

COMPLICATIONS: None apparent

DESCRIPTION OF OPERATION:
The patient was brought to the main operating room and positioned supine. After general anesthesia was adequately obtained, a tourniquet was placed around the right proximal thigh. 1 gm Ancef was given IV. The right lower extremity was prepped and draped in the usual sterile fashion. The limb was elevated and the tourniquet inflated.

The arthroscope was placed through the standard inferolateral portal, with outflow through the superolateral portal, and instrumentation from the inferomedial portal. No effusion was noted upon entering the joint. The patella revealed an osteochondral flap roughly in the central portion of the patella, lining up with the trochlea. It was very unstable, barely being attached in one corner only. It was felt to be irreparable as it was nearly displaced. There was also some fraying of the cartilage surrounding this region. There was also relatively thickened plica (though it did not feel pathologic) noted in the

GODFREY REGIONAL HOSPITAL
123 Main Street • Aldon, FL 77714 • (407) 555-1234

Continued

OPERATIVE REPORT

Patient information:	
Patient name: DOB: MR#:	Date: Surgeon: Anesthetist:

Preoperative diagnosis:

Postoperative diagnosis:

Procedure(s) performed:

Anesthesia:

Assistant surgeon:

Description of procedure:

superomedial corner. Gutters otherwise clear; no loose bodies were identified. Medial and lateral compartments were pristine as well as ACL and PCL.

A shaver was placed within the joint and margins were debrided back and again noted to be a very unstable OCD-type lesion. Therefore a grabber was used to remove the two fragments basically falling out of the crater. I then beveled the crater back with the shaver. Through a small stab incision over the dorsum of the patella, I placed multiple .045 drill holes directly into the lesion, visualizing it through the arthroscope. After this, I placed the shaver back in the joint and cleaned out debris and completed the beveling. Then I irrigated out the knee and removed the arthroscopic equipment. I instilled 0.25% Marcaine as we removed the arthroscope. A sterile compression bandage was applied, and the tourniquet was deflated.

The patient was awakened and returned to PAR in stable condition without apparent complication.

Patrick Chug MD

GODFREY REGIONAL HOSPITAL
123 Main Street • Aldon, FL 77714 • (407) 555-1234

EXERCISE 29

Level II

OPERATIVE REPORT

Patient information:

Patient name: Date:
DOB: Surgeon:
MR#: Anesthetist:

Preoperative diagnosis:

Displaced fracture, distal left radius and ulna

This is a 15-year-old white male who came to the emergency room with a displaced fracture of his distal left radius and ulna that was attempted to be reduced with Versed and morphine in the emergency room, but was unable to have good reduction and subsequently was brought back to the operating room for general anesthesia reduction.

Postoperative diagnosis:

Same

Procedure(s) performed:

Closed reduction of distal left radius and ulna

Anesthesia:

Assistant surgeon:

Description of procedure:

With the patient under general anesthesia, traction made on his distal radius and ulna, and countertraction placed into his upper arm; finally after the fifth attempt, satisfactory reduction was achieved after manipulating the fracture with the thumbs pushing the distal fragment palmarly and ulnarly. Subsequently, the fracture then showed satisfactory reduction. The arm was then wrapped with a Webril and then a plaster cast sufficient enough to hold it in position. The arm was placed in mild pronation and slight ulnar deviation with some mild flexion to the wrist. A significant flexion was not done, because previously when this was tried when he was awake, he would get numbness along the distribution of the median nerve.

The patient tolerated this procedure well. He will be kept overnight to watch the neurovascular status, and if there is any compromise, he may need to have the cast split, but this will be watched quite closely.

GODFREY REGIONAL HOSPITAL
123 Main Street • Aldon, FL 77714 • (407) 555-1234

EXERCISE 30

Level II

OPERATIVE REPORT

Patient information:	
Patient name: DOB: MR#:	Date: Surgeon: Anesthetist:

Preoperative diagnosis:

1. Comminuted, markedly displaced fracture of the distal mid 1/3 junction of the left tibia and fibula with associated bacterial infection, and delayed union
2. Status post multiple debridement and insertion of antibiotic impregnated methyl methacrylate beads

Postoperative diagnosis:

Same

Procedure(s) performed:

Operative, multicultures of fracture site, removal of methyl methacrylate and antibiotic beads from distal lower leg fracture site, wound irrigation, local debridement, and lysis of adhesions

Anesthesia:

Assistant surgeon:

Description of procedure:

The patient was brought to the operating room and placed under spinal anesthesia without episode. Tourniquet was applied high on the proximal aspect of the left thigh. The extremity was then prepped and draped in the usual sterile fashion from the tourniquet level distally. The extremity was elevated for exsanguination of venous blood and tourniquet inflated to 300 mm of mercury pressure. Following this, approach was made to the distal anterior aspect of the lower leg, utilizing previous old surgical scar in a slightly curvilinear fashion; the most posterior aspect of the distal incision was extended anteriorly to the most medial portion of the old scar in an extensile fashion. This allowed access to both the anteromedial methyl methacrylate antibiotic beads and the direct anterior methyl methacrylate impregnated antibiotic bead.

Sharp dissection was taken down through the skin and subcutaneous tissue. Care was taken to protect neurovascular and tendinous structures. The previous open wound area, measuring approximately 1 1/2 cm in widest diameter, directly over one of the methyl methacrylate beads, was quite easily discernible. Utilizing meticulous sharp and blunt dissection, the entire anteromedial antibiotic impregnated methacrylate bead construct was removed. There did not appear to be any gross drainage/infection at the site of bead placement or at the site of the fracture. Multiple cultures were obtained, including Gram stain of the area, and cultures for aerobic and anaerobic organisms.

Following this, dissection was continued directly medial, that is anteriorly, where the second antibiotic impregnated methyl methacrylate bead construct was easily discernible, and it likewise was removed. The latter was directly anteriorly placed over the periosteum at the distal fracture site. Again, this area did not disclose any gross evidence of pus. The area was further developed to allow release of adhesions

GODFREY REGIONAL HOSPITAL
123 Main Street • Aldon, FL 77714 • (407) 555-1234

Continued

OPERATIVE REPORT

Patient information:

Patient name: Date:
DOB: Surgeon:
MR#:   Anesthetist:

Preoperative diagnosis:

Postoperative diagnosis:

Procedure(s) performed:

Anesthesia:

Assistant surgeon:

Description of procedure:

between the ankle dorsiflexor tendons and the overlying skin. Following mobilization of this fibrous tissue, passive mobilization of the ankle could be facilitated; inversion/eversion motion was also facilitated without the persistence of cutaneous periosteal adhesions.

Following extensive irrigation of the area utilizing copious amounts of sterile saline mixed with vancomycin and tobramycin solution, the wound was subsequently closed in layers using widely spaced interrupted simple sutures of 4-0 nylon. A Penrose drain was left percutaneously exposed through the site of the previous small open wound to allow for egress of any seroma or drainage from the operative field. Tourniquet was released prior to skin closure with excellent and immediate return of distal circulation, excellent capillary refill, and pink toes. Following application of sterile Adaptic gauze and multiple layers of sterile 4 × 4s and sterile soft roll cast padding, the extremity was subsequently immobilized in a knee-high fiberglass splint overwrapped with an Ace bandage.

The patient tolerated the procedure quite well, was taken to postoperative recovery, and subsequently returned to the medical-surgical unit in good condition. No intraoperative or immediate postoperative difficulties were noted.

GODFREY REGIONAL HOSPITAL
123 Main Street • Aldon, FL 77714 • (407) 555-1234

EXERCISE 31

Level I

OPERATIVE REPORT

Patient information:

Patient name:
DOB:
MR#:

Date:
Surgeon:
Anesthetist:

Preoperative diagnosis:

Internal derangement to right knee; osteoarthritis, right knee

Postoperative diagnosis:

Grade 2 to 4 articular defects, medial tibial plateau; degenerative border, medial meniscus; intact anterior cruciate ligament; grade 2 to 4 articular defects, lateral tibial plateau; grade 2 to 4 articular defects under surface of patella and anterior femoral sulcus

Procedure(s) performed:

Right knee arthroscopy and arthroscopic chondroplastic shaving of medial, lateral, and patellar femoral compartments

Anesthesia:

Assistant surgeon:

Description of procedure:

After informed consent and complete discussion of the alternatives, potentials, and complications, and no guarantees implied or given, the patient was taken to the operating room. After an adequate level of regional and IV anesthesia had been obtained, the patient's lower extremity was surgically scrubbed with Hibiclens and prepped with Hibiclens solution and draped in the usual sterile fashion. A special knee arthroscopy pack was utilized. The instrument was placed through the anterolateral portal. Visualization immediately revealed an attenuated degenerative border of the medial meniscus beneath the meniscus; in the central portion of the medial tibial plateau were grade 2 to 4 articular changes with some areas down to subchondral bone on probing. Following this, the full radial shaving units were utilized for performing extensive chondroplastic shaving of the medial tibial plateau, medial femoral condyle, and debridement of the border of the meniscus. Visualization of anterior cruciate ligament was normal. Visualization of the lateral compartment revealed mild degenerative changes of the border of the lateral meniscus and grade 2 to 3 articular changes with probing some areas down to subchondral bone. On this arthroscopic foray, shaving instruments were utilized to perform extensive shaving of the lateral tibial plateau area and the degenerative margin of the meniscus. Visualization of the patella femoral joint revealed grade 2 to 4 articular changes with marked fibrillation and fissure formation and loose articular cartilage and anterior femoral sulcus.

GODFREY REGIONAL HOSPITAL
123 Main Street • Aldon, FL 77714 • (407) 555-1234

Continued

OPERATIVE REPORT

Patient information:	
Patient name: DOB: MR#:	Date: Surgeon: Anesthetist:

Preoperative diagnosis:

Postoperative diagnosis:

Procedure(s) performed:

Anesthesia:

Assistant surgeon:

Description of procedure:

A full radial shaving instrument was utilized to perform extensive debridement of the patellofemoral joint. Following this, thorough lavage of the joint was performed. Then 0.5% Marcaine and Decadron were instilled. A bulky Robert Jones dressing was applied. Benzoin and Steri-strips were applied.

The patient tolerated the operative procedure and anesthesia satisfactorily. No breaks in technique occurred. No complications occurred.

[signature]

GODFREY REGIONAL HOSPITAL
123 Main Street • Aldon, FL 77714 • (407) 555-1234

EXERCISE 32

Level II

OPERATIVE REPORT

Patient information:	
Patient name: DOB: MR#:	Date: Surgeon: Anesthetist:

Preoperative diagnosis:

Malposition of right both-bone forearm fracture

INDICATIONS FOR PROCEDURE: This is a 10-year-old female who sustained a both-bone forearm fracture and was treated with closed reduction and casting initially. She had gone on to malposition, despite appropriate casting, and the patient states that she had been wrestling with her brother, hitting her brother on top of the head with her cast. After discussion of the options, risks, and benefits of the surgical procedure, all questions were answered and consents were signed. The patient was taken to the operating room.

Postoperative diagnosis:

Malposition of right both-bone forearm fracture

Procedure(s) performed:

Closed reduction, intermedullary nailing radius

Anesthesia:

General

Assistant surgeon:

Description of procedure:

COMPLICATIONS: None

TOURNIQUET TIME: 36 minutes

The patient was taken to the operating room and placed supine on the operating room table. General anesthesia was obtained. The cast was then removed from the upper extremity. Obvious deformity was identified. Closed reduction was then able to be obtained with C-arm to verify adequacy of reduction. We then made a 1-cm incision over the area of Lister's tubercle, just proximal to the distal growth plate. We placed a 2.0-mm titanium flexible rod into the intermedullary canal with a radius and passed this past the fracture site. It was then bent and cut off. This was then sewed up with 3-0 Monocryl after irrigation with Bacitracin saline solution. The patient was placed into a well-padded long-arm cast after dressing it with Xeroform and 4 × 4s and sterile Webril. She was then extubated in the operating room, transferred from the operating room to her bed, and taken to the postanesthesia recovery room in stable condition.

Patrick Chung, MD

GODFREY REGIONAL HOSPITAL
123 Main Street • Aldon, FL 77714 • (407) 555-1234

EXERCISE 33

Level I

OPERATIVE REPORT

Patient information:

Patient name: Date:
DOB: Surgeon:
MR#: Anesthetist:

Preoperative diagnosis:

Left knee ACL tear, probable meniscal tear

Postoperative diagnosis:

1. Left knee ACL tear
2. Complex tear of the posterior horn of the medial meniscus
3. Flap tear and degenerative fraying of the free edge of the lateral meniscus
4. Large area of grade IV chondromalacia of the weight area of the medial femoral condyle

Procedure(s) performed:

1. Left knee arthroscopy
2. Partial medial meniscectomy
3. Partial lateral meniscectomy
4. Medial femoral condyle chondroplasty

Anesthesia:

Assistant surgeon:

Description of procedure:

The patient is under general anesthesia and LMA. He is supine. He received Ancef IV in holding. Lachman test is positive 21. Pivot shift test is positive. Medial and lateral laxities are within normal limits. The right lower extremity is placed in a well leg holder. A tourniquet is applied around the mid thigh on the affected left lower extremity. A low-profile leg holder is applied around the tourniquet. The left lower extremity is exsanguinated with an Esmarch. The tourniquet is inflated to 300 mm Hg. Total tourniquet time was 57 minutes. Prep and drape of the left lower extremity in the usual manner.

Knee arthroscopy was done using two portals, anterolateral and anteromedial. The arthroscope was inserted anterolaterally. Instrumentation is through the anteromedial portal. Inflow is through the sheath of the arthroscope. There is a very small amount of normal appearing synovial fluid inside the knee joint.

There is a mild amount of cartilage debris inside the joint. The suprapatellar pouch looks normal. The patellofemoral joint has normal tracking. There are very mild degenerative changes in the patellofemoral joint with fraying of the articular cartilage. In the medial gutter there is a plica extending towards the fat pad, making visualization of the medial compartment somewhat difficult. The 4.5 resector is inserted through the anterior medial portal and the medial plica is excised. A partial debridement of the fat pad is performed to improve visualization. The anterior cruciate ligament is completely torn mid substance. The posterior cruciate ligament looks normal. The tibial stump of the anterior cruciate ligament is excised. In the lateral compartment the articular cartilage looks normal. There is a flat horn of the lateral meniscus. There is also

GODFREY REGIONAL HOSPITAL
123 Main Street • Aldon, FL 77714 • (407) 555-1234

OPERATIVE REPORT

Patient information:

Patient name: Date:
DOB: Surgeon:
MR#:   Anesthetist:

Preoperative diagnosis:

Postoperative diagnosis:

Procedure(s) performed:

Anesthesia:

Assistant surgeon:

Description of procedure:

some degenerative fraying of the tree edge of the lateral meniscus. The popliteus tendon looks normal. A basket is used to excise the flap tear and the degenerative fraying of the free edge of the lateral meniscus. Next the edge of the meniscus is smoothed using an Oratec chondroplasty probe. In the medial compartment there is a very complex tear of the posterior horn of the medial meniscus. There is significant thinning of the articular cartilage of the medial tibial plateau. There is a large area of grade IV chondromalacia involving the weight-bearing area of the medial femoral condyle. This area is weight bearing at 45 degrees flexion. The complex tear of the posterior horn of the medial meniscus is excised using baskets. The free edge of the meniscus is smoothed using the Oratec chondroplasty probe. The large area of grade IV chondromalacia is treated next. The unstable articular cartilage flaps are completely debrided. The area is almost 4 cm in diameter. A microfracture technique is used to treat the area of grade IV chondromalacia.

The knee is thoroughly irrigated, removing all soft tissue and cartilage debris. The cannulas are removed. The skin portals are closed with 4-0 nylon. 30 cc of Marcaine with epinephrine are injected inside the knee joint. Each portal is also injected with a few ccs of Marcaine without epinephrine.

The patient was transferred to the recovery room and is in good condition.

GODFREY REGIONAL HOSPITAL
123 Main Street • Aldon, FL 77714 • (407) 555-1234

EXERCISE 34

Level II

OPERATIVE REPORT

Patient information:

Patient name:	Date:
DOB:	Surgeon:
MR#:	Anesthetist:

Preoperative diagnosis:

Left ankle extensor retinacular tear

INDICATIONS: Patient is a 36-year-old white male with persistent pain and swelling over the lateral aspect of his ankle. After alternatives, risks, and possible complications were carefully discussed, the patient desired surgical intervention. Consent was obtained.

Postoperative diagnosis:

1. Left superior extensor retinacular tear
2. Left peroneus brevis tendon tear
3. Low-lying muscle belly, left peroneus brevis tendon

Procedure(s) performed:

1. Repair of peroneus brevis tendon, left foot
2. Excision of low-lying muscle belly, left peroneus brevis tendon
3. Repair of superior extensor retinaculum

Anesthesia:

Assistant surgeon:

Description of procedure:

The patient was brought to the main operating room and positioned supine. After general anesthesia was adequately obtained, a tourniquet was placed around the left calf. 1 gm Ancef was given IV. The left lower extremity was prepped and draped in the usual sterile fashion. The limb was elevated and the tourniquet inflated.

A curvilinear incision was made posterior to the lateral malleolus, subcutaneous tissue was bluntly spread, and small bleeders were controlled with cautery as they were identified. The peroneal sheath was opened and noted to be filled with serous fluid; this was evacuated. The tendons were brought out of the groove. It was obvious that the extensor retinaculum had been avulsed off of the tip of the fibula with the peroneus brevis tendon overlying the tip of the fibula itself out of the groove. The tendon itself was splayed apart with obvious longitudinal tearing measuring approximately 5–6 cm. The peroneus longus tendon was otherwise in excellent condition. It was also obvious that he had a very-low-lying muscle belly all of the way in through the fibular groove on the peroneus brevis tendon.

We extended the incision proximally and distally to get good visualization of the peroneus brevis tendon and excised surrounding scar tissue and excess synovium. I then tubularized the peroneus brevis tendon with 3-0 Prolene, also excising the low-lying muscle belly up out of the fibular groove.

GODFREY REGIONAL HOSPITAL
123 Main Street • Aldon, FL 77714 • (407) 555-1234

Continued

OPERATIVE REPORT

Patient information:

Patient name: Date:
DOB: Surgeon:
MR#:   Anesthetist:

Preoperative diagnosis:

Postoperative diagnosis:

Procedure(s) performed:

Anesthesia:

Assistant surgeon:

Description of procedure:

Once this had been performed, we roughened up the lateral aspect of the fibula, removing synovial epithelialization down to good bleeding cancellous bone. I likewise roughened up the undersurface of the superior retinaculum with a curette, then placed two G2 Mitek anchors within the tip of the fibula and reapproximated the superior retinaculum down with sutures. I then repaired the remainder of the superior retinaculum, holding the tendon back within its groove utilizing #2 Ethibond sutures. We had excellent repair at this point; therefore we irrigated out the wound and closed the subcutaneous tissue with 2-0 Vicryl sutures and completed closure with 3-0 nylon. 0.25% Marcaine was instilled within the wound. A sterile compression bandage was applied as the tourniquet was deflated. The patient was placed into a plaster splint.

The patient was awoken and returned to PAR in stable condition without apparent complication.

Patrick Chung MD

GODFREY REGIONAL HOSPITAL
123 Main Street • Aldon, FL 77714 • (407) 555-1234

EXERCISE 35

Level II

OPERATIVE REPORT

Patient information:

Patient name:	Date:
DOB:	Surgeon:
MR#:	Anesthetist:

Preoperative diagnosis:

Severe right heel abscess

INDICATIONS: The patient is a 54-year-old immune-suppressed rheumatoid who had presented with a severe abscess of his right heel. The patient returned today for the possibility of tobramycin bead removal and possibility for wound closure. Consent was obtained.

Postoperative diagnosis:

Severe right heel abscess

Procedure(s) performed:

1. Tobramycin bead removal
2. Irrigation and debridement
3. Wound closure

Anesthesia:

Assistant surgeon:

Description of procedure:

The patient was brought to the main operating room and positioned supine. After general anesthesia was adequately obtained, bandages were removed. The outside of the wound was noted to be healed up nicely. Therefore the right lower extremity was prepped and draped in the usual sterile fashion.

Sutures were cut, and serous fluid was identified within the wound; however, there was no evidence of purulence, no aroma. No evidence of necrosis either. Tobramycin beads were removed. The wound was again inspected, and again there was no evidence for infection. Therefore we ran 3000 cc of pulse-lavaged fluid throughout the wound. Small areas of devitalized tissue were sharply removed. Noted good granulation tissue throughout the bed. Again no evidence of osteomyelitis. After final irrigation was performed, we then reapproximated deep tissues with 3-0 Prolene, subcutaneous tissue with 3-0 Prolene, and closed the skin with 3-0 nylon. A sterile compression bandage was applied.

The patient was awakened and returned to PAR in stable condition without apparent complication.

Robert Chung, MD

GODFREY REGIONAL HOSPITAL
123 Main Street • Aldon, FL 77714 • (407) 555-1234

EXERCISE 36

Level II

OPERATIVE REPORT

Patient information:

Patient name: Date:
DOB: Surgeon:
MR#:   Anesthetist:

Preoperative diagnosis:

Left knee internal derangement

Postoperative diagnosis:

1. Left knee radial and horizontal tear of the posterior horn and middle third of the lateral meniscus
2. Flap tear of the posterior horn of the medial meniscus
3. Grade II chondromalacia of the medial femoral condyle
4. Excessive lateral pressure syndrome

Procedure(s) performed:

1. Left knee arthroscopy
2. Partial lateral meniscectomy
3. Partial medial meniscectomy
4. Chondroplasty of the medial femoral condyle
5. Lateral retinacular release

Anesthesia:

Assistant surgeon:

Description of procedure:

The patient is under general anesthesia and endotracheal intubation. She received Ancef IV in holding. She is positioned supine. Knee laxity examination under general anesthesia is normal. The right lower extremity is placed in a well leg holder. A tourniquet is applied around the mid-thigh on the affected left lower extremity. A low-profile leg holder is applied around the tourniquet. The left lower extremity is exsanguinated with an Esmarch and the tourniquet is inflated to 300 mm Hg. Total tourniquet time was 60 minutes. Prep and drape of the left lower extremity in the usual manner.

Knee arthroscopy was done using two portals, anterolateral and anteromedial. The arthroscope was inserted anterolaterally. Instrumentation is through the anteromedial portal. Inflow is through the sheath of the arthroscope. The suprapatellar pouch looks normal. The medial and lateral gutters look normal. There is some fraying of the articular cartilage of the patella and trochlea. The patella is tilted laterally. Even beyond 60 degrees flexion, the patella remains tilted laterally. The cruciate ligaments are intact. In the lateral compartment there is a radial tear and a horizontal tear of the posterior horn and middle third of the lateral meniscus. The popliteus tendon looks normal. There is significant softening of the body of the meniscus. The articular cartilage of the lateral compartment is normal. A partial lateral meniscectomy is performed. The radial tear of the lateral meniscus is excised with baskets. The horizontal tear is sealed using an Oratec chondroplasty probe.

In the medial compartment there is a small sized flap tear of the posterior horn of the medial meniscus. The remaining meniscus is normal. The articular cartilage of the medial tibial plateau is normal. There is an area of grade II chondromalacia of the medial femoral condyle in its

GODFREY REGIONAL HOSPITAL
123 Main Street • Aldon, FL 77714 • (407) 555-1234

Continued

OPERATIVE REPORT

Patient information:

Patient name:
DOB:
MR#:

Date:
Surgeon:
Anesthetist:

Preoperative diagnosis:

Postoperative diagnosis:

Procedure(s) performed:

Anesthesia:

Assistant surgeon:

Description of procedure:

weight-bearing area at 45 degrees flexion. This area is 1.5 cm in size. A partial medial meniscectomy is performed with baskets, excising the small-sized flap tear of the posterior horn of the medial meniscus. The body of the meniscus is somewhat soft. A chondroplasty of the medial femoral condyle is performed, excising the unstable articular cartilage flaps with a 4.5 curved resector.

Finally, an arthroscopic lateral retinacular release is performed. The arthroscope is placed into the anteromedial portal. Patellar tracking is re-examined. The patella is tilted laterally even beyond 60 degrees flexion. A 4.5 resector is used to resect the fat pad anterolaterally. An Oratec chisel probe is next used to perform a limited lateral retinacular release. The release starts at the superior pole of the patella and extends towards the anterolateral portal. After the release is completed, the patella can be everted to 70 degrees. The patella tracks very nicely. Beyond 30 degrees flexion, the patella is well centered in the trochlear groove.

The knee is thoroughly irrigated, removing all soft tissue, cartilage, and meniscal debris. The arthroscopic cannulas are removed. The skin portals are closed with 4-0 nylon. 30 cc of Marcaine with epinephrine is injected inside the knee joint. Each portal is also injected with a few ccs of Marcaine without epinephrine. A bulky Jones dressing is applied. The tourniquet is released.

Surgery was well tolerated. The patient left the operating room to recovery in stable condition.

GODFREY REGIONAL HOSPITAL
123 Main Street • Aldon, FL 77714 • (407) 555-1234

EXERCISE 37

Level II

OPERATIVE REPORT

Patient information:	
Patient name: DOB: MR#:	Date: Surgeon: Anesthetist:

Preoperative diagnosis:

Tenosynovitis, left extensor pollicis longus tendon

INDICATIONS: Gary is a 48-year-old gentleman with persistent presence of a painful mass over the left wrist. There appeared to be a tenosynovioma around the extensor pollicis longus. After failing conservative treatment, alternatives, risks, and possible complications were carefully discussed. The patient desired surgical intervention. Consent was obtained.

Postoperative diagnosis:

Tenosynovitis, left extensor pollicis longus tendon

Procedure(s) performed:

Extensor pollicis longus tenosynovectomy

Anesthesia:

Local

Assistant surgeon:

Description of procedure:

EBL: Minimal

TOURNIQUET TIME: 9 minutes at 225 mm Hg

COMPLICATIONS: None apparent

The patient was brought to the main operating room and positioned supine. The left upper extremity was prepped and draped in the usual fashion. A linear longitudinal incision was made along the course of the extensor pollicis longus tendon, and subcutaneous tissue was carefully spread. A small Weitlaner retractor was placed. Small bleeders were controlled with cautery as they were identified. I then opened the sheath of the EPL, noting a mildly proliferative synovium/ganglion cyst in this location. It did not appear to be grossly pathologic, such as seen with rheumatoid arthritis. It was carefully peeled off of the tendon with small tenotomy scissors. The tourniquet was inflated during this portion of the procedure for better visualization. The tendon itself underlying it was in excellent condition. The sheath was mostly left open, other than just as it went around the radial styloid; I did close the sheath at this location with interrupted 2-0 Vicryl sutures. I then closed the subcutaneous tissue with 2-0 Vicryl sutures and completed closure with 4-0 nylon. A sterile compression bandage was applied. The tourniquet was deflated.

The patient was returned to PAR in stable condition without complication.

Patrick Chung md

GODFREY REGIONAL HOSPITAL
123 Main Street • Aldon, FL 77714 • (407) 555-1234

EXERCISE 38

Level II

OPERATIVE REPORT

Patient information:	
Patient name:	Date:
DOB:	Surgeon:
MR#:	Anesthetist:

Preoperative diagnosis:

Hallux limitus with possible fixation irritation or osteochondral defect

HISTORY:
This patient had a previous hallux limitus surgery on the right side. She has continued to have joint pain. She presented last month and was scheduled for surgery to explore the toe joint and remove the hardware.

Postoperative diagnosis:

Same

Procedure(s) performed:

Curettage of osteochondral lesion; removal of fixation

Anesthesia:

Assistant surgeon:

Description of procedure:

ESTIMATED BLOOD LOSS: Minimal

COMPLICATIONS: None

PROCEDURE: The patient was placed on the operating table in the supine position. She was sedated and local anesthesia was obtained using Marcaine. The foot was prepped and draped in a standard fashion. An incision was made over the previous incision. This was carried down to the capsular tissue that was incised linearly. Subperiosteal dissection was performed to expose the base of the phalanx and the head of the metatarsal. The screw and K-wire were removed. A central to lateral osteochondral defect was noted in the head of the metatarsal. This was extending beyond the subchondral bone plate and into the cancellus bone. The lesion measured approximately 4 cm wide by 8 mm long. The remaining cartilage was in pristine condition. Periarticular bone was hypertrophic and that was remodeled using a saw and rongeur. The area was irrigated and closed using Dexon and Prolene. The patient is to follow up in my clinic next month for final follow-up. She was given Vicodin for pain.

Robert Chung, MD

GODFREY REGIONAL HOSPITAL
123 Main Street • Aldon, FL 77714 • (407) 555-1234

EXERCISE 39

Level I

OPERATIVE REPORT

Patient information:	
Patient name:	Date:
DOB:	Surgeon:
MR#:	Anesthetist:

Preoperative diagnosis:

Avulsive crush injury, right long and ring fingers

INDICATIONS: Patient is a 33-year-old right-hand–dominant white male who caught his right hand in a brake press at work. The wounds were examined. Consent was obtained for shortening of the fingers and partial wound closure.

Postoperative diagnosis:

Same

Procedure(s) performed:

Irrigation, debridement, bone shortening, and partial closure, left long and ring fingers

Anesthesia:

Local

Assistant surgeon:

Description of procedure:

EBL: Minimal

TOURNIQUET TIME: 0

COMPLICATIONS: None apparent

The patient was brought to the main operating room and positioned supine. After anesthesia placed a digital block under sterile conditions, the left upper extremity was prepped and draped in the usual sterile fashion. Ragged ends of bone that were protruding through the wound were trimmed back with a rongeur, and on the right finger, it was taken back to the level of the DIPJ as it was marked comminuted. Devitalized tissue was excised with a #15 blade and tenotomy scissors as appropriate.

I then reapproximated the flexor and extensor tendons over the tip of the bone with 2-0 Ethibond sutures. I then utilized 4-0 nylon to loosely approximate the edges, leaving the central portion open to further granulate into place. Bacitracin was applied as well as a sterile light compression bandage.

The patient was returned to PAR in stable condition without apparent complication.

GODFREY REGIONAL HOSPITAL
123 Main Street • Aldon, FL 77714 • (407) 555-1234

Continued

OPERATIVE REPORT

Patient information:	
Patient name:	Date:
DOB:	Surgeon:
MR#:	Anesthetist:

Preoperative diagnosis:

Postoperative diagnosis:

Procedure(s) performed:

Anesthesia:

Assistant surgeon:

Description of procedure:

IMMUNIZATION: The patient was given tetanus prophylaxis as well as 3.1 gm Timentin IV.

DISCHARGE INSTRUCTIONS: The patient will be discharged to home. He is to keep the wound clean and dry. He is also given outpatient antibiotics and pain medications. He should follow up with myself in 48 hours for a wound check.

[signature]

GODFREY REGIONAL HOSPITAL
123 Main Street • Aldon, FL 77714 • (407) 555-1234

EXERCISE 40

Level I

OPERATIVE REPORT

Patient information:	

Patient name: Date:
DOB: Surgeon:
MR#:   Anesthetist:

Preoperative diagnosis:

1. Grade 2 open fracture of left distal radius and ulnar shafts
2. Fracture of left radial head

INDICATIONS FOR OPERATION: This 7-year-old young man fell out of a box on the back of a 4-wheeler where he lives. The patient fell on his left outstretched arm. He had pain around the wrist and elbow with deformity of the wrist. X-rays revealed a

Postoperative diagnosis:

1. Grade 1 open fracture of left distal radius and ulnar shafts
2. Fracture of left radial head

Procedure(s) performed:

1. Open treatment of left distal radius and ulnar shaft fractures with debridement, irrigation, and closed reduction of radius and ulna
2. Closed reduction (closed treatment with manipulation), left radial head
3. Application of long-arm cast

Anesthesia:

Assistant surgeon:

Description of procedure:

The patient was taken to the operating room and placed supine on the operating table. General anesthesia was administered and achieved and he was intubated. Initially, traction was applied to the left forearm through the flexed elbow, and manipulation of the radial head was carried out through the skin, and actually, a fairly good reduction of this was carried out. It was not felt that open treatment of that would improve that significantly enough to warrant it. A majority of the translation and angulation was corrected. It was felt that there was acceptable position. Traction was further applied and a closed reduction of the distal radius and ulna was obtainable.

At this point the left upper extremity was scrubbed, prepped, and draped free and in standard fashion. No tourniquet was used. The open wound in the distal forearm measured about 1 cm or slightly less in width. It was extended both radially and ulnarly and the soft tissues were bluntly dissected. The wound went down to the radius. The entire area was copiously irrigated with antibiotic saline solution. A small portion of the skin edge was debrided. There was no gross contamination of the wound. I did not explore for the median nerve.

Fluoroscopic visualization of both fractures was satisfactory. The forearm wound was closed with interrupted 4-0 nylon sutures and a sterile dressing was applied. At this point the patient was placed in finger trap traction and further traction was

GODFREY REGIONAL HOSPITAL
123 Main Street • Aldon, FL 77714 • (407) 555-1234

Continued

OPERATIVE REPORT

Patient information:	
Patient name:	Date:
DOB:	Surgeon:
MR#:	Anesthetist:

Preoperative diagnosis:

rather significantly displaced radial head fracture at the elbow, and a rather significantly displaced distal forearm fracture with the radius overriding in the ulna 45° angulated volarly. There was an open wound in the distal forearm that was initially thought to be greater than 1 cm in length, but at the time of surgery was found to be less than 1 cm in length. Probably the spike of the radius came through this. The patient was taken to the operating room for treatment of his fractures. Please see my History and Physical for the considerations discussed with the parents.

Postoperative diagnosis:

Procedure(s) performed:

Anesthesia:

Assistant surgeon:

Description of procedure:

carried out to reduce as close as possible the radial head and the distal radius and ulna. A well-padded long-arm cast was applied, with the forearm in some pronation and the elbow flexed to 90 degrees.

There were no complications and the patient tolerated the procedure well. He was awakened in the operating room and transported to Recovery in good condition.

Patrick Chung md

GODFREY REGIONAL HOSPITAL
123 Main Street • Aldon, FL 77714 • (407) 555-1234

EXERCISE 41

Level II

OPERATIVE REPORT

Patient information:

Patient name: Date:
DOB: Surgeon:
MR#:   Anesthetist:

Preoperative diagnosis:

Hammer digit syndrome, 4th and 5th digits, right foot

INDICATIONS FOR PROCEDURE: The patient is a 52-year-old white female who has painful hammer toes with associated keratotic lesions on 4th and 5th digits of right foot. She has failed conservative therapy that has included soaking her foot as well as periodic debridement and the use of corn pads. She is here today for surgical correction. We discussed the

Postoperative diagnosis:

Hammer digit syndrome, 4th and 5th digits, right foot

Procedure(s) performed:

1. PIPJ resection arthroplasty, 4th digit, right foot
2. Exostosectomy, distal medial 5th toe, right foot

Anesthesia:

Assistant surgeon:

Description of procedure:

The patient was brought to the operating room and placed on the operating table in the supine position. Under IV sedation, local anesthesia was obtained using 3 ccs of a 1:1 mix of 1% plain lidocaine and 0.25% plain Sensorcaine in a digital block fashion. The foot was then prepped and draped in the usual sterile manner. An ankle tourniquet was inflated to 250 mm Hg after the foot was exsanguinated using an Esmarch bandage. Attention was then directed to the dorsal aspect of the 4th digit where a 1.5 cm dorsal linear incision was made, beginning at the mid shaft of the proximal phalanx and extending distally to the mid shaft of the middle phalanx. The incision was deepened via sharp and blunt dissection with care to identify and retract all neurovascular structures. Hemostasis was obtained as needed. The incision was deepened down to the level of the extensor tendon, which was then transected at the level of the PIPJ. The medial and lateral collateral ligaments were released. The extensor tendon was reflected proximally. Using a sagittal saw, the distal third of the proximal phalanx was resected. The wound was irrigated with sterile saline. The extensor tendon was reapproximated with 3-0 Vicryl. The skin was reapproximated with 5-0 nylon.

Attention was then directed to the dorsal distal and medical aspects of the 5th digit, right foot, where a 1-cm dorsal medial linear incision was made over the distal phalanx. The incision was deepened down to the level of the distal and medial

GODFREY REGIONAL HOSPITAL
123 Main Street • Aldon, FL 77714 • (407) 555-1234

Continued

OPERATIVE REPORT

Patient information:	

Patient name: Date:
DOB: Surgeon:
MR#:   Anesthetist:

Preoperative diagnosis:

procedure, postoperative course, as well as potential risks and complications, which include but are not limited to prolonged pain, swelling, numbness, infection, undercorrection, overcorrection, the possibility of recurrence, and the possibility that additional procedures may be needed in the future. All of her questions were answered. Consent was obtained.

Postoperative diagnosis:

Procedure(s) performed:

Anesthesia:

Assistant surgeon:

Description of procedure:

condyles. Using a handheld rasp, this bone prominent area was resected. The wound was irrigated with sterile saline. The skin was reapproximated with 5-0 nylon. A dry sterile forefoot compressive dressing consisting of Betadine, adaptic gauze, and Kling was applied.

She tolerated the procedure and anesthesia well and was discharged to the Anesthesia Department in good condition with vital signs stable and profusion noted to all digits. She was given written and oral postoperative instructions and will return to clinic in two weeks for postoperative check, sooner if she has any other problems.

GODFREY REGIONAL HOSPITAL
123 Main Street • Aldon, FL 77714 • (407) 555-1234

EXERCISE 42

Level II

OPERATIVE REPORT

Patient information:

Patient name: Date:
DOB: Surgeon:
MR#:   Anesthetist:

Preoperative diagnosis:

1. Calcaneal navicular tarsal coalition, left foot
2. Flat foot deformity, left foot

Postoperative diagnosis:

1. Calcaneal navicular tarsal coalition, left foot
2. Flat foot deformity, left foot

Procedure(s) performed:

1. Resection of calcaneal navicular tarsal coalition, left foot
2. Achilles tendon lengthening, left foot
3. Young's tenosuspension, left foot
4. First cuneiform osteotomy with bone graft, left foot
5. Evan's calcaneal osteotomy with bone graft, left foot

Anesthesia:

General

Assistant surgeon:

Description of procedure:

ESTIMATED BLOOD LOSS: Less than 10 cc

CONDITION: Stable

PROCEDURE:
The patient was taken to the OR and placed on the operating table in supine position. General anesthetic was administered by anesthesiologist. The patient received a local anesthetic block to the left foot consisting of 20 cc of 1:1 mix of 1% lidocaine plain with 0.5% Marcaine plain. The left lower extremity was then prepped and draped in usual sterile manner. The patient was placed in prone position prior to draping. An Esmarch bandage was used to exsanguinate the left lower extremity and the tourniquet was inflated to 350 mm Hg.

Attention was directed over the posterior aspect of the left leg just medial to the midline. A linear incision was made, approximately 8 cm in length. The incision was dissected, meticulously maintaining tissue layers down to the level of the Achilles tendon in which a frontal plane Achilles tendon lengthening was performed. A Z-plasty lengthening of the plantaris tendon was performed. The Achilles tendon was sutured using 0 Ticron and 2-0 Vicryl. Peritenon was reapproximated and sutured using 4-0 Vicryl. Subcutaneous tissues were reapproximated using 4-0 Vicryl. Skin was closed using 4-0 nylon.

The tourniquet was released after 37 minutes. The patient was repositioned in supine position. The patient was re-prepped and draped. Theleg was exsanguinated and a thigh tourniquet inflated to 350 mm Hg.

GODFREY REGIONAL HOSPITAL
123 Main Street • Aldon, FL 77714 • (407) 555-1234

Continued

OPERATIVE REPORT

Patient information:	
Patient name: DOB: MR#:	Date: Surgeon: Anesthetist:

Preoperative diagnosis:

Postoperative diagnosis:

Procedure(s) performed:

Anesthesia:

Assistant surgeon:

Description of procedure:

Attention was directed over the lateral aspect of the left foot, inferior to the lateral malleolus in which a curvilinear incision was made, coming up along the calcaneal cuboid joint over the cuneiforms up to the lateral aspect of the talus. The incision was deepened down to the level of the extensor digitorum brevis muscle belly in which care was taken to avoid all neurovascular structures in the area. Superficial bleeders were bovied as necessary. The muscle was then incised at its level of origin and retracted distally. The incision was deepened down to the level of bone. The area of calcaneal navicular bar was identified through fluoroscopy in which the bar was then excised with osteotome and mallet removing a centimeter of bone from the coalition site. Bone edges were rasped smooth with copious amounts of sterile saline. The flexor digitorum brevis muscle belly was sutured with 2-0 Vicryl and sutured to the defect where the coalition had been excised in which the suture was passed out through the medial plantar aspect of the foot and tied with a button at this level, maintaining the muscle in the area of defect. The wound was flushed with copious amounts of sterile saline.

Attention was then directed over the lateral aspect of the calcaneus in which the incision was deepened down to level of bone. Using power instrumentation, an Evans calcaneal osteotomy was then performed. Approximately 0.8 cm bone graft along the lateral aspect tapering down to 2 mm was then placed in the calcaneus. The osteotomy was fixated with two 0.062 K wires. Fluoroscopy was used to assess position of the K wires. The anterior K wire was repositioned and further fluoroscopy noted that the K wires were in good position. The proximal aspects of the K wires were then bent, cut, and K wire caps placed on the end. The osteotomy site was flushed with copious amounts of sterile saline. Subcutaneous tissues were reapproximated and sutured using 4-0 Vicryl. Skin was closed using 4-0 nylon in horizontal mattress stitches. The

GODFREY REGIONAL HOSPITAL
123 Main Street • Aldon, FL 77714 • (407) 555-1234

Continued

OPERATIVE REPORT

Patient information:	
Patient name: DOB: MR#:	Date: Surgeon: Anesthetist:

Preoperative diagnosis:

Postoperative diagnosis:

Procedure(s) performed:

Anesthesia:

Assistant surgeon:

Description of procedure:

tourniquet was then released for ten minutes. The foot was re-exsanguinated and the tourniquet re-inflated.

Attention was directed over the medial aspect of the left foot in which an incision was made, curving dorsally from the inferior aspect of the medial malleolus and extending over to the plantar aspect of the mid shaft of the first metatarsal. The incision was deepened down to the level of deep fascia. Care was taken to avoid all neurovascular structures in the area. Superficial bleeders were bovied as necessary. Further dissection identified the tibial os anterior tendon. The navicular was identified and a drill hole placed through the navicular. Using power instrumentation with the power saw, a channel was created on the medial aspect of the navicular to re-route the tibial os anterior tendon through. It was noted that the tendon would not stay in the channel. The tendon was approximated in the drill hole, the wedge of bone taken out to create the channel was replaced, and bone staple along the plantar medial aspect of the navicular was put into place. Fluoroscopy was obtained and was noted that the staple was in good position.

Attention was directed to the first cuneiform in which using power instrumentation, an osteotomy was performed dorsally. A wedge of bone graft was placed into plantar flex at the first ray. A bone staple was placed anteriorly and with fluoroscopy was noted to be in good position. The wound was flushed with copious amounts of sterile saline. It was noted that increased subtalar joint motion was obtained. With the subtalar joint in neutral, it was noted that there had been an increase in the longitudinal medial arch and that the forefoot varus had been corrected. Subcutaneous tissues were then reapproximated and sutured using 4-0 Vicryl. Skin was closed using 4-0 nylon and horizontal mattress stitches.

GODFREY REGIONAL HOSPITAL
123 Main Street • Aldon, FL 77714 • (407) 555-1234

Continued

OPERATIVE REPORT

Patient information:	
Patient name:	Date:
DOB:	Surgeon:
MR#:	Anesthetist:

Preoperative diagnosis:

Postoperative diagnosis:

Procedure(s) performed:

Anesthesia:

Assistant surgeon:

Description of procedure:

Postoperative injection consisted of 30 cc of a 1:1 mix of 1% lidocaine plain with 0.5% Marcaine plain. Dressings consisted of Betadine solution–impregnated Adaptic. Xeroform was placed between the button for the suturing of the flexor digitorum brevis muscle, 4 × 4s, Kling, and Coban.

The tourniquet was deflated and noted normal vascular status returned to digits 1 through 5 on the left foot.

The patient had received 2 grams of Ancef, one preop and one postop.

A below-the-knee fiberglass cast with ankle at 90 degrees was placed on the patient.

The patient appeared to tolerate the procedure and anesthesia well and left the OR to recovery room with vital signs stable and normal vascular status to digits one through five of the left foot.

[signature]

GODFREY REGIONAL HOSPITAL
123 Main Street • Aldon, FL 77714 • (407) 555-1234

EXERCISE 43

Level II

OPERATIVE REPORT

Patient information:

Patient name: Date:
DOB: Surgeon:
MR#:   Anesthetist:

Preoperative diagnosis:

Gout versus osteomyelitis

Postoperative diagnosis:

Same

Procedure(s) performed:

Bone biopsy with arthroplasty of interphalangeal joint, right hallux

Anesthesia:

Assistant surgeon:

Description of procedure:

HEMOSTASIS: None

MATERIALS: 3-0 and 4-0 PDS and 5-0 nylon

COMPLICATIONS: None

DESCRIPTION OF PROCEDURE:
The patient was taken to the OR by OR staff, and the patient was placed on the operating room table in the supine position. Once given a small amount of IV sedation, a ring block of the hallux was made using approximately 12 cc of 1% lidocaine plain. The foot was then prepped and draped using sterile technique.

Attention was then directed to the dorsal hallux and the area of the interphalangeal joint where anesthesia was tested and then a linear incision was made using a #15 blade. Using both blunt and sharp dissection, the incision was deepened to the level of the interphalangeal joint. It became evident at this point that there was a large amount of gouty tophi in the area. As much of this was removed as possible and the area flushed throughout the procedure.

The most distal aspect of the proximal phalanx was identified. The head of the proximal phalanx, however, appeared

GODFREY REGIONAL HOSPITAL
123 Main Street • Aldon, FL 77714 • (407) 555-1234

Continued

OPERATIVE REPORT

Patient information:	
Patient name: DOB: MR#:	Date: Surgeon: Anesthetist:

Preoperative diagnosis:

Postoperative diagnosis:

Procedure(s) performed:

Anesthesia:

Assistant surgeon:

Description of procedure:

completely eroded and impregnated with gouty tophi. There were no clinical signs of any purulence in the area. The bone proximal to the head of the phalanx was hard to touch and appeared intact. The most distal aspect of the head of the proximal phalanx was resected using a bone saw and sent to Pathology for gross anatomy and culture. The incision was again flushed with copious amounts of sterile saline, and any large gouty tophi were excised at this time and sent to Pathology as well.

At this time, fluoro scan imaging was taken of the foot to ensure that a clean surface had been created with this cut. I was satisfied with the amount of bone resection and satisfied with the sample taken for the biopsy. The incision was again flushed with copious amounts of sterile saline and closed using 3-0 and 4-0 PDS for deep closure and 5-0 nylon for skin closure.

The patient tolerated the surgery well with vital signs stable and no complications. He will follow up in my office in one week.

Patrick Chung, M.D.

GODFREY REGIONAL HOSPITAL
123 Main Street • Aldon, FL 77714 • (407) 555-1234

EXERCISE 44

Level I

OPERATIVE REPORT

Patient information:

Patient name: Date:
DOB: Surgeon:
MR#:   Anesthetist:

Preoperative diagnosis:

Medial meniscal tear, left knee

Postoperative diagnosis:

Medial meniscal tear and marked synovitis, medial compartment notch in lateral compartment, left knee

Procedure(s) performed:

Left knee arthroscopy, partial arthroscopic medial and lateral meniscectomy, synovectomy of medial compartment notch and lateral compartment, left knee

Anesthesia:

Assistant surgeon:

Description of procedure:

After suitable general anesthesia had been achieved, the patient's left knee was prepped and draped in the usual manner. Prior to prepping, a thigh tourniquet was applied, and after draping, inflated to 300 mm of mercury. No inflow cannula was used. Arthroscope was inserted through an anteromedial portal. Lateral compartment was examined first. There were noted to be intact articular surfaces and a stable intact lateral meniscus. There were noted to be synovial polyps in the lateral compartments. These were cauterized with the radiofrequency probe. Examination of the notch revealed marked inflammatory synovitis. There is marked hypertrophy of the fat pad. Using combination punch and shaver, the thickened synovial tissue was excised. Synovial bleeders were cauterized with a radiofrequency probe. Examination of the medial compartment revealed a complex flap tear of the posterior horn of the medial meniscus. Articular surfaces were in good shape. There was noted to be a complex tear of the anterior horn. There was noted to be marked synovial hypertrophy over the anterior horn. Using combination punch and shaver, the unstable meniscus of the posterior and anterior horn was excised and contoured. Thickened synovium over the anterior horn of the medial meniscus was excised. Examination of the patellofemoral joint revealed good articular surface. There was noted to be thickened hypertrophic synovium surrounding medial synovial plica. Using combination punch and shaver, this was excised. Synovial bleeders were cauterized. Knee joint was then thoroughly irrigated and the arthroscope removed. Stab wounds were closed with 4-0 nylon. Dressing was then applied. Tourniquet was released. Following tourniquet release, good circulation was noted to return to the foot.

The patient tolerated the procedure well and returned to the recovery room in a stable condition.

GODFREY REGIONAL HOSPITAL
123 Main Street • Aldon, FL 77714 • (407) 555-1234

EXERCISE 45

Level II

OPERATIVE REPORT

Patient information:

Patient name:
DOB:
MR#:

Date:
Surgeon:
Anesthetist:

Preoperative diagnosis:

1. Hallux varus, left foot
2. Hammer toe deformity with contracture, second toe, left foot
3. Hammer toe deformity with contracture, third toe, left foot
4. Hammer toe deformity with contracture, fourth toe, left foot

Postoperative diagnosis:

1. Hallux varus, left foot
2. Hammer toe deformity with contracture, second toe, left foot
3. Hammer toe deformity with contracture, third toe, left foot
4. Hammer toe deformity with contracture, fourth toe, left foot

Procedure(s) performed:

1. Abductor hallucis tenotomy with medial capsulotomy of first metatarsal phalangeal joint, left foot
2. Reverse Austin bunionectomy, left foot
3. DIPJ arthroplasty, second toe, left foot, with second metatarsal phalangeal joint tenotomy and capsulotomy

extensor digitorum longus Z-plasty tendon lengthening
4. DIPJ arthroplasty, third toe, with third MPJ tenotomy and capsulotomy extensor digitorum longus Z-plasty tendon lengthening, left foot
5. DIPJ arthroplasty, fourth toe, left foot

Anesthesia:

MAC

Assistant surgeon:

Description of procedure:

ESTIMATED BLOOD LOSS: Less than 3 cc

CONDITION: Stable

PROCEDURE:
Patient was taken to OR and placed on OR table in supine position, and IV sedation was administered by the anesthesiologist. The left foot was then anesthetized with local anesthetic comprising 15 cc of 1 to 1 mix of 1% lidocaine plain with 25% Marcaine plain.

The left lower extremity was then prepped and draped in the usual sterile manner. An Esmarch bandage was used to exsanguinate the left foot. A pneumatic ankle tourniquet was inflated to 250 mm Hg. The total tourniquet time was 103 minutes. The Esmarch bandage was removed, and the left lower extremity lowered into sterile field.

Attention was directed over the dorsal medial aspect of the first metatarsal phalangeal joint, over which an appropriate linear incision was made. Incision was deepened down to the level of the abductor hallucis tendon, which was identified and incised. A medial capsulotomy was then performed and still the hallux was within varus position. Continuation of the capsulotomy exposed the first metatarsal head, in which a Chevron osteotomy was made with dorsal and plantar wings at 60 degrees through and through, from the medial to lateral direction with the apex approximately 1 cm to the articular cartilage of the first metatarsal head. Scar tissue was freed from around the joint, and the capital

GODFREY REGIONAL HOSPITAL
123 Main Street • Aldon, FL 77714 • (407) 555-1234

Continued

OPERATIVE REPORT

Patient information:	
Patient name: DOB: MR#:	Date: Surgeon: Anesthetist:

Preoperative diagnosis:

Postoperative diagnosis:

Procedure(s) performed:

Anesthesia:

Assistant surgeon:

Description of procedure:

fragment was transposed medially. In doing so, it was noted that the varus deformity was corrected, and a smooth 0.045 K-wire was introduced across the osteotomy site. Several attempts were made before ideal positioning of the hallux and stability of the capital fragment. The K-wire was then bent, cut, and twisted to be flush with the bone. Using power instrumentation, the medial aspect of the first metatarsal head was made flush. No rough bone edges were remaining. The wound was flushed with copious amounts of sterile saline. Capsule was sutured with 3-0 Vicryl. Subcutaneous tissue was reapproximated with sutures using 4-0 Vicryl. Skin was closed using 5-0 nylon while maintaining hallux in rectus position.

Attention was directed over the dorsal aspect of the second metatarsal phalangeal joint in which a curvilinear incision was made. The incision was deepened down to the level of the second metatarsal phalangeal joint. Care was taken to avoid all neurovascular structures in the area. The extensor hood was freed along with scar tissue at this level. A Z-plasty extensor tendon lengthening was performed and a dorsal capsulotomy was made. Using the McClamary elevator, the flexor plate was freed, and with the forefoot loaded, it was noted that the contracture at this level had been reduced.

Attention was directed over the dorsal aspect of the proximal dorsal phalangeal joint in which an appropriate linear incision was made. The incision was deepened down to the level of the extensor tendon, which was incited transversely. Medial and lateral collateral ligaments were incised, and the head of the intermediate phalanx was exposed. Using power instrumentation, the head of the intermediate phalanx was

GODFREY REGIONAL HOSPITAL
123 Main Street • Aldon, FL 77714 • (407) 555-1234

Continued

OPERATIVE REPORT

Patient information:

Patient name: Date:
DOB: Surgeon:
MR#:   Anesthetist:

Preoperative diagnosis:

Postoperative diagnosis:

Procedure(s) performed:

Anesthesia:

Assistant surgeon:

Description of procedure:

excised. Rough bone edges were rongeured and rasped smooth. The wound was flushed with copious amounts of sterile saline. The extensor tendon was reapproximated and sutured using 4-0 Vicryl with forefoot loaded. It was noted that the second digit was in rectus position. Prior to closure of the tendon, a smooth 0.045 K-wire was introduced across the intermediate distal phalanx and retrograded across the proximal phalanx and across the metatarsal phalangeal joint with the forefoot loaded, maintaining the digit in rectus position. The tendon was repaired with 4-0 Vicryl, and the skin was closed using 5-0 nylon in horizontal mattress and simple interrupted stitches along both incision sites at this level.

Attention was directed to the third digit. The same procedures that were performed on the second were then performed on the third. The same intraoperative course and postoperative results were found.

Attention was directed to the fourth digit. Two converging semi-elliptical incisions along the distal interphalangeal joint were made in transverse fashion. The ellipse of skin was excised. Incision was deepened down to level of the extensor tendon that was incised transversely. Medial and lateral collateral ligaments were incised. The tendon was retracted proximally, and the head of the intermediate phalanx was exposed. Using power instrumentation, the head of the phalanx was excised. The wound was flushed with copious amounts of sterile saline. No rough bone edges remained. Repair of the extensor tendon was done with 4-0 Vicryl with forefoot loaded. It was noted that the fourth digit was in rectus position. The skin was closed with 5-0 nylon and simple interrupted stitches. With the forefoot loaded, it was

GODFREY REGIONAL HOSPITAL
123 Main Street • Aldon, FL 77714 • (407) 555-1234

Continued

OPERATIVE REPORT

Patient information:	
Patient name:	Date:
DOB:	Surgeon:
MR#:	Anesthetist:

Preoperative diagnosis:

Postoperative diagnosis:

Procedure(s) performed:

Anesthesia:

Assistant surgeon:

Description of procedure:

noted that the hallux was rectus along with digits 2, 3, and 4 of the left foot.

Postoperative injection consisted of 7 cc of 5% Marcaine sling with 2 cc of dexamethasone phosphate per cc infiltrated around the surgical site.

Dressings consisted of Betadine solution–impregnated Adaptic, Betadine solution–impregnated gauze sponges, 4 × 4, Kling, and Coban.

Tourniquet was deflated, and it was noted that normal vascular status returned to digits 1 through 5 of the left foot.

The patient appeared to tolerate the procedure and anesthesia well and left the OR to recovery room with vital signs stable. Normal vascular status was present in digits 1 through 5 of the left foot.

Patrick Chug MD

GODFREY REGIONAL HOSPITAL
123 Main Street • Aldon, FL 77714 • (407) 555-1234

EXERCISE 46

Level II

OPERATIVE REPORT

Patient information:	
Patient name: DOB: MR#:	Date: Surgeon: Anesthetist:

Preoperative diagnosis:

Left small finger proximal phalanx fracture

INDICATIONS FOR PROCEDURE: The patient is a 29-year-old white male who reports suffering a crush injury to his left non-dominant hand in a press at work. This resulted in small wounds over the hand that have now healed, as well as a fracture of the proximal aspect of the proximal phalanx of the left small finger. He now presents for elective repair of his fracture.

Postoperative diagnosis:

Same

Procedure(s) performed:

Open reduction and K-wire fixation of left small finger proximal phalanx fracture

Anesthesia:

Assistant surgeon:

Description of procedure:

The patient underwent an axillary block and was then brought to the operating room and placed supine on the operating room table. After adequate sedation, the patient's left arm was prepped and draped in the usual sterile fashion. A tourniquet had been placed over the upper arm. The left hand and forearm were exsanguinated with an Esmarch bandage and the tourniquet was deflated to 250 mm Hg pressure. Please note that the tourniquet time for the operation was 25 minutes.

Next, using a zigzag pattern over the proximal aspect of the left small finger, a 15-blade scalpel was used to make a skin incision. Blunt dissection was carried out with tenotomy scissors. Small crossing veins were cauterized with a bipolar cautery. Further dissection identified the extensor tendon over the proximal phalanx. This was incised longitudinally with a fresh 15-blade scalpel. Then with the use of a periosteal elevator, the underlying fracture site was defined.

Using dissection with the periosteal elevator, the fibrous tissue hematoma within the fracture site and a small piece of bone were removed. After this was removed, the area was irrigated with saline solution mixed in with Bacitracin. Next, the fracture site was reduced by rotating the fracture and pulling on the finger. Once there was good reduction of the fracture fragment, K-wires were passed to keep the fracture reduced. Then 0.035 K-wires were used, crossing each other from the ulnar and radial aspects of the finger. The K-wire positions were confirmed using fluoroscopy. After good reduction was achieved, the

GODFREY REGIONAL HOSPITAL
123 Main Street • Aldon, FL 77714 • (407) 555-1234

Continued

OPERATIVE REPORT

Patient information:

Patient name: Date:
DOB: Surgeon:
MR#:   Anesthetist:

Preoperative diagnosis:

Postoperative diagnosis:

Same

Procedure(s) performed:

Open reduction and K-wire fixation of left small finger proximal phalanx fracture

Anesthesia:

Assistant surgeon:

Description of procedure:

K-wires were cut. The tourniquet was deflated and hemostasis was achieved with bipolar cautery. The extensor tendon was repaired with running 4-0 Vicryl sutures. Next, the skin was closed with interrupted 4-0 nylon sutures. The wound was then cleaned. Caps were placed on the K-wires. Xeroform and Bacitracin were placed over the K-wires and incision, and 4×4 fluffs were placed in between the fingers and around the K-wire pins for padding. The hand was wrapped in cast padding and two 10-plys of 4-inch plaster were applied along the volar and ulnar aspects of the hand to maintain the fingers and hand in reduction. This was then wrapped with 3-inch and 4-inch Ace wraps.

The patient tolerated the procedure well. He was then taken to the PACU for recovery in stable condition.

[signature] Patrick Chung MD

GODFREY REGIONAL HOSPITAL
123 Main Street • Aldon, FL 77714 • (407) 555-1234

EXERCISE 47

Level I

OPERATIVE REPORT

Patient information:	
Patient name:	Date:
DOB:	Surgeon:
MR#:	Anesthetist:

Preoperative diagnosis:

Right trigger thumb

Postoperative diagnosis:

Same

Procedure(s) performed:

Right trigger thumb release

Anesthesia:

Assistant surgeon:

Description of procedure:

After suitable general anesthesia had been achieved, the patient's right hand was prepped and draped. Prior to prepping the arm, a tourniquet was applied, and after draping, it was inflated to 250 mm Hg. A 2.5-cm transverse incision was made at the base of the thumb. Digital nerve was carefully identified. Digital nerve was retracted radially to expose the Al pulley, and under direct vision, the Al pulley was cut. There was noted to be a small fusiform nodule in the tendon, which was causing the triggering. After cutting the pulley, the triggering no longer occurred. The incision was then closed with 5-0 nylon simple sutures. A bulky hand dressing was then applied. The tourniquet was released. Following tourniquet release, good circulation was noted to return to the hand.

The patient tolerated the procedure well and was returned to the recovery room in stable condition.

Patrick Chung MD

GODFREY REGIONAL HOSPITAL
123 Main Street • Aldon, FL 77714 • (407) 555-1234

EXERCISE 48

Level II

OPERATIVE REPORT

Patient information:

Patient name:
DOB:
MR#:

Date:
Surgeon:
Anesthetist:

Preoperative diagnosis:

1) Underlapping second digit, left foot
2) Hallux valgus with bunion, right foot
3) Hammertoe, 2nd through 4th digits of right foot

Postoperative diagnosis:

Same

Procedure(s) performed:

1) Syndactylization of digits 2 and 3 on the left foot
2) Bunionectomy, right foot
3) First metatarsal osteotomy with screw fixation, right foot

4) Arthroplasty, 2nd PIPJ, right foot
5) Arthroplasty, 3rd PIPJ, right foot with K-wire fixation
6) Arthroplasty, 4th PIPJ, right foot with K-wire fixation

Anesthesia:

Assistant surgeon:

Description of procedure:

The patient was placed in the supine position on the operating table. A tourniquet was applied to the level of the left malleolus. Attention was directed to the second and third digits on the left foot. Incision was made to remove interdigital skin. The skin was resected in toto. The wound was flushed with copious amounts of sterile saline and closed in a single layer. Skin was reapproximated with 4-0 nylon simple interrupted sutures. Xeroform gauze was applied plus a sterile gauze bandage for compression and hemostasis. The tourniquet was let down and blood flow returned immediately.

Attention was then directed to the right foot where a 6-cm curvilinear incision was made, coursing medial and parallel to the extensor hallucis longus tendon. Incision was deepened, with care taken to clamp and ligate all superficial bleeders as they were encountered. All neurovascular and tendinous structures were carefully identified and retracted. An inverted L-capsulotomy was performed. Hypertrophic bone was delivered from the wound and resected in toto from the dorsomedial and medial aspects of the first metatarsal head. The wound was flushed with copious amounts of sterile saline.

Attention was directed to the proximal aspect of the incision where a periosteal incision was made at the base of the first metatarsal down to bone. All periosteal structures were reflected from bone, and a base wedge osteotomy was performed, with the base of the osteotomy lateral and the apex proximal and medial. The resultant wedge of bone was removed. This was closed and fixated with two compression screws. The wound was flushed with copious amounts of sterile saline and then closed in layers with periosteal reapproximation using 2-0 Polysorb simple interrupted sutures. This was followed by subcutaneous reapproximation with 3-0 Polysorb simple interrupted sutures, followed by skin

GODFREY REGIONAL HOSPITAL
123 Main Street • Aldon, FL 77714 • (407) 555-1234

Continued

OPERATIVE REPORT

Patient information:	
Patient name:	Date:
DOB:	Surgeon:
MR#:	Anesthetist:

Preoperative diagnosis:

Postoperative diagnosis:

Procedure(s) performed:

Anesthesia:

Assistant surgeon:

Description of procedure:

reapproximation with 4-0 nylon simple interrupted sutures.

Attention was then directed to the second digit on the right foot where a 3-cm linear incision was made over the PIPJ. Incision was carried down to the level of the joint where transverse tenotomy was performed. All tendinous and capsular structures were reflected from the head of the proximal phalanx and were delivered from the wound. The head of the proximal phalanx was resected in toto with care taken to rasp smooth all bony edges. The wound was flushed with copious amounts of sterile saline. The wound was closed with tendon reapproximation using 3-0 Polysorb simple interrupted sutures, followed by skin reapproximation with 4-0 nylon simple interrupted sutures.

Attention was directed to the third digit on the right foot where a 3-cm linear incision was made, coursing proximal and distal over the PIP joint. Transverse tenotomy was performed. All tendinous and capsular structures were reflected from the head of the proximal phalanx. The head of the proximal phalanx was delivered from the wound and resected in toto. Care was taken to rasp smooth all raw bony edges. The third digit was then closed and fixated with a single 0.045-inch K-wire. Tendon reapproximation was achieved with 3-0 Polysorb simple interrupted sutures, followed by skin reapproximation with 4-0 nylon simple interrupted sutures.

Attention was directed to the fourth digit of the right foot where the same exact procedure was performed as on the third, up to and including wound closure.

Dexamethasone phosphate was instilled into each surgical site. This was followed by Xeroform gauze, followed by sterile gauze bandage for

GODFREY REGIONAL HOSPITAL
123 Main Street • Aldon, FL 77714 • (407) 555-1234

Continued

OPERATIVE REPORT

Patient information:	
Patient name: DOB: MR#:	Date: Surgeon: Anesthetist:

Preoperative diagnosis:

Postoperative diagnosis:

Procedure(s) performed:

Anesthesia:

Assistant surgeon:

Description of procedure:

compression and hemostasis. All digits were splinted in rectus position.

The tourniquet was let down and blood flow returned immediately to all digits on the right foot.

The patient tolerated the procedure and anesthesia well and was transported to the recovery room with vital signs stable and in good condition.

Patrick Chong MD

GODFREY REGIONAL HOSPITAL
123 Main Street • Aldon, FL 77714 • (407) 555-1234

EXERCISE 49

Level I

OPERATIVE REPORT

Patient information:

Patient name: Date:
DOB: Surgeon:
MR#:   Anesthetist:

Preoperative diagnosis:

Chronic anterior cruciate ligament deficiency, right knee; meniscal tear, right knee

Postoperative diagnosis:

Chronic ACL deficiency, right knee. Tear anterior middle and posterior thirds of medial meniscus and posterior horn tear lateral meniscus, right knee.

Procedure(s) performed:

Right knee arthroscopy and partial arthroscopic medial and lateral meniscectomy.

Anesthesia:

Assistant surgeon:

Description of procedure:

After suitable general anesthesia had been achieved, the patient's right knee was prepped and draped in the usual manner. Prior to prepping, a thigh tourniquet was applied and, after draping, inflated to 300 mm of mercury. No inflow cannula was used. Arthroscope was inserted through an anterior medial portal. The lateral compartment was examined first. There was noted to be a flap tear of the medial aspect of the posterior horn of the lateral meniscus. Using combination of punch and shaver, the unstable meniscus was excised and contoured. Examination of the notch revealed some residual ACL tissue, but this represented probably only about 10% to 20% of his ACL and this tissue was somewhat lax. Examination of the articular surfaces, medially and laterally, revealed these were in good shape. Examination of the medial meniscus revealed a large flap tear of the middle third. There are horizontal cleavage tears of the posterior third and flap tear of the anterior third. Using combination of punch and shaver, the unstable meniscus was excised and contoured. The patient had a thickened medial synovial plica and this was excised so that it wouldn't cause him problems. Synovial bleeders were cauterized using the radiofrequency probe. Knee joint was then thoroughly irrigated. Arthroscope was removed. Stab wounds were closed with 4-0 nylon. Dressing was then applied. Tourniquet was released. Following tourniquet release, good circulation was noted to return to the foot.

Patient tolerated the procedure well and returned to the recovery room in stable condition.

[signature] MD

GODFREY REGIONAL HOSPITAL
123 Main Street • Aldon, FL 77714 • (407) 555-1234

EXERCISE 50

Level I

OPERATIVE REPORT

Patient information:

Patient name: Date:
DOB: Surgeon:
MR#:   Anesthetist:

Preoperative diagnosis:

Chondromalacia patellae, left knee (post-traumatic)

Postoperative diagnosis:

Same plus post-traumatic hypertrophy of fat pad

Procedure(s) performed:

Left knee arthroscopy. Arthroscopic chondroplasty of patella. Excision of hypertrophic fat pad.

Anesthesia:

Assistant surgeon:

Description of procedure:

After suitable general anesthesia had been achieved, the patient's left knee was prepped and draped in the usual manner. Prior to prepping, a thigh tourniquet was applied and, after draping, inflated to 300 mm of mercury. No inflow cannula was used. Arthroscope was inserted through an anterior lateral portal. Medial compartment was examined first. There was noted to be some hypertrophic synovium overgrowing the anterior horn of the medial meniscus. This was excised with the shaver and synovial bleeders cauterized using the radiofrequency probe. Examination of the medial meniscus, after shaving the hypertrophic synovium, revealed intact stable meniscus and intact articular surfaces. Examination of the notch revealed intact ACL and PCL. Examination of the lateral compartment revealed intact articular surfaces and a stable intact meniscus. Examination of the patellofemoral joint revealed localized grade II chondromalacia at the inferior pole of the patella. This was smoothed using the radiofrequency probe. Trochlea looked in good shape. Patient was noted to have hypertrophic fat pad, which is impinging between the patella and the trochlea. The remaining fat pad was excised with the shaver. Bleeders were cauterized using the radiofrequency probe. The knee joint was then thoroughly irrigated and the arthroscope was removed. Stab wounds were closed with 4-0 nylon. Dressing was then applied. Tourniquet was released. Following tourniquet release, good circulation was noted to return to the foot.

Patient tolerated the procedure well and returned to the recovery room in stable condition.

[signature] MD

GODFREY REGIONAL HOSPITAL
123 Main Street • Aldon, FL 77714 • (407) 555-1234

EXERCISE 51

Level I

OPERATIVE REPORT

Patient information:	
Patient name:	Date:
DOB:	Surgeon:
MR#:	Anesthetist:

Preoperative diagnosis:

Left carpal tunnel

Postoperative diagnosis:

Left carpal tunnel

Procedure(s) performed:

Laparoscopic carpal tunnel release

Anesthesia:

Monitored anesthesia care, local

Assistant surgeon:

Description of procedure:

The patient was taken to the operating room. The left upper extremity was prepped and draped in the usual sterile fashion. The arm was elevated and the tourniquet inflated to 250 mm Hg. The portals were marked out per routine and anesthetized with local infiltration of 1% lidocaine.

The proximal portal was opened with a 15-blade. Blunt spreading exposed the retinaculum, which was opened, allowing instrumentation to be placed in the canal and brought out distally through the distal portal that was opened with a 15-blade. A scope was placed within the cannula and the undersurface of the retinaculum was cleared, confirmed, and sectioned with good spreading of the retinaculum.

Instrumentation was removed. The portal was closed with Steri-strips. Compressive Ace was applied. Pressure was held and the tourniquet was dropped.

The patient was removed from the operating room in satisfactory condition.

Patrick Chrug MD

GODFREY REGIONAL HOSPITAL
123 Main Street • Aldon, FL 77714 • (407) 555-1234

EXERCISE 52

Level II

OPERATIVE REPORT

Patient information:	
Patient name:	Date:
DOB:	Surgeon:
MR#:	Anesthetist:

Preoperative diagnosis:

Hallux abducto valgus to the left foot and overlapping hammertoe, left second

Postoperative diagnosis:

Hallux abducto valgus to the left foot and overlapping hammertoe, left second

Procedure(s) performed:

Keller bunionectomy and arthroplasty of the second and capsulotomy of the left second metacarpophalangeal joint

Anesthesia:

Local with monitored anesthesia care

Assistant surgeon:

Description of procedure:

HEMOSTASIS: Well padded ankle tourniquet inflated to 250 mm of mercury

ESTIMATED BLOOD LOSS: Less than 20 cc

MATERIALS: 0.45 K-wire, injectable 20 ccs of 1:1 mix of 1% lidocaine and 0.5% Marcaine

PROCEDURE:
The patient was brought to the operating room and placed in a supine position. Intravenous sedation was administered. Local block was performed at the left first and second metacarpophalangeal joints using 20 ccs of 1:1 mix of 1% lidocaine and 0.51 Marcaine. Well padded pneumatic tourniquet was applied 1 cm above the medial malleolus. The patient was prepped and draped in the usual sterile manner. The foot was exsanguinated with an Esmarch bandage and the previously applied ankle tourniquet was inflated to 250 mm of mercury. Anesthesia was checked and found to be adequate.

Attention was then drawn to the left first metacarpophalangeal joint. A 5-cm dorsal linear incision was made, being in the midshaft of the first metatarsal and extending midshaft to the proximal phalanx. This incision was deepened to the level of the joint capsule and all veins were cauterized. The capsular structures were reflected from the head of the first metatarsal and the base of the proximal phalanx. A small 1 cm × 1 cm flap was fashioned out of the medial aspect of the capsule and was reserved for future use. A sagittal saw was then used to remove the base of the proximal phalanx, and approximately 1 cm of bone was removed. We looked for sharp bony edges; none were found. The flexor

GODFREY REGIONAL HOSPITAL
123 Main Street • Aldon, FL 77714 • (407) 555-1234

Continued

OPERATIVE REPORT

Patient information:	
Patient name: DOB: MR#:	Date: Surgeon: Anesthetist:

Preoperative diagnosis:

Postoperative diagnosis:

Procedure(s) performed:

Anesthesia:

Assistant surgeon:

Description of procedure:

tendons were found to be intact and undamaged. The flap that was previously fashioned was then placed between the metatarsal head and the proximal phalanx and was sutured into place with 3-0 absorbable suture attaching it to the lateral capsule. The rest of the capsule was then closed with 4-0 Dexon. The skin was then closed with 4-0 nylon in an interlocking suture.

Attention was then drawn to the second toe. A linear incision was made, beginning just proximal to the metacarpophalangeal joint and extending just past the proximal interphalangeal joint. The incision was deepened to the level of the joint capsule at the proximal interphalangeal joint. The capsule was entered with a transverse linear incision, and the capsular structures were reflected from the head of the proximal phalanx. The sagittal saw was then used to resect the head of the proximal phalanx at the surgical neck. This allowed the toe to come into a more rectus position, but it was inadequate. The extensor tendon was extremely shortened and contracted because of the longstanding deformity. Decision was made that capsulotomy and tendon lengthening would need to be performed. The dissection was carried down to the metacarpophalangeal joint. The dorsal, medial, and lateral aspects of that capsule were transected. This still did not allow the toe to go into a rectus position. Z-tendon lengthening was then performed on the extensor tendon, lengthening it approximately 1 cm. It was re-sutured with 4-0 Dexon, and also, the extensor tendon at the proximal interphalangeal joint was re-approximated with 4-0 Dexon. The area was flushed with saline, and a K-wire was driven through all three of the phalanges and was then anchored into the head of the second metatarsal. The skin incision was closed with nylon in an interlocking fashion. Both incisions were then covered with Adaptic 4 × 4 Kling and Ace wrap in a moderately compressive fashion.

GODFREY REGIONAL HOSPITAL
123 Main Street • Aldon, FL 77714 • (407) 555-1234

Continued

OPERATIVE REPORT

Patient information:	
Patient name: DOB: MR#:	Date: Surgeon: Anesthetist:

Preoperative diagnosis:

Postoperative diagnosis:

Procedure(s) performed:

Anesthesia:

Assistant surgeon:

Description of procedure:

The ankle tourniquet was deflated and vascular status returned to all digits. The patient was sent to the recovery room with vital signs stable.

She was given both written and oral postoperative instructions. She had been previously dispensed a prescription for Darvocet and a postop shoe. The instruction sheet includes phone numbers to call if she has questions before her next appointment which is 21st of June with Dr. Carter in his office.

[signature]

GODFREY REGIONAL HOSPITAL
123 Main Street • Aldon, FL 77714 • (407) 555-1234

EXERCISE 53

Level I

OPERATIVE REPORT

Patient information:	
Patient name: DOB: MR#:	Date: Surgeon: Anesthetist:

Preoperative diagnosis:

Osteofibrosis post total knee arthroplasty

Postoperative diagnosis:

Same

Procedure(s) performed:

Right knee manipulation and injection

Anesthesia:

Assistant surgeon:

Description of procedure:

After suitable anesthesia had been achieved, the patient's knee was gently manipulated. Surprisingly, with her asleep, the knee easily flexed to about 85°. It was then gently manipulated so that it flexed to about 125°. Scar tissue bands were heard to be popping with the gentle manipulation. Following this, the knee passively flexed to its gravity to 115°. Full extension was achieved with the manipulation. The knee was then sterilely prepped and draped and then was injected with 80 mg of Kenalog and 15 cc of 0.5% Marcaine. A bandage was then applied.

The patient tolerated the procedure well and returned to the recovery room in stable condition.

[signature] MD

GODFREY REGIONAL HOSPITAL
123 Main Street • Aldon, FL 77714 • (407) 555-1234

EXERCISE 54

Level I

OPERATIVE REPORT

Patient information:	
Patient name:	Date:
DOB:	Surgeon:
MR#:	Anesthetist:

Preoperative diagnosis:

Comminuted fracture, left distal radius, closed

Postoperative diagnosis:

Comminuted fracture, left distal radius, closed

Procedure(s) performed:

Closed reduction with external fixation, fracture, left distal radius utilizing fluoroscopy

Anesthesia:

Assistant surgeon:

Description of procedure:

The patient was placed supine on the operating room table and a satisfactory general anesthetic was given. Preoperative intravenous cephalosporin antibiotic was given. Pneumatic tourniquet was placed high about the left arm but did not require inflation during this procedure. The left hand, wrist, and forearm to proximal to the elbow were prepped sterilely with DuraPrep, and the left wrist and hand were draped in the usual sterile fashion. Pins were placed in the usual fashion via full-thickness skin incisions and spreading of the subcutaneous tissue down to bone. Drilling was performed within a soft tissue protector that was placed all the way down to bone. Pins were then placed. Two pin sites needed to be revised because of the soft bone in these areas. Two pins were proximal to the fracture and two pins were distal. Each pin was placed on the radial aspect of either the radius or second metacarpal. External fixator was applied and a closed reduction of the fracture was performed and the bolts of the fixator were tightened down. The fracture was lengthened as needed. Fluoroscopy was used to view the fracture site in AP and lateral views, and it was extremely close to anatomic position with good restoration of the articular joint surface, as well as the alignment of the distal radius on the AP and lateral views.

The pin sites were copiously irrigated with normal saline antibiotic solution and closed over the pins as needed with 3-0 nylon. Neosporin ointment and dry sterile dressings were applied.

GODFREY REGIONAL HOSPITAL
123 Main Street • Aldon, FL 77714 • (407) 555-1234

Continued

OPERATIVE REPORT

Patient information:	
Patient name: DOB: MR#:	Date: Surgeon: Anesthetist:

Preoperative diagnosis:

Postoperative diagnosis:

Procedure(s) performed:

Anesthesia:

Assistant surgeon:

Description of procedure:

The patient tolerated the procedure well. There were no complications. She was awakened in the operating room and transported to the recovery room in stable condition.

Patrick Chen, MD

GODFREY REGIONAL HOSPITAL
123 Main Street • Aldon, FL 77714 • (407) 555-1234

EXERCISE 55

Level I

OPERATIVE REPORT

Patient information:

Patient name:	Date:
DOB:	Surgeon:
MR#:	Anesthetist:

Preoperative diagnosis:

Right knee pain

Postoperative diagnosis:

1. Right knee osteoarthritis; posterior horn lateral meniscal tear with degenerative fraying of the medial meniscus
2. Posterior cruciate ligament tear

Procedure(s) performed:

Diagnostic arthroscopy of right knee with arthroscopic debridement of the posterior horn lateral meniscus tear; debridement of degenerative fraying of the medial meniscus; chondroplasty (three-compartment).

Anesthesia:

Assistant surgeon:

Description of procedure:

The patient was taken to the operating room where, after general anesthesia was administered, the right lower extremity was prepped and draped in a sterile fashion. Standard anterolateral and anteromedial arthroscopic portals were made. Diagnostic arthroscopy was performed. The undersurface of the patella had some fibrillation and fraying. The corresponding femoral groove did not have any significant changes. The medial joint line was visualized and there was some degenerative fraying of the meniscus and some fibers of the PCL that were caught within the medial joint line as well. The meniscal edges and the PCL area of tearing were debrided as needed. The articular surface had some softening as well as some fibrillations but no full-thickness defects. The notch was further visualized and the PCL had some significant tearing.

The synovium here appeared to be normal, and there was not felt to be any kind of synovial lesion that was questioned after visualizing the MRI. The lateral joint line was visualized and there was significant tearing of the posterior horn of the lateral meniscus as well as degenerative fraying around the rest of the meniscus. There were full-thickness defects along the lateral tibial plateau as well as the lateral femoral condyle. All of this was debrided back as needed. The knee was irrigated out copiously and drained. The wounds were closed with Biosyn and Steri-strips. A sterile dressing was applied.

The patient was taken to the recovery room in stable condition. There were no complications.

Patrick Chung, md

GODFREY REGIONAL HOSPITAL
123 Main Street • Aldon, FL 77714 • (407) 555-1234

EXERCISE 56

Level I

OPERATIVE REPORT

Patient information:	
Patient name: DOB: MR#:	Date: Surgeon: Anesthetist:

Preoperative diagnosis:

Stiffness post-total knee arthroplasty, right knee

Postoperative diagnosis:

Same

Procedure(s) performed:

Right knee manipulation under anesthesia and injection

Anesthesia:

Assistant surgeon:

Description of procedure:

After suitable general anesthesia had been achieved, a gentle manipulation was performed on the right knee. Pressure was applied on the proximal tibia and the knee gradually flexed. Prior to the manipulation, knee flexion was 65° and after manipulation went to 115°. Scar tissue bands were noted to pop while this manipulation was performed.

Using sterile technique, the patient's right knee was then injected with 18 cc of Marcaine and 80 mg of Kenalog.

The patient tolerated the procedure well and returned to the recovery room in stable condition.

Patrick Chung MD

GODFREY REGIONAL HOSPITAL
123 Main Street • Aldon, FL 77714 • (407) 555-1234

EXERCISE 57

Level I

OPERATIVE REPORT

Patient information:	
Patient name:	Date:
DOB:	Surgeon:
MR#:	Anesthetist:

Preoperative diagnosis:

Right ring finger mass

Postoperative diagnosis:

Same

Procedure(s) performed:

Excisional biopsy of right ring finger mass

Anesthesia:

Assistant surgeon:

Description of procedure:

The patient was taken to the operating room, and after IV sedation was administered, her right upper extremity was prepped and draped in a sterile fashion. A mixture of 1% lidocaine and 0.5% Marcaine without epinephrine was used for digital block anesthesia. The mass was located over the dorsolateral aspect of the middle phalanx distally. An incision was made dorsolaterally. Sharp and blunt dissection around the mass were performed. The mass did shell out fairly easily. It appeared to be somewhat fixed to the underlying DIP joint. Care was taken to try to stay out of the mass itself and dissect around it. Once the mass was fully excised, the wound was irrigated out copiously. The mass was cut in half in the operating room, and it appeared to be a fibrous type mass. There was no fluid within the mass. The wound was closed with simple nylon sutures. A sterile tube gauze-type dressing was applied. The Ace wrap that had been used to exsanguinate the arm and as a tourniquet around the upper forearm was removed. There was no significant bleeding encountered. This was done prior to wound closure.

The patient was taken to the recovery room in stable condition; there were no complications. The specimen was sent to Pathology for permanent examination.

GODFREY REGIONAL HOSPITAL
123 Main Street • Aldon, FL 77714 • (407) 555-1234

EXERCISE 58

Level I

OPERATIVE REPORT

Patient information:	
Patient name: DOB: MR#:	Date: Surgeon: Anesthetist:

Preoperative diagnosis:

Displaced fracture, left distal radius, extra-articular, closed

Postoperative diagnosis:

Displaced fracture, left distal radius, extra-articular, closed

Procedure(s) performed:

Closed reduction of fracture, left distal radius with percutaneous pinning, utilization of fluoroscopy, application short-arm cast

Anesthesia:

Assistant surgeon:

Description of procedure:

The patient was placed supine on the operating room table and a satisfactory general anesthetic was given. Preoperative intravenous cephalosporin antibiotic was given. No pneumatic tourniquet was used. The left hand, wrist, and forearm to proximal to the elbow were prepped sterilely with DuraPrep, and the left wrist area was draped in the usual sterile fashion. A closed reduction of the left distal radius was performed and visualized fluoroscopically. It was in essentially anatomic reduction on AP and lateral views and showed minimal instability. The decision, therefore, was made to perform percutaneous pinning rather than external fixation. Two smooth K-wires were drilled from the radial styloid across the fracture site to engage the proximal fracture fragment cortex. There was excellent stability at the fracture. It was viewed fluoroscopically with stress and was noted to be quite stable. Neosporin ointment was applied to the pin sites, followed by Jergen balls with the pins cut at appropriate lengths. Dry, sterile dressings were applied, followed by sterile circumferential cast padding. All drapes were removed. Cast padding was applied for short-arm cast application and a short-arm fiberglass cast was applied.

The patient tolerated the procedure well. There were no complications. He was awakened in the operating room and transported to the recovery room in stable condition.

GODFREY REGIONAL HOSPITAL
123 Main Street • Aldon, FL 77714 • (407) 555-1234

EXERCISE 59

Level I

OPERATIVE REPORT

Patient information:

Patient name:
DOB:
MR#:

Date:
Surgeon:
Anesthetist:

Preoperative diagnosis:

Partial ACL tear and posterior horn tear, lateral meniscus, left knee

Postoperative diagnosis:

Partial ACL tear and post-traumatic synovitis, left knee

Procedure(s) performed:

Left knee arthroscopy and major synovectomy

Anesthesia:

Assistant surgeon:

Description of procedure:

After suitable general anesthesia had been achieved, the patient's left knee was prepped and draped in the usual manner. Prior to prepping, a thigh tourniquet was applied and after draping was inflated to 300 mm Hg. The arthroscope was inserted through an interior medial portal. Operative anterolateral and operative accessory anterior medial portals were established.

The lateral compartment was examined first. There was noted to be some scuffing of the posterior horn of the lateral meniscus on its medial aspect, but no definite tears were noted. The meniscus was carefully probed, and no hidden tears were noted. The posterior horn was stable. Articular surfaces looked in good shape laterally.

Examination of the notch revealed marked synovial hypertrophy and inflamed synovial tissue. This thickened synovial tissue was excised with a shaver and synovial bleeders were cauterized. The ACL was examined. There was noted to be at least a 50% tear, and the remaining ACL tissue was slightly lax when probed. PCL was intact. Examination of the medial compartment revealed intact articular surfaces. There was noted to be some thickened synovium over the anterior horn of the medial meniscal, and this was excised with a shaver.

Examination of the patellofemoral joint revealed a small area of focal scuffing on the inferior pole of the patella. There was minimal loose articular cartilage flap. The trochlear looked in good shape. There was a thickened medial synovial plica,

GODFREY REGIONAL HOSPITAL
123 Main Street • Aldon, FL 77714 • (407) 555-1234

Continued

OPERATIVE REPORT

Patient information:

Patient name: Date:
DOB: Surgeon:
MR#:   Anesthetist:

Preoperative diagnosis:

Postoperative diagnosis:

Procedure(s) performed:

Anesthesia:

Assistant surgeon:

Description of procedure:

which was excised. There was also a kissing lesion on the femur where the plica was rubbing, and some frayed articular cartilage was smoothed in this area as well. There was a small suprapatellar plica, and this was also excised.

The knee joint was then thoroughly irrigated, and the arthroscope removed. Stab wounds were closed with 4-0 nylon. A knee OA was then performed. The patient had a negative pivot shift, an 11 Lachman, and an 11 anterior drawer. The dressing was then applied. The tourniquet was released. Following tourniquet release, good circulation was noted to return to the foot.

The patient tolerated the procedure well and returned to the recovery room in stable condition.

GODFREY REGIONAL HOSPITAL
123 Main Street • Aldon, FL 77714 • (407) 555-1234

EXERCISE 60

Level II

OPERATIVE REPORT

Patient information:

Patient name: Date:
DOB: Surgeon:
MR#:   Anesthetist:

Preoperative diagnosis:

Internal derangement, right knee

Postoperative diagnosis:

1. Grade 3 to grade 4 chondromalacia, medial femoral condyle, right knee
2. Grade 2 to grade 3 chondromalacia, femoral groove, right knee

Procedure(s) performed:

Diagnostic arthroscopy of chondroplasty, medial femoral condyle and femoral groove, right knee

Anesthesia:

Assistant surgeon:

Description of procedure:

The patient was brought to the operating room and general anesthetic was induced. The right lower extremity was exsanguinated and tourniquet inflated to 300 mm Hg for 35 minutes. The leg was placed in a leg holder, prepped with Betadine, and draped in a sterile fashion. The inlet cannula was inserted through the superior and medial portions and the otoscope into the inferolateral portal. Suprapatellar pouch was well visualized for inferior pathology. Along the medial parapatellar region, there was plica evident, and this was trimmed down with a Striker shaver. The patellofemoral joint showed central chondromalacia of grade 2 variety of the patella, and this was trimmed down lightly with a shaver and also with the thermal probe. In the femoral groove there was significant chondromalacia of grade 3 and a few small areas of grade 4 chondromalacia, and this was also trimmed down with the shaver and the thermal probe. Within the medial compartment there were significant and major changes on the medial femoral condyle with loss of cartilage over large areas of about 2 × 3 cm with grade 3 chondromalacia changes. The medial meniscus was entirely intact, and the tibial plateau appeared excellent with only a grade 1 chondromalacia changes. Within the notch a synovectomy was performed, and the underlying anterior cruciate ligament was normal. In the lateral compartment, the lateral meniscus was intact and there was no chondromalacia laterally.

GODFREY REGIONAL HOSPITAL
123 Main Street • Aldon, FL 77714 • (407) 555-1234

Continued

OPERATIVE REPORT

Patient information:

Patient name:	Date:
DOB:	Surgeon:
MR#:	Anesthetist:

Preoperative diagnosis:

Postoperative diagnosis:

Procedure(s) performed:

Anesthesia:

Assistant surgeon:

Description of procedure:

We used the thermal probe in the femoral groove and the medial femoral condyle to shave down some of the loose cartilage. Some loose debris within the joint was also evacuated. At the conclusion of this, we drained the knee of all fluid and injected the knee with 80 mg of Kenalog. The arthroscopy portals were closed with interrupted 3-0 nylon sutures, and gauze dressings and an Ace wrap were applied. The tourniquet was released. Good circulation returned to the leg.

The patient tolerated the procedure well. She went to the recovery room in excellent condition and will be dismissed as an outpatient today with plans for follow-up at the office in 2 weeks for suture removal.

DISCHARGE MEDICATIONS: Darvocet N-100, #25 tablets

[signature]

GODFREY REGIONAL HOSPITAL
123 Main Street • Aldon, FL 77714 • (407) 555-1234

EXERCISE 61

Level II

OPERATIVE REPORT

Patient information:

Patient name:
DOB:
MR#:

Date:
Surgeon:
Anesthetist:

Preoperative diagnosis:

Hallux abducto valgus, left hammertoe, left second, third

Postoperative diagnosis:

Hallux abducto valgus, left hammertoe, left second, third

Procedure(s) performed:

Keller bunionectomy of the left first, arthroplasty of the left second and third proximal interphalangeal joints, and capsulotomy of the left second metatarsophalangeal joint

Anesthesia:

Local with monitored anesthesia care

Assistant surgeon:

Description of procedure:

HEMOSTASIS: Well padded ankle tourniquet at 250 mm Hg

ESTIMATED BLOOD LOSS: Less than 20 ml

MATERIAL: 0.45 K-wire and 3-0 and 4-0 Dexon and Vicryl

INJECTABLES: 20 ccs of 1:1 mix of 1% lidocaine and 0.5% Marcaine preoperatively
PROCEDURE:
The patient was brought to the operating room and placed in the supine position. Intravenous sedation was administered. Local block was performed at the first, second, and third metatarsophalangeal joints using 20 ccs of 1:1 mix of 1% lidocaine and 0.5% Marcaine. A well padded pneumatic tourniquet was applied 1 cm above the medial malleolus. The patient was prepped and draped in the usual sterile fashion.

The foot was exsanguinated with an Esmarch bandage and the previously applied ankle tourniquet was inflated to 250 mm Hg. Attention was then drawn to the left first metatarsophalangeal joint. A 5-cm linear incision was made, beginning mid shaft of the first metatarsal and extending to mid shaft of the proximal phalanx. This incision was carried to the capsule and

GODFREY REGIONAL HOSPITAL
123 Main Street • Aldon, FL 77714 • (407) 555-1234

Continued

OPERATIVE REPORT

Patient information:

Patient name: Date:
DOB: Surgeon:
MR#:   Anesthetist:

Preoperative diagnosis:

Postoperative diagnosis:

Procedure(s) performed:

Anesthesia:

Assistant surgeon:

Description of procedure:

vessels were cauterized.

The capsule was then entered with a dorsolinear incision. A flap was fashioned of the medial aspect of the metatarsophalangeal joint capsule, which was approximately 1 cm in all directions. A sagittal saw was then used to resect the base of the proximal phalanx. A rasp was used to smooth rough edges, and the area was flushed with saline.

The flap, which had been previously fashioned, was then inserted between the first metatarsal head and the base of the proximal phalanx and was sutured firmly to the lateral side of the capsule with 3-0 absorbable sutures. The rest of the capsule was then closed with 3-0 Dexone sutures. The skin was closed with 3-0 nylon in a running interlocking fashion.

Attention was then drawn to the second and third digits on the left foot. A linear incision was made over the proximal interphalangeal joints. This was carried down to the level of the joint capsule. Both the joints were entered with a transverse linear incision, and the capsular structures were reflected from the head of the proximal phalanx. A sagittal saw was then used to remove the head at the surgical neck, and this was done on both toes.

After this procedure was done, the left third toe lay down in a very nice rectus position, but the right one still was dorsiflexed.

GODFREY REGIONAL HOSPITAL
123 Main Street • Aldon, FL 77714 • (407) 555-1234

Continued

OPERATIVE REPORT

Patient information:	
Patient name:	Date:
DOB:	Surgeon:
MR#:	Anesthetist:

Preoperative diagnosis:

Postoperative diagnosis:

Procedure(s) performed:

Anesthesia:

Assistant surgeon:

Description of procedure:

We carried our dissection down to the metatarsophalangeal joint on the second toe and performed a dorsomedial and lateral capsulotomy at the metacarpophalangeal joint. We also loosened the extensor tendon from the dorsal aspect of the proximal phalanx, and this allowed the toe to lay in a nice rectus fashion.

For the second toe, we applied a 0.45 K-wire through the distal intermediate and proximal phalanges, and we anchored it about 1 cm into the second metatarsal head. The extensor tendons on both the second and the third toes were then reapproximated in their new repaired positions using 4-0 Dexon. The skin was closed with 4-0 nylon in a simple interrupted and running fashion.

All of the incisions were then covered with Adaptic and 4 × 4s, Kling, and Ace wrap in a moderately compressive fashion. The ankle tourniquet was deflated and vascular status returned to all digits.
The patient was sent to the recovery room with vital signs stable and capillary refill at preoperative levels. She was given an instruction sheet for postoperative care. This instruction sheet includes phone numbers to call if she has questions before her appointment, which is October 5. X-rays were taken as the patient left the hospital.

GODFREY REGIONAL HOSPITAL
123 Main Street • Aldon, FL 77714 • (407) 555-1234

EXERCISE 62

Level I

OPERATIVE REPORT

Patient information:	
Patient name:	Date:
DOB:	Surgeon:
MR#:	Anesthetist:

Preoperative diagnosis:

Symptomatic hardware of the right knee

Postoperative diagnosis:

Symptomatic hardware of the right knee and ganglion cyst

Procedure(s) performed:

Excision of symptomatic hardware and ganglion cyst

Anesthesia:

Assistant surgeon:

Description of procedure:

The patient was taken to the operating room, and after IV sedation was administered, her right lower extremity was prepped and draped in sterile fashion. A mixture of 1% lidocaine and 1/2% Marcaine without epinephrine was used for local anesthesia. Approximately a 3-cm skin incision was made, with sharp dissection and blunt dissection down to bone being performed. A ganglion cyst was encountered. It was not a discrete cyst, but the fluid in it was definitely that of a ganglion cyst. This was opened up and cauterized as needed.

The hardware was identified and the screws removed. The bone had grown over the edges of the washer and some bone resection was required to get the washer out. Once this washer had been retrieved, the wound was irrigated out copiously and the screw hole was curetted. Copious amounts of antibiotic irrigation were used. The wound was closed in layers with Vicryl for the subcutaneous tissue, and Biosyn and Steri-strips were applied to the skin.

Sterile dressing was applied. The patient was taken to the recovery room in good condition.

[signature] MD

GODFREY REGIONAL HOSPITAL
123 Main Street • Aldon, FL 77714 • (407) 555-1234

EXERCISE 63

Level II

OPERATIVE REPORT

Patient information:	
Patient name:	Date:
DOB:	Surgeon:
MR#:	Anesthetist:

Preoperative diagnosis:

Left slipped capital femoral epiphysis

Postoperative diagnosis:

Same

Procedure(s) performed:

Pinning of left slipped capital femoral epiphysis

Anesthesia:

Assistant surgeon:

Description of procedure:

The patient was taken to the operating room, and after general anesthesia was administered, he was placed on the fracture table. No traction or manipulation was done to the hip. Fluoroscopy was used to visualize the hip in AP and lateral planes as well as multiple other planes. The hip was then prepped and draped in a sterile fashion. An anterior lateral thigh incision was made with blunt dissection down to the deep fascia. It was divided, and blunt dissection down to the femoral neck was performed. A guide pin was inserted through the anterior lateral femoral neck and into the epiphysis. Multiple views were taken to ensure appropriate positioning of the pin. The pin depth was measured and an 80-mm screw selected. It was put in place after drilling. After the screw was placed, intraoperative x-rays were taken in AP and lateral planes that showed what appeared to be appropriate hardware position. Several threads were across the epiphysis.

The wound was irrigated out copiously and closed in layers. Vicryl sutures were used for the deep fascia, Vicryl for the subcutaneous tissue, and Biosyn and Steri-strips for the skin. A sterile dressing was applied.

The patient was taken to the recovery room in stable condition. There were no complications.

Patrick Chung MD

GODFREY REGIONAL HOSPITAL
123 Main Street • Aldon, FL 77714 • (407) 555-1234

EXERCISE 64

Level II

OPERATIVE REPORT

Patient information:	
Patient name: DOB: MR#:	Date: Surgeon: Anesthetist:

Preoperative diagnosis:

Tear, quadriceps tendon, right knee

Postoperative diagnosis:

Same

Procedure(s) performed:

Repair of tear, quadriceps tendon, right knee

Anesthesia:

Assistant surgeon:

Description of procedure:

The patient was placed supine on the operating room table and a satisfactory general anesthetic was given. Preoperative intravenous cephalosporin antibiotic was given. Pneumatic tourniquet was placed high about the right thigh. Right leg was prepped sterilely from the tourniquet to the foot and the right knee was draped in the usual sterile fashion. Knee was fully flexed and the tourniquet was inflated to 350 mm Hg. Longitudinal skin incision was made over the upper pole of the patella, extending proximally over the quadriceps tendon in the midline. The incision was carried through subcutaneous tissue. Hemostasis was achieved as necessary. Full-thickness skin flaps were raised. There were two separate vertically oriented tears in the quadriceps tendon, one fairly central and one on its lateral aspect. These were sharply debrided to healthy tissue. The wound and knee joint were copiously irrigated with normal saline antibiotic solution. The quadriceps tendon was reapproximated full thickness with interrupted figure-of-eight sutures of 0 Ethibond. The wound again was copiously irrigated with normal saline antibiotic solution. The knee was fully flexed and the tendon repair was holding quite well and was quite strong. The skin was closed full thickness with staples. Dry sterile dressings were applied followed by sterile circumferential cast padding. Tourniquet was deflated. All drapes were removed including the tourniquet. Ace bandage was applied about the knee area.

GODFREY REGIONAL HOSPITAL
123 Main Street • Aldon, FL 77714 • (407) 555-1234

Continued

OPERATIVE REPORT

Patient information:		
Patient name: DOB: MR#:		Date: Surgeon: Anesthetist:

Preoperative diagnosis:

Postoperative diagnosis:

Procedure(s) performed:

Anesthesia:

Assistant surgeon:

Description of procedure:

The patient tolerated the procedure well. There were no complications. He was awakened in the operating room and transported to the recovery room in stable condition.

[signature]

GODFREY REGIONAL HOSPITAL
123 Main Street • Aldon, FL 77714 • (407) 555-1234

EXERCISE 65

Level II

OPERATIVE REPORT

Patient information:	
Patient name: DOB: MR#:	Date: Surgeon: Anesthetist:

Preoperative diagnosis:

Nonhealing diabetic ulcer, plantar surface of the right 5th MP

Postoperative diagnosis:

Same

Procedure(s) performed:

Resection of distal right 5th metatarsal head and debridement of plantar ulcer

Anesthesia:

Assistant surgeon:

Description of procedure:

After sterile preparation of the right foot, infiltration of 1% plain Xylocaine was carried out, digital block was made, and incision was made laterally over the right MP joint and up on to the 5th metatarsal, carried down to the metatarsal. A periosteal elevator was used to isolate this area. Then using a rongeur, the entire metatarsal head was removed. Sizable bleeders that could be noted were cauterized, and attention was directed to the plantar surface where this was debrided. Following this, the wound was closed with interrupted 4-0 nylon, and a bulky dressing was placed.

The patient was given routine postoperative instructions. Darvocet-N 100, 1-2 q4h prn pain. She will be seen in the clinic for dressing change on Monday.

Patrick Chung MD

GODFREY REGIONAL HOSPITAL
123 Main Street • Aldon, FL 77714 • (407) 555-1234

EXERCISE 66

Level I

OPERATIVE REPORT

Patient information:	
Patient name: DOB: MR#:	Date: Surgeon: Anesthetist:

Preoperative diagnosis:

Left distal radius fracture

Postoperative diagnosis:

Same

Procedure(s) performed:

Open reduction, internal fixation of left distal radius fracture; long-arm splinting; fluoroscopy

Anesthesia:

Assistant surgeon:

Description of procedure:

The patient was taken to the operating room, and after general anesthesia was administered, her left upper extremity was examined under fluoroscopy. It was noted that the fracture was unstable and would slide back into the volarly displaced position after reduction. The decision was made to do an open reduction internal fixation at that point. The arm was prepped and draped in a sterile fashion. A well padded pneumatic tourniquet had been applied around the upper arm, and after exsanguination of the extremity with an Esmarch, it was inflated to 200 mm Hg.

Standard volar approach to the distal forearm was made. The brachioradialis was palpated and a longitudinal incision was made. The radial artery was identified and protected. It was taken laterally. Dissection down to the pronator was done and it was divided off its insertion on the radius. The fracture site was identified. The fracture was reduced, and a small T plate off of the small fragment set was used to hold the fracture on the volar surface using buttressing type effect. One screw was placed in the sliding hole and fluoroscopy was used to assess the fracture position as well as hardware placement. Each of these was felt to be acceptable, and therefore additional cortical screws were placed proximally. A single cancellous screw was placed distally. Care was taken to remain out of the growth plate. The hardware being in place, the fracture site was identified under fluoroscopy using AP and lateral views. It was felt that hardware position as well as fracture reduction were

GODFREY REGIONAL HOSPITAL
123 Main Street • Aldon, FL 77714 • (407) 555-1234

Continued

OPERATIVE REPORT

Patient information:	
Patient name:	Date:
DOB:	Surgeon:
MR#:	Anesthetist:

Preoperative diagnosis:

Postoperative diagnosis:

Procedure(s) performed:

Anesthesia:

Assistant surgeon:

Description of procedure:

acceptable. The wound was irrigated out copiously. The pronate was closed back down with 2-0 Vicryl. The subcutaneous tissue was closed with 2-0 Vicryl. The skin was closed with 4-0 Biosyn and Steri-strips. A sterile dressing and long arm sugar tong type splint were applied.

The patient was taken to the recovery room in stable condition. Of note, the tourniquet was deflated prior to wound closure and the wound had minimal bleeding. The radial artery was pulsating and had good flow.

[signature]

GODFREY REGIONAL HOSPITAL
123 Main Street • Aldon, FL 77714 • (407) 555-1234

EXERCISE 67

Level I

OPERATIVE REPORT

Patient information:	
Patient name: DOB: MR#:	Date: Surgeon: Anesthetist:

Preoperative diagnosis:

Foreign body, left long finger

Postoperative diagnosis:

Foreign body, left long finger

Procedure(s) performed:

Removal, foreign body, left long finger

Anesthesia:

Assistant surgeon:

Description of procedure:

The patient was placed supine on the operating room table and a satisfactory general anesthetic was given. Preoperative intravenous cephalosporin antibiotic was given. Pneumatic tourniquet was placed high about the left arm. The left hand, wrist, and forearm to proximal to the elbow were prepped sterilely with DuraPrep. The left hand was draped in the usual sterile fashion. Tourniquet was inflated to 250 mm of mercury. Oblique skin incision was made over the proximal phalanx of the left long finger on the volar surface. The incision was carried through subcutaneous tissue. Hemostasis was achieved as necessary. Full-thickness skin flaps were raised. Flexion creases were not crossed. Gentle blunt dissection was performed deeply. The entrance site of the three BBs was found and the three BBs were gently delivered into the wound and removed. The wound was copiously irrigated with normal saline antibiotic solution. The skin was reapproximated full thickness with interrupted simple sutures of 3-0 Ethilon. Dry, sterile dressings were applied, followed by a tube gauze-type bandage.

The patient tolerated the procedure well and there were no complications. Tourniquet was deflated. All drapes were removed, including the tourniquet. He was transported to the recovery room in stable condition.

Robert Cherry MD

GODFREY REGIONAL HOSPITAL
123 Main Street • Aldon, FL 77714 • (407) 555-1234

EXERCISE 68

Level II

OPERATIVE REPORT

Patient information:

Patient name: Date:
DOB: Surgeon:
MR#:   Anesthetist:

Preoperative diagnosis:

Left foot second interspace neuroma

Postoperative diagnosis:

Same

Procedure(s) performed:

Excision of left foot second interspace neuroma

Anesthesia:

Assistant surgeon:

Description of procedure:

The patient was taken to the operating room, and after IV sedation was administered, her left foot was prepped and draped in a sterile fashion. The foot was wrapped with an Esmarch after administering local anesthesia using 1% lidocaine. The Esmarch was used as a tourniquet around the lower calf.

A standard longitudinal incision was made in the second interspace, and blunt dissection down into the interspace was performed. Care was taken to protect the superficial vessels. The neurovascular bundle was identified and the nerve selected. It was dissected out into each toe and clipped off sharply. It was also dissected down into the foot to the furthest point available and it was transected there. This tissue was sent to Pathology for examination. The tourniquet was removed. There was minimal bleeding encountered. The wound was irrigated out copiously and closed with nylon sutures. Sterile dressing was applied.

The patient was taken to the recovery room in stable condition. Her toes were pink and warm after completion of the procedure.

GODFREY REGIONAL HOSPITAL
123 Main Street • Aldon, FL 77714 • (407) 555-1234

EXERCISE 69

Level I

OPERATIVE REPORT

Patient information:

Patient name:	Date:
DOB:	Surgeon:
MR#:	Anesthetist:

Preoperative diagnosis:

Nonunion of medial malleolar fracture fragment and symptomatic hardware of the tibia and fibula

Postoperative diagnosis:

Same

Procedure(s) performed:

Resection of nonunion fragment of the medial malleolus, hardware removal of the tibia, hardware removal of the fibula, fluoroscopy, short-leg splinting

Anesthesia:

Assistant surgeon:

Description of procedure:

The patient was taken to the operating room, and after general anesthesia was administered, her left lower extremity was prepped and draped in a sterile fashion. Standard medial approach through the prior incision was made to the distal tibia. Blunt and sharp dissection down to the bone was performed. The plate was identified and a periosteal elevator was used to dissect the soft tissue away from the plate. The plate was removed without difficulty along with the screws. The nonunion fragment at the anterior-most aspect of the medial malleolus was identified. It was dissected along the bone and resected without difficulty. It appeared that most of the deltoid ligament remained intact. The area of resection of soft tissue here was closed with Vicryl sutures.

Attention was then turned to the lateral aspect of the ankle. The prior incision was used, with blunt and sharp dissection down to the bone being performed. The hardware was identified and removed without difficulty. Both wounds were irrigated out copiously with antibiotic irrigation solution and closed in layers with 2-0 Vicryl for the subcutaneous tissue and 3-0 nylon for the skin. Sterile dressing and a short-leg splint were applied. Of note, the fracture fragment along the medial aspect was visualized with fluoroscopy, and fluoroscopy was used to confirm removal of all of the portions of that fragment.

Patrick Choy, MD

GODFREY REGIONAL HOSPITAL
123 Main Street • Aldon, FL 77714 • (407) 555-1234

EXERCISE 70

Level II

OPERATIVE REPORT

Patient information:	
Patient name:	Date:
DOB:	Surgeon:
MR#:	Anesthetist:

Preoperative diagnosis:

Chronic nonhealing neuropathic ulceration, left hallux toe

Postoperative diagnosis:

Same

Procedure(s) performed:

Partial first ray amputation, left lower extremity

Anesthesia:

Assistant surgeon:

Description of procedure:

PATHOLOGY: Bone and culture and sensitivity from postop wound

DESCRIPTION OF PROCEDURE:
Under local with IV sedation, the patient was prepped and draped in the usual aseptic manner. OpSite was placed over the left hallux wound. Two converging circumferential incisions were made about the first ray. The left hallux toe was removed. Bleeders were identified and cauterized. Next, partial first ray amputation was performed about the mid shaft of the first metatarsal. The wound was flushed with copious amounts of sterile saline. A culture was taken. A 7-mm Jackson-Pratt was instilled, and the skin was reapproximated utilizing interspersed 3-0 nylon and 4-0 nylon vertical mattress stitches and simple interrupted stitches. The previously placed ankle tourniquet was released. Blood flow returned immediately. The Jackson-Pratt was activated. Postop boot was applied.

The patient tolerated procedure and anesthesia well.

[signature] MD

GODFREY REGIONAL HOSPITAL
123 Main Street • Aldon, FL 77714 • (407) 555-1234

EXERCISE 71

Level I

OPERATIVE REPORT

Patient information:	
Patient name: DOB: MR#:	Date: Surgeon: Anesthetist:

Preoperative diagnosis:

CC: Elbow injury
Patient suffered extremity injury as a result of a fall on arm. Patient sustained additional injuries stating she feel off back of 1-ft step, hitting the back of her head on the concrete. She is complaining of altered vision in the left eye, but denies headache, nausea, or vomiting.

Postoperative diagnosis:

TREATMENT:
OCL splint applied. Device is fit appropriately and neurovascular exam remains intact.

Laceration is repaired with 3 sutures through the subcutaenous with 3-0 Nylon. Wound was covered with sterile dressing. Antibiotic ointment was applied over suture line.

Procedure(s) performed:

Partial first ray amputation, left lower extremity

Anesthesia:

Assistant surgeon:

Description of procedure:

REVIEW OF SYSTEMS:
Neuro: Negative headache, dizziness, confusion, numbness, tingling, weakness

MS: Positive joint pain, negative back pain, neck pain

GI: Negative nausea, vomiting, chills

Eyes: Positive visual changes, negative pain

EXAM:
General, well-nourished 47-year-old in no acute distress. Vital signs are reviewed.

HEENT: PERRLA. EOMI

Chest: No visibile signs of trauma.

CV: Regular rate and rhythm.

GI: Abdoment, no signs of trauma

GODFREY REGIONAL HOSPITAL
123 Main Street • Aldon, FL 77714 • (407) 555-1234

Continued

OPERATIVE REPORT

Patient information:	
Patient name:	Date:
DOB:	Surgeon:
MR#:	Anesthetist:

Preoperative diagnosis:

Symptoms are contained to the left elbow and are described by the patient as severe.

Allergies: Aspirin, Codeine

Postoperative diagnosis:

Procedure(s) performed:

Anesthesia:

Assistant surgeon:

Description of procedure:

MS: 1-cm laceration, left elbow. No active bleeding, no foreign bodies noted.
  Range of motion decreased secondary to pain. Moderate amount of tissue.
  Swelling. Severe tenderness to palpation.

Skin: Intact throughout without significant abrasion.

Neuro: Alert and oriented ×3

X-Ray: Left elbow, positive proximal olecranon fracture

Robert Rai MD

GODFREY REGIONAL HOSPITAL
123 Main Street • Aldon, FL 77714 • (407) 555-1234

EXERCISE 72

Level I

EMERGENCY ROOM RECORD

Name:		Age:	ER physician:
		DOB:	

Allergies/type of reaction:	Usual medications/dosages:

Triage/presenting complaint:

CC: Left thumb injury

Initial assessment:

Time	T	P	R	BP	Other:					

Medication orders:

Lab work:

X-Ray:

X-ray of left thumb was reviewed and was negative for fracture. Possible minimal degenerative joint disease.

Physician's report:

HPI: Patient reports jamming thumb into wall last night and woke up this AM with bruising, pain, and decreatesed range of motion at the interphalangeal joint. Minimal pain per patient. He denies numbness, tingling, or weakness.

ROS: Positive extremity pain, no fevers, all other symptoms reviewed are negative.

PMH/SH: Unremarkable

EXAM:
Vital signs are stable, well-nourished, and in no acute distress

Respiratory: Clear to auscultation

Extremity: Left thumb, bruising of thumb pad with decreased extension of IP joint secondary to pain. Possibly minimal tenderness to palpation at IP joint. Neurovascular intact. Other fingers and extremities without injury.

Metal splint was applied to left thumb.

Diagnosis:	Physician sign/date
IMPRESSION: Left thumb contusion	*Robert Rai MD*
Discharge Transfer Admit Good Satisfactory Other:	

GODFREY REGIONAL HOSPITAL
123 Main Street • Aldon, FL 77714 • (407) 555-1234

RESPIRATORY EXERCISES

EXERCISE 1

Level II

OPERATIVE REPORT

Patient information:

Patient name: Date:
DOB: Surgeon:
MR#: Anesthetist:

Preoperative diagnosis:

Chronic left maxillary and ethmoid sinusitis, left middle turbinate hypertrophy

CLINICAL NOTE:
The patient is a 54-year-old white female with chronic left maxillary and ethmoid sinusitis, not responding to conservative medical treatment. Preoperatively on CT scan, post treatment she was found to have complete opacification. The patient

Postoperative diagnosis:

Chronic left maxillary and ethmoid sinusitis, left middle turbinate hypertrophy

OPERATIVE FINDINGS:
There is chronic mucosal thickening of the left maxillary sinuses. Right middle turbinate was partially removed to prevent postoperative synechia/scarring and obstruction of the ostiomeatal complex, which was opened surgically.

Procedure(s) performed:

Endoscopic left total ethmoidectomy. Left middle meatal enterostomy. Left partial middle turbinectomy.

Anesthesia:

General

Assistant surgeon:

Description of procedure:

The patient was brought to the operating room and placed in the supine position. General endotracheal anesthesia was administered. The nose was vasoconstricted with topical Afrin and injected with 6 cc 1% lidocaine with 1:100,000 parts of epinephrine into the left middle turbinate and lateral nasal wall mucosa.

Using a two-view monitor for visualization, the 0 degree sinus endoscope was placed in the left nasal cavity and the left middle turbinate was lateralized with a Freer elevator. Using the sharp edge of the Freer, the anterior ethmoid air cells were entered and bone and mucosa were removed with straight and upbiting Blakesley forceps. The left maxillary sinus ostia was identified and an enterostomy, approximately 1 cm in diameter, was made with the upbiting forceps and power microdebrider. The left maxillary sinus cavity was examined with a 30- and 70-degree sinus endoscope and it showed chronic, thickened mucosa with no evidence of fungus or mucopurulent discharge. The left total ethmoidectomy was completed with Blakesley forceps and the power microdebrider. The specimen was sent to Pathology for permanent section. An anterior inferior portion of the left middle turbinate was incised with turbinate scissors.

Upon completion of the procedures, the left ethmoid sinus cavity was packed with MeroGel and two Kennedy nasal

GODFREY REGIONAL HOSPITAL
123 Main Street • Aldon, FL 77714 • (407) 555-1234

Continued

OPERATIVE REPORT

Patient information:

Patient name: Date:
DOB: Surgeon:
MR#:   Anesthetist:

Preoperative diagnosis:

had opacification of the left maxillary sinus and left chronic ethmoid sinusitis.

Postoperative diagnosis:

Procedure(s) performed:

Anesthesia:

Assistant surgeon:

Description of procedure:

tampons. A 9-cm standard tampon was placed along the floor of the nose, which was impregnated with Bacitracin ointment. The sutures of the tampon were tied together, and a nasal turbinate pad was placed. The oropharynx was suctioned. There was adequate hemostasis present. The patient was awakened from general anesthesia, extubated, and brought to the recovery room in stable condition, having tolerated the procedure well.

ESTIMATED BLOOD LOSS: Less than 10 cc

Maurice Doater, MD

GODFREY REGIONAL HOSPITAL
123 Main Street • Aldon, FL 77714 • (407) 555-1234

EXERCISE 2

Level II

OPERATIVE REPORT

Patient information:	
Patient name:	Date:
DOB:	Surgeon:
MR#:	Anesthetist:

Preoperative diagnosis:

Chronic right maxillary/ethmoid sinusitis

CLINICAL NOTE:
The patient is a 27-year-old white female with chronic right cheek tenderness and pain that has not responded to conservative medical treatment. Preoperative CT scan showed opacification of the maxillary sinus with obstruction of the osteomeatal complex. The remaining sinuses were clear.

Postoperative diagnosis:

Mucocele of the right maxillary sinus with obstruction of the osteomeatal complex

Procedure(s) performed:

1. Endoscopic right anterior ethmoidectomy
2. Right meatal antrostomy with removal of right maxillary sinus mucocele

Anesthesia:

General

Assistant surgeon:

Description of procedure:

The patient was brought in to the operating room and placed on the operating room table in a supine position. General endotracheal anesthesia was performed. The right nose was vasoconstricted with topical Afrin and injected with 3 cc of 1% lidocaine with 1:100,000 parts epinephrine to the right middle turbinate and lateral nasal wall mucosa adjacent. After the face was prepped and draped, a TV monitor was used for visualization attached to a zero-degree sinus endoscope. The mucosa around the hiatus, semiluminaris, and the middle meatus was removed with straight biting forceps. Using a Bolger probe, the antrum of the right maxillary sinus was entered. Using a power microdebrider and Blakesley forceps, anterior ethmoidectomy and 1-cm maxillary antrostomy were performed. Using 30- and 70-degree sinus endoscopes, the right maxillary sinus was examined, and there was no evidence of fungus or mucopurulent debris present. It appeared that there was a large right mucous retention cyst completely filling the right maxillary sinus that was removed upon entering the right maxillary sinus. Large curved suction was placed into the sinus and was irrigated copiously with normal saline and suctioned dry. MeroGel was placed into the right anterior ethmoid sinus cavity, followed with a slim Kennedy nasal tampon into the right middle meatal region. The posterior nasal cavity and oropharynx were suctioned dry, and there was adequate hemostasis present.

The patient was awakened from general anesthesia, extubated, and brought to the recovery room in stable condition, having tolerated the procedure well.

Maurice Doater, MD

ESTIMATED BLOOD LOSS: Less than 10 cc

GODFREY REGIONAL HOSPITAL
123 Main Street • Aldon, FL 77714 • (407) 555-1234

EXERCISE 3

Level II

OPERATIVE REPORT

Patient information:	
Patient name:	Date:
DOB:	Surgeon:
MR#:	Anesthetist:

Preoperative diagnosis:

1. Nasal fracture
2. Deviated nasal septum
3. Bilateral inferior turbinate hypertrophy

Postoperative diagnosis:

Same

Procedure(s) performed:

1. Open reduction of nasal fracture
2. Septoplasty
3. Bilateral inferior turbinate reduction

Anesthesia:

General

Assistant surgeon:

Description of procedure:

The patient was taken to the operating room and placed in the usual supine position. After the induction of general anesthesia via endotracheal intubation, the patient was prepped and draped in the usual fashion for a clean, uncontaminated procedure.

We first began by decongesting the nose with 4% cocaine on cottonoids. We then injected both sides of the septum as well as the inferior turbinates and the skin of the nose with 1% lidocaine with epinephrine. We first began the procedure by performing the septoplasty. We used a #15 blade knife to make a left hemitransfixion incision and elevated the mucoperichondrial flap off of the cartilage and bone of the septum. We removed and/or replaced in the midline the deviated portions of the septum. After this was completed, we moved to the bony nasal pyramid of the nose. We performed lateral and medial osteotomies on the nose because of the significant deviation of the nose to the left as well as the large dorsal hump. We also used a rasp to smooth out the dorsal surface of the nose. After this was completed, we were able to reduce the inferior turbinates by first outfracturing them and then reducing them with the bipolar electrocautery. The bony nasal work was done via intercartilaginous incisions, which were made between the upper lateral and the lower lateral cartilages of the nose. These were all sutured back together at the end of the procedure using 4-0 chromic gut sutures.

GODFREY REGIONAL HOSPITAL
123 Main Street • Aldon, FL 77714 • (407) 555-1234

Continued

OPERATIVE REPORT

Patient information:	
Patient name: DOB: MR#:	Date: Surgeon: Anesthetist:

Preoperative diagnosis:

Postoperative diagnosis:

Procedure(s) performed:

Anesthesia:

Assistant surgeon:

Description of procedure:

Doyle splints were placed in the nose. An Aquaplast splint was placed on the dorsum of the nose.

The patient tolerated both procedures well and there were no complications. The patient was thus removed directly to recovery room in stable condition.

ESTIMATED BLOOD LOSS: 50 cc

COMPLICATIONS: None. Instrument count correct at the end of the procedure.

Maurice Doater, MD

GODFREY REGIONAL HOSPITAL
123 Main Street • Aldon, FL 77714 • (407) 555-1234

EXERCISE 4
Level II

OPERATIVE REPORT

Patient information:	
Patient name: DOB: MR#:	Date: Surgeon: Anesthetist:

Preoperative diagnosis:

Nasal septal deformity with nasal obstruction due to extensive nasal polyposis, chronic bilateral ethmoid sinusitis. Polypoid degeneration in the middle turbinates bilaterally. Chronic left maxillary sinusitis.

CLINICAL NOTE:
The patient is a 75-year-old white male with severe left nasal septal deviation. He has extensive bilateral nasal polyps and

Postoperative diagnosis:

Nasal septal deformity with nasal obstruction due to extensive nasal polyposis, chronic bilateral ethmoid sinusitis. Polypoid degeneration in the middle turbinates bilaterally. Myosteoma of the left maxillary sinus.

Procedure(s) performed:

Septoplasty, endoscopic bilateral total ethmoidectomies, left middle meatal antrostomy with removal of left maxillary sinus myosteoma, bilateral turbinate resection. Bilateral extensive nasal polypectomies.

Anesthesia:

General

Assistant surgeon:

Description of procedure:

The patient was brought to the operating room and placed on the operating table in supine position. General endotracheal anesthesia was performed. He received Ancef 1 gram IV perioperatively. Nose was prepped and draped after being injected with 12 cc 1% lidocaine with 1:100,000 parts epinephrine into the nasal septal mucosa, middle turbinates, and lateral nasal mucosa bilaterally. Nose was vasoconstricted with topical Afrin.

Left hemitransfixion incision was made on the nasal septum and elevated with Freer elevator to expose the deviated cartilage and bone. The inferior half of the cartilaginous septum was removed, preserving the nasal spine and caudal septum. This was removed off the maxillary crest. The bony cartilaginous septum was separated with a Freer elevator, and the mucoperiosteum was elevated off the bony septum bilaterally. Using open Jansen-Middleton rongeurs, the mid inferior portions of the bony septum were removed. Further removal with Takahashi forceps of the vomer bone was performed. Using a 3-mm osteotome and mallet, the maxillary crest bone that was deviated severely into the left nasal cavity was removed along the anterior and mid portions of the septum. This completed removal of the deviated bone and cartilage. The left hemitransfixion incision was closed with interrupted 4-0 chromic sutures.

Using straight and biting Blakesley forceps, polyps were removed from the left nasal cavity. Left total ethmoidectomy was performed with the same instruments. The degenerated middle turbinate due to polyposis was removed with same instrumentation as well. After completion of total ethmoidectomy and middle turbinectomy and nasal polypectomy, a Bolger probe was used to bluntly enter the left maxillary sinus. Antrostomy was made with the biting forceps to approximately 1 cm in diameter. Using curved suction and cochlea curets, the myosteoma

GODFREY REGIONAL HOSPITAL
123 Main Street • Aldon, FL 77714 • (407) 555-1234

Continued

OPERATIVE REPORT

Patient information:	
Patient name:	Date:
DOB:	Surgeon:
MR#:	Anesthetist:

Preoperative diagnosis:

chronic sinusitis. He does not respond to conservative medical treatment. He is being brought to the operating room for these operative procedures. Operative findings showed extensive polyposis filling the left nasal cavities bilaterally and into the ethmoid sinuses bilaterally. The left ostial medial complex was obstructed both by the nasal septal spur from the deviation and by a myosteoma found in the left maxillary sinus. Both middle turbinates showed extensive polypoid degeneration.

Postoperative diagnosis:

Procedure(s) performed:

Anesthesia:

Assistant surgeon:

Description of procedure:

was removed. Specimen was taken through the Lukens trap and sent to Microbiology for fungal culture. A large curved suction was placed in maxillary sinus and irrigated copiously with normal saline and suctioned through a Frazier suction positioned in the posterior nasal pharynx. Approximately 150 cc was irrigated through the left maxillary sinus until effluent was clear.

Total ethmoidectomy, polypectomy, and middle turbinectomy were performed in similar fashion in the right nasal cavity. After this was completed, Silastic sheeting was cut to size and placed on both sides in the nasal septum and sutured into place with 3-0 silk mattress sutures. MeroGel was placed in the posterior ethmoid cavities bilaterally, followed by small Merocel nasal tampons. 10-cm flat nasal tampons impregnated with Bacitracin ointment were placed at the floor of the left and right nasal airways. I sutured the tampons tight across the columella of the nose. Nasal dripper pad was placed. Oropharynx was suctioned. There was adequate hemostasis present.

The patient was awakened from general anesthesia, extubated, and brought to the recovery room in stable condition, having tolerated the procedure well.

ESTIMATED BLOOD LOSS: 200 cc

Maurice Doater, MD

GODFREY REGIONAL HOSPITAL
123 Main Street • Aldon, FL 77714 • (407) 555-1234

EXERCISE 5

Level II

OPERATIVE REPORT

Patient information:

Patient name: Date:
DOB: Surgeon:
MR#:   Anesthetist:

Preoperative diagnosis:

1. Chronic maxillary sinusitis
2. Chronic ethmoid sinusitis
3. Deviated nasal septum
4. Nasal polyps

Postoperative diagnosis:

1. Chronic maxillary sinusitis
2. Chronic ethmoid sinusitis
3. Deviated nasal septum
4. Nasal polyps

Procedure(s) performed:

1. Bilateral endoscopic maxillary antrostomies with tissue removal
2. Bilateral endoscopic anterior ethmoidectomies
3. Septoplasty
4. Bilateral endoscopic nasal polypectomies

Anesthesia:

General

Assistant surgeon:

Description of procedure:

The patient was taken to the operating room and placed in the usual supine position. After induction of general anesthesia via endotracheal intubation, the patient was prepped and draped in the usual fashion for a clean uncontaminated procedure.

We first began by decongesting the nose with 4% cocaine on cottonoids. We then injected both sides of the nasal septum as well as the lateral nasal walls with 1% lidocaine with epinephrine.

We first performed the endoscopic sinus surgery on the left side because there were some very large polyps, in fact, some antral choanal polyps on the left side. The polyps were removed using the microdebrider. The uncinate process, the anterior ethmoid cells, and the natural ostium of the maxillary sinuses as well as a thick mucoid tissue within the sinus itself were all removed using the microdebrider. We then directed our attention to the septum where a left hemitransfixion incision was made. We performed a standard septoplasty with particular removal of the cartilage and bone that was compressing the right middle turbinate and obstructing the middle meatus on the right side. After this was done, we then resumed the sinus surgery, this time on the right side, and performed the exact same procedure with removal of the polyps, the anterior ethmoid cells, and the natural ostium of the maxillary sinus on the right-hand side.

GODFREY REGIONAL HOSPITAL
123 Main Street • Aldon, FL 77714 • (407) 555-1234

Continued

OPERATIVE REPORT

Patient information:	
Patient name: DOB: MR#:	Date: Surgeon: Anesthetist:

Preoperative diagnosis:

Postoperative diagnosis:

Procedure(s) performed:

Anesthesia:

Assistant surgeon:

Description of procedure:

After all this was done, the sinuses were thoroughly irrigated with normal saline solution. The left hemitransfixion incision on the septum was closed with a 5-0 plain gut suture. The mucoperichondrial flaps of the septum were closed with 4-0 plain gut in a basting suture fashion. The middle meatus on each side were packed with MeroGel packing. Doyle nasal splints were placed on each side of the septum, and 8-cm Merocel packs were placed on each side of the nose.

The patient tolerated the procedures well. There were no complications. The patient was subsequently moved directly to the recovery room in stable condition.

ESTIMATED BLOOD LOSS: 250 cc

COMPLICATIONS: None

COUNTS: Instrument count correct at the end of the procedure

Maurice Doater, MD

GODFREY REGIONAL HOSPITAL
123 Main Street • Aldon, FL 77714 • (407) 555-1234

EXERCISE 6

Level II

OPERATIVE REPORT

Patient information:	
Patient name:	Date:
DOB:	Surgeon:
MR#:	Anesthetist:

Preoperative diagnosis:

1. Traumatic nasoseptal deformity
2. Septal perforation
3. Nasal obstruction

Postoperative diagnosis:

Same

Procedure(s) performed:

1. Septoplasty utilizing an external columella approach
2. Columella reconstruction utilizing cartilage graft
3. Repair of nasoseptal perforation

Anesthesia:

Assistant surgeon:

Description of procedure:

After consent was obtained, the patient was taken to the operating room and was placed on the operating room table in a supine position. After an adequate level of IV sedation was obtained, the patient was draped in an appropriate manner for nasal surgery. The patient's nose was prepped with Betadine prep and then draped in a sterile manner. The nose was packed with cotton pledgets soaked with 4% cocaine. After several minutes, intranasal and external nasal injection of 1% Xylocaine with 1:100,000 units epinephrine was made. Nasal hairs were trimmed. Then utilizing the columella incision, the skin and subcutaneous tissue were elevated off the lower lateral cartilages. The soft tissue between the lower lateral cartilage and the medial crura of the lower lateral cartilages was removed. Subsequently, the septum was isolated and bilateral mucoperichondrial and mucoperiosteal flaps were elevated. The perforation was encountered and the edges freshened. The cartilaginous septum was then removed in its entirety except for a dorsal strip. Subsequently, the deviated portion of the bony septum, as well as the maxillary crest, was removed. Subsequently, the perforation was closed on both sides with interrupted 4-0 chromic sutures. The septal cartilage that was removed was then shaved to straighten the cartilage out. This was then brought anteriorly between the perforation repair and the lower lateral cartilage to restore nasal tip support. This was secured between the medial crura with 4-0 clear nylon sutures. A quilting suture of 4-0 plain gut was then performed. The columella incision was closed with interrupted 6-0 nylon sutures. Sinolastic splints were then placed on

GODFREY REGIONAL HOSPITAL
123 Main Street • Aldon, FL 77714 • (407) 555-1234

Continued

OPERATIVE REPORT

Patient information:	
Patient name: DOB: MR#:	Date: Surgeon: Anesthetist:

Preoperative diagnosis:

INDICATION:
55-year-old male with prior history of nasal trauma. He also underwent some sort of nasal surgery. Subsequent to that, he was left with a septal perforation and continued to have nasal obstruction. Examination reveals a significant septal deformity around the perforation with the anterior perforation of approximately 2–3 cm in size.

Postoperative diagnosis:

Procedure(s) performed:

Anesthesia:

Assistant surgeon:

Description of procedure:

both sides of the nasal septum and secured with nylon suture. The nose was then packed bilaterally with Merocel sponges coated with Bacitracin ointment and inflated with local solution. Nasal dressing was applied.

The patient tolerated the procedure well; there was no break in technique. The patient was awakened and taken to the recovery room in good condition.

Fluids administered: 1000 cc RL

Estimated blood loss: less than 25 cc

Preoperative medication: 12 mg Decadron and 1 gram Ancef IV

Maurice Doater, MD

GODFREY REGIONAL HOSPITAL
123 Main Street • Aldon, FL 77714 • (407) 555-1234

EXERCISE 7

Level II

OPERATIVE REPORT

Patient information:

Patient name:	Date:
DOB:	Surgeon:
MR#:	Anesthetist:

Preoperative diagnosis:

Primary hyperparathyroidism secondary to parathyroid adenoma

INDICATIONS:
The patient had presented to her local physician with an elevated calcium level. She had seen Dr. Smith, endocrinologist, and was found to have elevated PTH as well as elevated calcium, and sestamibi scan was consistent with an adenoma of

Postoperative diagnosis:

Same

Procedure(s) performed:

Excision of parathyroid adenoma with guided techniques

Anesthesia:

Assistant surgeon:

Description of procedure:

The patient was then brought to the operating room and placed under sedation. She was prepped and draped over the neck, and after this was completed and sedation was adequate, the neck was investigated with the navigator probe. I used a small calumniated probe. There was an area just lateral and slightly below the level of the cricoid. At this point, I did get the highest reading, which was around 417 counts. This was just static counts, not a 10-second count. The standard background seemed to be around 300 to 350. I thought this was most likely the position. I went ahead and planned my incision transversely and made a skin incision through a field of injected anesthetic, elevated platysma flaps for just about a centimeter, placed a self-retaining retractor, and divided the straps in the midline after injection of further lidocaine.

I then began my dissection, exposing the thyroid. There was a nodule on the thyroid that I did remove, feeling it was probably thyroid. It was on the inferior aspect and did come back as thyroid. Attempts to rotate the parathyroid adenoma initially were unsuccessful. The patient became uncomfortable. I went ahead and had the Anesthesia Department put her under general anesthesia and extended my incision. With the incision then larger, I was able to immediately get the probe deeper in the neck and identified the position of the adenoma. This was located in the tracheo-esophageal groove, not consistent with an inferior pole gland but with a superior pole gland that had become heavy and fallen posteriorly into the tracheo-esophageal groove. This was lying adjacent to the inferior thyroid artery where it crosses the recurrent laryngeal nerve.

GODFREY REGIONAL HOSPITAL
123 Main Street • Aldon, FL 77714 • (407) 555-1234

Continued

OPERATIVE REPORT

Patient information:	
Patient name:	Date:
DOB:	Surgeon:
MR#:	Anesthetist:

Preoperative diagnosis:

the inferior pole position. The patient was sent to my office for evaluation of surgical excision. The patient underwent injection with sestamibi again here at our facility. She did have images done again, which were consistent with adenoma of the right inferior pole position.

Postoperative diagnosis:

Procedure(s) performed:

Anesthesia:

Assistant surgeon:

Description of procedure:

Blunt dissection was used to deliver this gland out of this position. It was teased up and its vascular pedicle was clipped carefully times two, and it was excised. We were careful to stay well away from and preserve the recurrent laryngeal nerve and the inferior thyroid artery in the process. The majority of the case was done with blunt dissection. We did occasionally use the Bovie to divide areolar tissue superficially in the neck. We did divide the middle thyroid vein between clips during the dissection process so that we could better expose the tracheo-esophageal groove.

After removing the gland from the neck and placing it on the tip of the probe, it had about 50% background count. The area of the excision of the gland also had decreased counts by about 50% after its removal. There were no other hot zones. Everything had essentially the same counts in that area, in all four quadrants of the thyroid.

At this point, the wound was irrigated. There was no bleeding. I closed the strap muscles with 3-0 Vicryl, the platysma with 3-0 Vicryl, and the skin with Prolene. The specimen was evaluated by Pathology and confirmed to be parathyroid. With the findings histologically, surgical findings, and radiographic findings as well as nuclear findings, I feel like this was the offending gland.

At this point, the procedure was terminated. The patient is stable in recovery.

GODFREY REGIONAL HOSPITAL
123 Main Street • Aldon, FL 77714 • (407) 555-1234

EXERCISE 8

Level II

OPERATIVE REPORT

Patient information:	
Patient name: DOB: MR#:	Date: Surgeon: Anesthetist:

Preoperative diagnosis:

1. Left septal deviation
2. Bilateral turbinate hypertrophy
3. Chronic pansinusitis
4. Nasal polyposis
5. Nasal airway obstruction

Postoperative diagnosis:

1. Left septal deviation
2. Bilateral turbinate hypertrophy
3. Chronic pansinusitis
4. Nasal polyposis
5. Nasal airway obstruction

Procedure(s) performed:

1. Functional endoscopy
2. Nasal polypectomy
3. Bilateral inferior turbinectomy
4. Endoscopic maxillary sinus antrostomies, bilateral
5. Bilateral endoscopic anterior ethmoidectomies

Anesthesia:

Assistant surgeon:

Description of procedure:

The patient was brought to the operating room and placed in the supine position. General endotracheal anesthesia was obtained without difficulty. The patient was prepped and draped in the usual standard fashion. The table was turned 180 degrees and the nose was Afrinized and cocainized. Examination of the nasal septum revealed an overall bending of the nasal septum that corresponded to what was seen on the CT scan. This was from right to left with what looked like bilateral middle turbinate impactions. Massive nasal mucosal fullness of both bilateral inferior turbinates and bilateral middle turbinates, obliteration of the middle meatus bilaterally due to mucosal thickening, and polyposis were seen. More polyposis was seen endoscopically on the right than left. We endoscopically scoped the inferior, middle, and superior meatus on the right side. We were unable to get a scope between the turbinates and septum, as there was such a deviation of the septum. We endoscopically started removing polyposis, starting from around the anterior aspect of the inferior portion of the middle turbinate all the way posterior into the nasopharyngeal area. This corresponded to the polyposis seen on CT scan. We then removed the mucosa overlying the uncinate process and part of that uncinate process, getting into the infundibulum and the anterior ethmoid air cells that were seen to be mucosally compromised. This again corresponded to what was seen on the CT scan. The maxillary sinus opening was noted to be obliterated. It was found with a seeking olive-tipped sucker. Once identified, the maxillary sinus opening was opened larger with an oscillating endoscopic shaver. This same shaver was utilized in the removal of excess mucosa and of the polyposis. Once I had enlarged the maxillary sinus opening to about a square centimeter, I noted there was diseased mucosa within the confines of the maxillary sinus cavity along with some fluid material. I did not enter the maxillary sinus cavity to any degree. I just suctioned out all the fluid with the olive-tipped seeker and turned my attention to other matters. Once I had removed the anterior ethmoid air cells, I then started to decrease the mucosal fullness on the

GODFREY REGIONAL HOSPITAL
123 Main Street • Aldon, FL 77714 • (407) 555-1234

Continued

OPERATIVE REPORT

Patient information:	
Patient name:	Date:
DOB:	Surgeon:
MR#:	Anesthetist:

Preoperative diagnosis:

Postoperative diagnosis:

Procedure(s) performed:

Anesthesia:

Assistant surgeon:

Description of procedure:

inferior aspect of the middle turbinate as well as using the Don Dennis depolarizer to reduce the mucosal hypertrophy inferior turbinate. Once I was satisfied that I had opened the airway as much as possible endoscopically, I then used a long nasal speculum to fracture medially the deviated septum anteriorly and posteriorly that was so posteriorly deviated back to the left. This was fractured back to the midline so as to even up the nasal passages in terms of airflow and volume.

We then turned our attention to the right side that was more diseased; inferior and middle turbinate hypertrophy was noted. The middle meatus mucosa was noted to be significant, which corresponded also to what was seen on the CT scan. This area was scoped through the inferior, middle, and superior meatus. Endoscopically, using the shaver, we removed the polyposis noted in the middle meatus and on the inferior surface of the nasal turbinate all the way back into the nasopharyngeal area. All this polyposis was removed with the shaver. Entering into the anterior ethmoid air cells, this was done following the polyposis into the anterior ethmoid air cells. Some of the uncinate bone was likewise removed on the left side. The maxillary sinus opening was noted to be obliterated. There were actually two entries into the maxillary sinus. We took the more posterior and inferior sinus ostium. Immediately when we opened the sinus up, purulent material bubbled out of the maxillary sinus as if it were under pressure. The polyposis surrounding the ostium was removed with the shaver and the ostium itself was enlarged to about 1 square centimeter, as was the case on the opposite side. The Don Dennis depolarizer was utilized to shrink and fulgurate the inferior turbinate on the right side. The shaver was utilized to reduce the fullness of the mucosa on the middle turbinate. We outwardly fractured the impacted middle turbinate on the right side that was impacted into the nasal septum so it again gained more volume

GODFREY REGIONAL HOSPITAL
123 Main Street • Aldon, FL 77714 • (407) 555-1234

Continued

OPERATIVE REPORT

Patient information:

Patient name:
DOB:
MR#:

Date:
Surgeon:
Anesthetist:

Preoperative diagnosis:

Postoperative diagnosis:

Procedure(s) performed:

Anesthesia:

Assistant surgeon:

Description of procedure:

and airflow in the right nasal airway. When I was satisfied that I had cleared the airway to my satisfaction, I packed the anterior ethmoid air cell area with Neosporin-impregnated Nu-Gauze. This was done on both sides to about an equal degree. The inferior nasal airway bilaterally was packed with Neosporin-impregnated Merocel injected with 1% Xylocaine with 1:100,000 epinephrine. About 200 cc blood loss ensued during the case.

The patient was awakened, extubated, and brought to the recovery room in stable condition.

PATHOLOGY:
Contents of left and right middle meatus in separate containers

Maurice Doater, MD

GODFREY REGIONAL HOSPITAL
123 Main Street • Aldon, FL 77714 • (407) 555-1234

EXERCISE 9

Level II

OPERATIVE REPORT

Patient information:	
Patient name: DOB: MR#:	Date: Surgeon: Anesthetist:

Preoperative diagnosis:

Chronic dacryocystitis with infection and tearing

INDICATIONS:
This elderly patient, who is 90 years old, has had chronic tearing and mattering on her right side. She normally has a very large cystic area that is very painful and expresses greenish-yellow purulent material. She currently is on Cipro 500 mg

Postoperative diagnosis:

Same

Procedure(s) performed:

Incision and drainage of a chronic dacryocystitis of the right eyelid

Anesthesia:

Local with moderate anesthesia care

Assistant surgeon:

Description of procedure:

The patient was taken to the operating room and prepped and draped. Large amounts of green purulent material were expressed from the right tear sac and this was sent for culture and sensitivity. I expressed until no further mucus was coming from the sac. IV sedation was given and a 2-cc volume of the standard mixture was injected in the upper and lower lid medially as well as the tear sac area near the nose. The patient was prepped with Betadine and draped. A 0 and a 1 Bowman probe were passed through the lower and the upper puncta. I used a 15 blade scalpel to cut down over the tear sac. I used a Westcott scissors to dissect as much of the tear sac to the bone as I could. Then the tear sac wall was incised. Irrigation was done and nothing passed beyond that tear sac obstruction. I did attempt to probe into the nose before cutting the tear sac and this was unsuccessful as far as any passage of irrigation. Cautery was used. Gentamicin-soaked packing was placed after the area was copiously irrigated with gentamicin. Both upper and lower puncta were cauterized completely shut in order to eliminate any inflow into the area. It is thought that with no inflow and outflow, this cyst will not reform. Antibiotic ointment was placed.

The patient tolerated the procedure well. She will be followed in the outpatient clinic in one day's time when her packing will be removed. She will continue on Cipro as well as triple antibiotic ointment to the area until it has healed in secondarily. I did

GODFREY REGIONAL HOSPITAL
123 Main Street • Aldon, FL 77714 • (407) 555-1234

Continued

OPERATIVE REPORT

Patient information:	
Patient name: DOB: MR#:	Date: Surgeon: Anesthetist:

Preoperative diagnosis:

twice a day and is doing better than she ever has. It is elected to try and probe this and see if anything can be passed through, and if nothing can, then to incise and drain and pack the area to let it heal secondarily. A consent was signed.

Postoperative diagnosis:

Procedure(s) performed:

Anesthesia:

Assistant surgeon:

Description of procedure:

close above and below with some 6-0 Vicryl in order to lessen the area that has to heal in secondarily as the initial incision was made approximately 10 millimeters. The patient was transferred in good condition.

ESTIMATED BLOOD LOSS: Less than 5 ccs

COMPLICATIONS: None

Maurice Doater, MD

GODFREY REGIONAL HOSPITAL
123 Main Street • Aldon, FL 77714 • (407) 555-1234

EXERCISE 10

Level II

OPERATIVE REPORT

Patient information:	
Patient name: DOB: MR#:	Date: Surgeon: Anesthetist:

Preoperative diagnosis:

1. Nasal polyposis
2. Chronic sinusitis

Postoperative diagnosis:

1. Nasal polyposis
2. Chronic sinusitis

Procedure(s) performed:

Functional endoscopic sinus surgery with bilateral Caldwell-Luc nasal antral windows; endoscopic anterior and posterior ethmoidectomies

Anesthesia:

Assistant surgeon:

Description of procedure:

The patient was brought to the operating room and placed in the supine position, and general endotracheal anesthesia was obtained without difficulty. The table was turned 180 degrees. The nose was examined. I Neo-Synephrinized his nose and injected his nasal polyps with 1% Xylocaine with 1:100,000 epinephrine after waiting about 10–15 minutes. We then started using the shaver and an endoscope to remove the polyps that were massive in nature and extended from anterior to posterior and inferior to superior inside the patient's nose. He has had previous nasal polypectomy and anterior and posterior ethmoidectomies, Caldwell-Luc and nasal antral windows in the past. There was complete obliteration of all anatomy due to the polyposis. I could identify, however, his nasal septum and it was hypersensitive—that is, swollen and very easy to bruise and start bleeding. In fact, all the structures in his nose were extremely vascular despite Neo-Synephrine and 1% Xylocaine with 1:100,000 epinephrine. I shaved the polyps out of the left side, following them from inferior to superior and identifying polyps medial to the middle turbinate and superior to the middle turbinate. They were lateral to the turbinate, inside the middle meatus, and I followed them into the anterior and posterior ethmoid air cells where I cleaned these areas out. Inspissated mucous was noted in the frontal sinus recess as well as in the anterior and posterior ethmoid air cells, and a large amount of inspissated mucous was in the left maxillary sinus. I enlarged the maxillary sinus opening endoscopically and could not get all the inspissated mucous out from this direction. I therefore injected the upper

GODFREY REGIONAL HOSPITAL
123 Main Street • Aldon, FL 77714 • (407) 555-1234

Continued

OPERATIVE REPORT

Patient information:	
Patient name: DOB: MR#:	Date: Surgeon: Anesthetist:

Preoperative diagnosis:

Postoperative diagnosis:

Procedure(s) performed:

Anesthesia:

Assistant surgeon:

Description of procedure:

canine fossa area and used cautery to cut down to the maxillary sinus opening where I identified the anterior maxillary sinus wall. I decided to make a more medial approach to my opening and, therefore, used a Kerrison rongeur to chisel my way into the maxillary sinus, removing that anterior half-dime-sized plate of bone (less than 1 cm in size). I identified massive polyposis and inspissated mucous inside the maxillary sinus. I cleaned it out completely and identified the nasal antral window enlarging it slightly. I packed this area, the maxillary sinus as well as the nasal area, and all the meatus with Neosporin-impregnated Nu-Gauze. I closed the initial incision with interrupted 2-0 chromic. I also packed the nose on that side with Merocel splint impregnated with Neosporin and injected with 1% Xylocaine with 1:100,000 epinephrine. I then turned my attention to the right side where an identical situation occurred and only more bleeding was encountered than on the left side. I removed massive polyposis on the right side and, again, I identified the nasal antral window on the right side. It was stenosed and I enlarged it, again removing inspissated mucous there and from the frontal sinus recess. A lot of bleeding from the anterior ethmoid artery was noted. It was very difficult to control. The septum appeared to be pretty much in the midline, and I decided not to do anything with it. The turbinates were of normal size. He had been on prednisone preoperatively, and I decided not to do anything with the turbinates. After packing the right maxillary sinus after having performed the Caldwell-Luc in an identical fashion to that on the left side, I packed it with Neosporin-impregnated

GODFREY REGIONAL HOSPITAL
123 Main Street • Aldon, FL 77714 • (407) 555-1234

Continued

OPERATIVE REPORT

Patient information:	
Patient name: DOB: MR#:	Date: Surgeon: Anesthetist:

Preoperative diagnosis:

Postoperative diagnosis:

Procedure(s) performed:

Anesthesia:

Assistant surgeon:

Description of procedure:

Nu-Gauze and packed the inferior middle meatus with Nu-Gauze. I placed a Merocel splint inside the nasal airway. It should be noted that an anterior-posterior ethmoidectomy was performed on the right, just merely following the massive polyposis into the anterior posterior ethmoid air cells. Previous surgery had been done on this area, removing the uncinate process so access was relatively easy.

Once I found that the patient was no longer bleeding, I awakened him and he was extubated and taken to the recovery room in stable condition.

PATHOLOGY:
1. Bilateral nasal polyps
2. Contents of both maxillary sinuses

Maurice Doater, MD

GODFREY REGIONAL HOSPITAL
123 Main Street • Aldon, FL 77714 • (407) 555-1234

EXERCISE 11

Level I

OPERATIVE REPORT

Patient information:

Patient name: Date:
DOB: Surgeon:
MR#:   Anesthetist:

Preoperative diagnosis:

Right thyroid cold nodule

INDICATIONS:
The patient presented to my office with a right thyroid cold nodule, which had grown over a ten-year or more period of time by 1 cm in diameter. After consultation with Endocrinology, removal was recommended.

Postoperative diagnosis:

Right thyroid cold nodule

Procedure(s) performed:

Right thyroid lobectomy

Anesthesia:

Assistant surgeon:

Description of procedure:

The patient was brought to the operating room and placed on the table in the supine position. After general anesthesia was achieved, he was prepped and draped sterilely over the neck and shoulder. A roll was then placed to hyperextend the neck, and we did make a transverse incision in the skin folds through the skin with the scalpel through the subcutaneous tissues with the Bovie through the platysma. Platysmal flaps were then elevated with the Bovie. Midline was opened with the Bovie and thyroid isthmus was identified. I then began my dissection over the right lobe. This was done with blunt and sharp dissection and right inguinal clamp. Vessels were either controlled with the Bovie or cut between vascular clips. The upper pole was taken down between clips. Large and small clips were used. The inferior pole was rolled off and vessels there were taken down between clips also. I stayed directly on the gland, did not encounter the parathyroid gland that I could see, and continued to roll the gland out at that point after freeing the superior and inferior poles. I divided the middle thyroid vein between clips; then the branches of the inferior thyroid artery were divided as they spread out onto the gland, being careful to control these between clips and divide. I did not see the recurrent laryngeal nerve, although it could be palpated. The ligament was taken down between clips. Then once we freed the thyroid up onto the isthmus, the isthmus was divided against the left lobe where the Kelly clamp passed across it, and the specimen was handed off to be evaluated by Pathology. I suture ligated beneath the Kelly clamp at the left isthmus. Hemostasis was excellent there. I then irrigated and

GODFREY REGIONAL HOSPITAL
123 Main Street • Aldon, FL 77714 • (407) 555-1234

Continued

OPERATIVE REPORT

Patient information:	
Patient name: DOB: MR#:	Date: Surgeon: Anesthetist:

Preoperative diagnosis:

Postoperative diagnosis:

Procedure(s) performed:

Anesthesia:

Assistant surgeon:

Description of procedure:

aspirated. There was no bleeding in the wound. A Penrose drain was placed on the right, 1/4 inch. I closed the strap muscles in the midline with Vicryl; the platysma flap was closed with 2-0 Vicryl, and the skin with staples. Drain was anchored in the skin with a single Prolene suture.

With the patient still under anesthesia, I went to Pathology and reviewed the frozen section with the pathologist. He felt it was benign by frozen-section criteria.

The patient was then discharged from the operating room to the recovery room in stable condition.

SPECIMEN: Right thyroid lobe, frozen section by Dr. Morris, benign

CONDITION: Stable in PACU; prognosis is excellent

Maurice Doater, MD

GODFREY REGIONAL HOSPITAL
123 Main Street • Aldon, FL 77714 • (407) 555-1234

EXERCISE 12

Level I

OPERATIVE REPORT

Patient information:	
Patient name: DOB: MR#:	Date: Surgeon: Anesthetist:

Preoperative diagnosis:

Traumatic external nasal and internal nasal septal deviation. Deficient nasal tip support. Nasal obstruction.

INDICATION:
69-year-old male who sustained nasal trauma several years ago. Subsequent to that he was left with nasal obstruction. This was never treated. Now present is significant nasal septal deviation with absent nasal tip support.

Postoperative diagnosis:

Same

Procedure(s) performed:

Septoplasty. Columella reconstruction with cartilage graft.

Anesthesia:

Assistant surgeon:

Description of procedure:

After consent was obtained, the patient was taken to the operating room and placed on the operating table in supine position. After an adequate level of general endotracheal anesthesia was obtained, the patient was draped in the appropriate manner for nasal surgery. The patient's nose was prepped with Betadine prep and then draped in a sterile manner. Patient's nose was packed with cotton pledgets soaked with 4% cocaine. After several minutes, an intranasal injection of 1% Xylocaine to 1:100,000 units epinephrine was made. In addition, infiltration was also done in the columella. Nasal hairs were trimmed. Then utilizing a right hemitransfixion incision, bilateral mucoperichondrial and mucoperiosteal flaps were elevated. There was a significant amount of scarring around the cartilaginous septum. There were several fractures in the septum. Portions of the cartilaginous septum were missing. As such, under dissection there were several tears in the mucoperichondrium. Remnants of the cartilaginous septum were removed except for a dorsal strip. Portions of the bony septum were then removed. Spurs off the maxillary crest were also removed. The tears in the mucoperichondrium were reapproximated as best as possible with 4-0 chromic sutures. Attention was then focused on the columella. Utilizing an interior columella incision, the excess tissue at the base of the columella was excised. Excessive scar tissue was excised. Subsequently, a tip support was reconstructed with cartilaginous graft obtained from removed cartilaginous septum remnants. The medial crura were reapproximated with the cartilage graft. The incision was closed with interrupted 4-0

GODFREY REGIONAL HOSPITAL
123 Main Street • Aldon, FL 77714 • (407) 555-1234

Continued

OPERATIVE REPORT

Patient information:	
Patient name: DOB: MR#:	Date: Surgeon: Anesthetist:

Preoperative diagnosis:

Postoperative diagnosis:

Procedure(s) performed:

Anesthesia:

Assistant surgeon:

Description of procedure:

chromic sutures. A hemitransfixion incision was then closed with 4-0 chromic sutures. Sinolastic splints were then placed on both sides of the nasal septum and secured with nylon sutures. The nose was then packed bilaterally with Merocel sponge coated with Bacitracin ointment–infiltrated local solution. Nasal dressings were applied. The patient tolerated the procedure well. There was no break in technique. The patient was extubated and taken to postanesthesia care in good condition.

Fluids administered: 50 cc of RL

Blood loss: Less than 50 cc

Preoperative medication: 12 mg Decadron and 1 gram Ancef IV

Maurice Doater, MD

GODFREY REGIONAL HOSPITAL
123 Main Street • Aldon, FL 77714 • (407) 555-1234

EXERCISE 13

Level I

OPERATIVE REPORT

Patient information:

Patient name: Date:
DOB: Surgeon:
MR#:   Anesthetist:

Preoperative diagnosis:

Chronic right ethmoid and maxillary sinusitis

INDICATION:
77-year-old female with chronic right ethmoid and maxillary sinusitis. This was confirmed on CT scan. Patient opted for surgical treatment.

Postoperative diagnosis:

Same

Procedure(s) performed:

1) Right endoscopic antral ethmoidectomy 2) Right endoscopic maxillary antrostomy with removal of polyp from maxillary sinus

Anesthesia:

Assistant surgeon:

Description of procedure:

After consent was obtained, the patient was taken to the operating room and placed on the operating room table in the supine position. After an adequate level of IV sedation was obtained, the patient was positioned for right-sided sinus surgery. The patient's nose was packed with cotton pledgets soaked with 4% cocaine. After several minutes, 1% Xylocaine with 1:100,000 units epinephrine was infiltrated into the inferior and middle turbinates, as well as in the lateral nasal wall anterior to the medial meatus. Then utilizing the 5° sinuscope, the middle turbinate was medialized. Additional local solution was then infiltrated into the uncinate process. Then, utilizing a sickle knife, biting forceps, and microdebrider, the uncinate process was removed. Hypertrophic mucosa was noted to be filling the area of the lateral nasal wall and the anterior wall of the ethmoid bulla. This was cleared with the microdebrider. This was cleared. Subsequently, the anterior wall of the ethmoid bulla was incised and then the anterior wall was removed with the microdebrider. Hypertrophic mucosa filling the anterior ethmoid air cells was then removed with the microdebrider. The frontal recess area was examined and was found to be clear. The maxillary sinus was then addressed. Thickened mucosa was affecting the ostia. This was incised and thickened polypoid mucosa was removed from the ostia as well as the sinus. The ostia was widened in a posterior-inferior direction. The area was then packed with cotton pledgets soaked with 1:50,000 units of epinephrine. After several minutes, re-inspection showed no active bleeding. The ethmoid cavity was then coated with FloSeal and then several strips of

GODFREY REGIONAL HOSPITAL
123 Main Street • Aldon, FL 77714 • (407) 555-1234

Continued

OPERATIVE REPORT

Patient information:	
Patient name:	Date:
DOB:	Surgeon:
MR#:	Anesthetist:

Preoperative diagnosis:

Postoperative diagnosis:

Procedure(s) performed:

Anesthesia:

Assistant surgeon:

Description of procedure:

Surgicel soaked with local solution. Bacitracin ointment was then applied. Nasal dressing was then applied. Patient tolerated procedure well, and there was no break in technique. Patient was awakened and taken to the recovery room in good condition.

Fluids administered: 500 cc RL

Estimated blood loss: Less than 25 cc

Preoperative medications: 12 mg Decadron IV

Maurice Doates, MD

GODFREY REGIONAL HOSPITAL
123 Main Street • Aldon, FL 77714 • (407) 555-1234

EXERCISE 14

Level I

OPERATIVE REPORT

Patient information:	
Patient name: DOB: MR#:	Date: Surgeon: Anesthetist:

Preoperative diagnosis:

1) Recurrent, and chronic ethmoid and maxillary sinusitis; 2) Bilateral inferior turbinate hypertrophy; 3) Septal deformity; 4) Nasal obstruction

INDICATION:
51-year-old female with history of recurrent and chronic sinusitis, confirmed on exam and CT scan. She also has a nasal

Postoperative diagnosis:

Same

Procedure(s) performed:

1. Bilateral endoscopic anterior ethmoidectomy
2. Bilateral endoscopic maxillary antrostomy
3. Bilateral inferior turbinate reduction with radiofrequency

Anesthesia:

Assistant surgeon:

Description of procedure:

After consent was obtained, the patient was taken to the operating room and placed on the operative table in a supine position. After an adequate level of IV sedation was obtained, the patient was draped in an appropriate manner for a nasal and sinus surgery. The patient's nose was packed with cotton pledgets soaked with 4% cocaine. After several minutes, intranasal injection of 1% Xylocaine with 1:100,000 units epinephrine was made. Nasal hairs were trimmed. Attention first focused on the right side. Utilizing the sinuscope, the middle turbinate was medialized. Local solution was then infiltrated into the uncinate process. A similar procedure was then performed on the left side. Attention then refocused on the right, where utilizing a sickle knife and microdebrider, the uncinate process was removed. The anterior ethmoids were then cleared of hypertrophic mucosa. The maxillary sinus ostia were then cleared of the hypertrophic mucosa and the ostia were widened in the posterior and inferior directions. Retained secretions were suctioned. The area was then packed with cotton pledgets soaked with 1:50,000 units epinephrine. A similar procedure then performed on the left uncinate process, anterior ethmoids, and maxillary sinus ostia. That area was also packed with cotton pledgets soaked with the epinephrine solution. Subsequently, the inferior turbinates were addressed. The anterior mucosa was treated with the radiofrequency to 400 joules on each side. With completion of this, there was an adequate nasal airway. As such, the septoplasty portion was not performed. She had some mild right anterior septal deformity, septal deflection, and also a left superior mid septal

GODFREY REGIONAL HOSPITAL
123 Main Street • Aldon, FL 77714 • (407) 555-1234

Continued

OPERATIVE REPORT

Patient information:	
Patient name:	Date:
DOB:	Surgeon:
MR#:	Anesthetist:

Preoperative diagnosis:

obstruction secondary to bilateral inferior turbinate hypertrophy and a traumatic septal deformity.

Postoperative diagnosis:

Procedure(s) performed:

Anesthesia:

Assistant surgeon:

Description of procedure:

deflection, which at this time did not appear to be obstructing the airway. As such, no further work was done. The ethmoid cavities were then packed lightly with Surgicel and Bacitracin ointment. Nasal dressing was then applied. Patient tolerated the procedure well, and there was no break in technique. Patient was awakened and taken to the recovery room in good condition.

Fluids administered: 800 cc of RL

Estimated blood loss: Less than 25 cc

Preoperative medications: 12 mg of Decadron IV

Maurice Doater, MD

GODFREY REGIONAL HOSPITAL
123 Main Street • Aldon, FL 77714 • (407) 555-1234

EXERCISE 15

Level II

OPERATIVE REPORT

Patient information:

Patient name: Date:
DOB: Surgeon:
MR#:   Anesthetist:

Preoperative diagnosis:

1) Pansinusitis. 2) Bilateral sinonasal polyposis.

INDICATION:
68-year-old male with a several-month history of chronic sinusitis. Examination reveals bilateral sinonasal polyposis. This was confirmed on CT scan with polypoid disease involving all sinuses. The patient also has a nasal deformity for which he does not wish to have revision surgery at this time.

Postoperative diagnosis:

Same

Procedure(s) performed:

1) Bilateral endoscopic nasal polypectomy. 2) Bilateral endoscopic total ethmoidectomy. 3) Bilateral endoscopic frontal sinusotomy. 4) Bilateral endoscopic sphenoidotomy. 5) Bilateral endoscopic maxillary antrostomy with removal of polyps and maxillary sinus.

Anesthesia:

Assistant surgeon:

Description of procedure:

After consent was obtained, the patient was taken to the operating room and placed on the operating room table in supine position. After an adequate level of general endotracheal anesthesia was obtained, the patient was turned and draped in the appropriate manner for sinus surgery. The patient's nose was packed with cotton pledgets soaked with 4% cocaine. After several minutes, 1% Xylocaine with 1:100,000 units of epinephrine was infiltrated into the nasal portion of the polyps bilaterally. Nasal hairs were then trimmed. Then utilizing the microdebrider, a portion of the nasal polyps was removed. Subsequently, local solution was infiltrated into the uncinate processes bilaterally. Then utilizing the sickle knife and microdebrider, the right uncinate process was removed. Subsequently, polyps were noted to be filling the anterior ethmoid air cells. These were removed with the microdebrider. This was followed posteriorly to the sphenoid sinus area. The polyps were cleared from the anterior wall of the sphenoid sinus in the skull base, once identified. Attention was then focused anteriorly where the frontal recess area was cleared of obstructive polyps. The frontal sinus was then cleared of thickened mucus. Attention was then focused on the maxillary sinus. The polyps obstructing the ostia were removed. Ostia were widened in posterior, inferior, and anterior directions. Polyps in the maxillary sinus were also removed. Attention was then focused medial to the middle turbinate where polyps coming from the sphenoid-ethmoid recess were cleared with the microdebrider. The ostia were identified and polyps cleared from the ostia. The ostia were then widened in a medial and inferior direction. Attention was then focused to the posterior ethmoid area, and the inferior portion of the superior turbinate was removed; then the ostia were widened in a lateral direction again inferiorly. The area was then packed with cotton pledgets soaked with 1:50,000 units epinephrine. Attention was then focused on the left side where a similar procedure was performed with removal of the uncinate process, followed by clearing of polyps from the anterior and posterior ethmoids, frontal recess area, and then the frontal sinus, maxillary

GODFREY REGIONAL HOSPITAL
123 Main Street • Aldon, FL 77714 • (407) 555-1234

Continued

OPERATIVE REPORT

Patient information:

Patient name: Date:
DOB: Surgeon:
MR#:   Anesthetist:

Preoperative diagnosis:

Postoperative diagnosis:

Procedure(s) performed:

Anesthesia:

Assistant surgeon:

Description of procedure:

sinus, and then sphenoid sinus. The area on the left was then packed with cotton pledgets soaked with the epinephrine solution. Re-inspection showed some oozing from the ethmoid cavity and sphenoid sinus area bilaterally. Recess area was coated with FloSeal. Surgicel soaked with local solution was then placed on top of this. The middle meatus was then packed bilaterally with Merocel middle meatus stents. This was infiltrated with local solution. Bacitracin ointment was then applied. Nasal dressing was then applied. The patient tolerated the procedure well; there was no break in technique. Patient was extubated and taken to postanesthesia care in good condition.

Fluids administered: 1400 cc RL

Blood loss: 150 cc

Preoperative medications: 12.5 mg Decadron IV

Maurice Doaters, MD

GODFREY REGIONAL HOSPITAL
123 Main Street • Aldon, FL 77714 • (407) 555-1234

EXERCISE 16

Level II

OPERATIVE REPORT

Patient information:	
Patient name:	Date:
DOB:	Surgeon:
MR#:	Anesthetist:

Preoperative diagnosis:

Nasal septal deformity with nasal obstruction due to extensive nasal polyposis, chronic bilateral ethmoid sinusitis. Polypoid degeneration in the middle turbinates bilaterally. Chronic left maxillary sinusitis.

CLINICAL NOTE:
The patient is a 75-year-old white male with severe left nasal septal deviation. He has extensive bilateral nasal polyps and

Postoperative diagnosis:

Nasal septal deformity with nasal obstruction due to extensive nasal polyposis, chronic bilateral ethmoid sinusitis. Polypoid degeneration in the middle turbinates bilaterally. Myosteoma of the left maxillary sinus.

Procedure(s) performed:

Septoplasty, endoscopic bilateral total ethmoidectomies, left middle meatal antrostomy with removal left maxillary sinus myosteoma, bilateral middle turbinate resection. Bilateral extensive nasal polypectomies.

Anesthesia:

General

Assistant surgeon:

Description of procedure:

The patient was brought to the operating room and placed on the operating table in supine position. General endotracheal anesthesia was performed. He received Ancef 1 gram IV perioperatively. Nose was prepped and draped after being injected with 12 cc 1% lidocaine with 1:100,000 parts epinephrine into the nasal septal mucosa, middle turbinates, and lateral nasal mucosa bilaterally. Nose was vasoconstricted with topical Afrin. Left hemitransfixion incision was made on the nasal septum and elevated with the Freer elevator to expose the deviated cartilage and bone. The inferior half of the cartilaginous septum was removed, preserving the nasal spine and caudal septum. This was removed off the maxillary crest. The bony cartilaginous septum was separated with the Freer elevator, and the mucoperiosteum was elevated off the bony septum bilaterally. Using open Jansen-Middleton rongeurs, the mid inferior portions of the bony septum were removed. Further removal with Takahashi forceps of the vomer bone was performed. Using a 3-mm osteotome and mallet, the maxillary crest bone that was deviated severely into the left nasal cavity was removed along the anterior and mid portions of the septum. This completed removal of the deviated bone and cartilage. The left hemitransfixion incision was closed with interrupted 4-0 chromic sutures. Using straight and biting Blakesley forceps, polyps were removed from the left nasal cavity. Left total ethmoidectomy was performed with the same instruments. The degenerated middle turbinate due to polyposis was removed with same instrumentation as well. After completion of total ethmoidectomy and middle turbinectomy and nasal polypectomy, a Bolger probe was used to bluntly enter the left maxillary sinus. Antrostomy was made with the biting forceps to approximately 1 cm in diameter. Using curved suction and cochlea curets, the myosteoma was removed. Specimen was taken through the Lukens trap and sent to Microbiology for fungal culture. A large curved suction was placed in maxillary sinus and irrigated copiously with normal saline and suctioned through a Frazier suction positioned in the posterior nasal pharynx. Approximately 150 cc was

GODFREY REGIONAL HOSPITAL
123 Main Street • Aldon, FL 77714 • (407) 555-1234

Continued

OPERATIVE REPORT

Patient information:	
Patient name:	Date:
DOB:	Surgeon:
MR#:	Anesthetist:

Preoperative diagnosis:

chronic sinusitis. He does not respond to conservative medical treatment. He is being brought to the operating room for these operative procedures. Operative findings showed extensive polyposis filling the left nasal cavities bilaterally and into the ethmoid sinuses bilaterally. The left ostial medial complex was obstructed both by the nasal septal spur from the deviation and by a myosteoma found in the left maxillary sinus. Both middle turbinates showed extensive polypoid degeneration.

Postoperative diagnosis:

Procedure(s) performed:

Anesthesia:

Assistant surgeon:

Description of procedure:

irrigated through the left maxillary sinus until effluent was clear.

Total ethmoidectomy, polypectomy, and middle turbinectomy were performed in similar fashion in the right nasal cavity. After this was completed, Silastic sheeting was cut to size and placed on both sides in nasal septum and sutured into place with 3-0 silk mattress sutures. MeroGel was placed in the posterior ethmoid cavities bilaterally, followed by small Merocel nasal tampons. 10-cm flat nasal tampons impregnated with Bacitracin ointment were placed at the floor of the left and right nasal airways. I sutured the tampons tight across the columella of the nose. Nasal dripper pad was placed. Oropharynx was suctioned. There was adequate hemostasis present.

The patient was awakened from general anesthesia, extubated, and brought to the recovery room in stable condition, having tolerated the procedure well.

ESTIMATED BLOOD LOSS: 200 cc

Maurice Dexter, MD

GODFREY REGIONAL HOSPITAL
123 Main Street • Aldon, FL 77714 • (407) 555-1234

EXERCISE 17

Level II

OPERATIVE REPORT

Patient information:	
Patient name: DOB: MR#:	Date: Surgeon: Anesthetist:

Preoperative diagnosis:

1) Recurrent and chronic ethmoid maxillary sinusitis. 2) Right concha bullosa.

INDICATION:
58-year-old female with chronic postnasal drainage from recurrent and chronic ethmoid and maxillary sinusitis. This was confirmed on CT scan. The patient is admitted now for surgical treatment.

Postoperative diagnosis:

Same

Procedure(s) performed:

1) Bilateral endoscopic antral ethmoidectomy. 2) Bilateral endoscopic maxillary antrostomy. 3) Right endoscopic resection of concha bullosa.

Anesthesia:

Assistant surgeon:

Description of procedure:

After consent was obtained, patient was taken to the operating room and placed on the operating room table in the supine position. After an adequate level of IV sedation was obtained, the patient was positioned and draped for sinus surgery. The patient's nose was packed with cotton pledgets soaked with 4% cocaine. After several minutes, 1% Xylocaine with 1:100,000 units epinephrine was infiltrated into the inferior turbinates bilaterally, middle turbinates bilaterally, and into the lateral wall of the nasal cavity bilaterally just anterior to the medial meatus. Attention was first focused on the right side. Utilizing a 5" sinuscope and the microdebrider, the right concha bullosa was resected in its lateral portion. Subsequently, the uncinate process was infiltrated with local solution. Attention then was focused on the left side where the middle turbinate was medialized and the uncinate process was also injected with local solution. Attention was then refocused on the right side. Utilizing a sickle knife, biting forceps, and microdebrider, the uncinate process was removed. Subsequently, the anterior wall of the ethmoid bulla was removed with the sickle knife and microdebrider; the frontal recess area was examined and was found to be clear of obstruction. Essentially no work was done there. The hypertrophic mucosa and the anterior ethmoid cells were then cleared with the microdebrider. Attention was now focused on the maxillary sinus ostia, which was obstructed by hypertrophic mucosa. This was cleared from the ostia, and the ostia were widened in the posterior inferior direction. Retained secretions were suctioned. The right middle meatus was then packed with cotton

GODFREY REGIONAL HOSPITAL
123 Main Street • Aldon, FL 77714 • (407) 555-1234

Continued

OPERATIVE REPORT

Patient information:	
Patient name:	Date:
DOB:	Surgeon:
MR#:	Anesthetist:

Preoperative diagnosis:

Postoperative diagnosis:

Procedure(s) performed:

Anesthesia:

Assistant surgeon:

Description of procedure:

pledgets soaked with 1:30,000 units of epinephrine. Attention was then focused on the left side. Again utilizing the sickle knife, biting forceps, and microdebrider, the uncinate process was removed. Subsequently, the anterior wall of the ethmoid bulla was also resected with sickle knife and microdebrider. The third frontal recess was examined and was found to be clear. Hypertrophic mucosa in the anterior ethmoid air cells was then cleared with a microdebrider. Attention was then focused on the maxillary sinus ostia, which were cleared of obstructive mucosa. The ostia were widened in a posterior inferior direction. Retained secretions were suctioned. The middle meatus was then packed with cotton pledgets soaked with the epinephrine solution. Re-inspection showed no active bleeding. FloSeal was coated into the ethmoid area bilaterally. Bacitracin ointment was applied. The middle meatus was then packed with the Merocel sponge coated Bacitracin ointment infiltrated in local solution. Nasal dressing was then applied. The patient tolerated the procedure well; there was no break in technique. Patient was awakened and taken to the recovery room in good condition.

Fluids administered: 800 cc of RL

Blood loss: Less than 10 cc

Preoperative medications: 12.5 mg Decadron IV

Maurice Doates, MD

GODFREY REGIONAL HOSPITAL
123 Main Street • Aldon, FL 77714 • (407) 555-1234

EXERCISE 18

Level I

PROCEDURE NOTE

Patient information:

Patient name: Date:
DOB: Surgeon:
MR#:   Anesthetist:

Preoperative diagnosis:

INDICATION:
Shortness of breath, recurrent right pleural effusion, history of bronchogenic carcinoma

The patient was identified by name bracelet prior to procedure. The Pharmaseal thoracentesis kit with catheter was used, sterile technique. 1% local lidocaine and Betadine scrub were used.

Postoperative diagnosis:

Procedure(s) performed:

Thoracentesis

Anesthesia:

Assistant surgeon:

Description of procedure:

FINDINGS:
The right posterior chest was prepped with Betadine, sterile technique. A Pharmaseal catheter was instilled into the right posterior clavicular line, 200 spaces below the scapula, and 1.2 liters of serosanguineous fluid was removed without difficulty. The patient had decreased shortness of breath prior to procedure. The patient tolerated the procedure well. Will check chest x-ray.

Maurice Doates, MD

GODFREY REGIONAL HOSPITAL
123 Main Street • Aldon, FL 77714 • (407) 555-1234

EXERCISE 19

Level I

PROCEDURE NOTE

Patient information:

Patient name: Date:
DOB: Surgeon:
MR#:   Anesthetist:

Preoperative diagnosis:

INDICATION:
Rule out recurrent bronchogenic carcinoma
Patient was identified by name bracelet prior to procedure. Patient had topical lidocaine via the nares and oropharynx prior to procedure. A total of 8 mg of IV Versed was given in 1 mg titrations. Video Olympus bronchoscope was used.

Postoperative diagnosis:

CONCLUSIONS:
1. No endobronchial lesions
2. Transbronchial biopsies and brushings obtained in the right upper lobe density

Procedure(s) performed:

Bronchoscopy

Anesthesia:

Assistant surgeon:

Description of procedure:

FINDINGS:
The bronchoscope was passed via the left naris without difficulty. The epiglottis and aryepiglottic folds were normal in appearance and color. The vocal cords moved equally and approximated with phonation. Bronchoscope was passed into the tracheobronchial tree. Right upper lobe, right middle lobe, and right lower lobe were all patent with no endobronchial lesions seen. Significant mucus was cleared. Left lower lobe and left upper lobe were also patent with no endobronchial lesions seen.

The bronchoscope was taken through the right upper lobe. Then with fluoroscopic guidance, brushings and biopsies were obtained of the density in the right upper lobe. Bleeding stopped spontaneously. The patient tolerated the procedure well.

Maurice Doater, MD

GODFREY REGIONAL HOSPITAL
123 Main Street • Aldon, FL 77714 • (407) 555-1234

EXERCISE 20

Level II

OPERATIVE REPORT

Patient information:

Patient name: Date:
DOB: Surgeon:
MR#:   Anesthetist:

Preoperative diagnosis:

Left vocal cord polyp and possible right vocal cord polyp

Postoperative diagnosis:

Polyps of both left and right vocal cords consistent with papillomas, pathology pending

Procedure(s) performed:

Microdirect laryngoscopy with CO2 laser excision of polyps/papilloma

Anesthesia:

Assistant surgeon:

Description of procedure:

The patient was taken to the operating room and placed in the usual supine position. After induction of general anesthesia via endotracheal intubation, the patient was prepped and draped in the usual fashion for a clean uncontaminated procedure. All precautions, set-up, and preparation of the patient for use with the CO2 laser were taken prior to initiation of the procedure.

The anterior commissure laryngoscope was entered into the oral cavity and passed down to the level of the vocal cords. It was placed into position using the Lewy suspension. The polyp on the left vocal cord was immediately visible. There was a small polyp on the left false vocal cord as well. The right true vocal cord had a small polyp in the very anterior-most region near the anterior commissure. A biopsy of these was taken and sent to Pathology. Grossly, these definitely appeared to be papillomas.

CO2 laser was used to carefully excise the papillomas without injuring the vocal cords themselves. Hemostasis was achieved with Afrin-soaked cottonoids.

The patient tolerated the above procedures well. There were no complications. The patient was subsequently moved directly to the recovery room in stable condition.

COUNTS: Instrument count correct at the end of the procedure

Maurice Doater, MD

GODFREY REGIONAL HOSPITAL
123 Main Street • Aldon, FL 77714 • (407) 555-1234

EXERCISE 21

Level I

PROCEDURE NOTE

Patient information:	
Patient name:	Date:
DOB:	Surgeon:
MR#:	Anesthetist:

Preoperative diagnosis:

HISTORY:
Right lower lobe mass

Postoperative diagnosis:

IMPRESSION:
CT guided biopsy of right lower lung mass

Procedure(s) performed:

CT guided lung biopsy

Anesthesia:

Assistant surgeon:

Description of procedure:

TECHNIQUE:
The patient was positioned supine and an appropriate area of puncture was made over the lower portion of the chest. An appropriate area was cleansed and anesthetized with 3 ccs of 1% Xylocaine. An 18-gauge spring-loaded needle was inserted approximately 4 cm to the right of the midline into a 6×5 cm mass in the right base medially. Three cores of tissue were removed using the co-axial spring-loaded 18-gauge biopsy needle. No bleeding could be seen in the chest after the study and there was no pneumothorax identified. The patient received 1 mg of Versed intravenously for sedation.

Maurice Doater, MD

GODFREY REGIONAL HOSPITAL
123 Main Street • Aldon, FL 77714 • (407) 555-1234

EXERCISE 22

Level I

PROCEDURE NOTE

Patient information:	
Patient name: DOB: MR#:	Date: Surgeon: Anesthetist:

Preoperative diagnosis:

INDICATIONS:
Large left symptomatic pleural effusion, history of breast carcinoma with widespread metastasis

Postoperative diagnosis:

Procedure(s) performed:

Thoracentesis

Anesthesia:

Assistant surgeon:

Description of procedure:

The patient was identified by name bracelet prior to the procedure. The procedure was done on the fourth floor in the hospital as an outpatient. A Pharmaseal thoracentesis kit was used with aspirating catheter. The patient was prepped in the posterior position with Betadine, and the catheter was advanced into the intercostal space, the mid clavicular line, two interspaces below the scapula after 1% local lidocaine anesthesia. 1 liter of cloudy amber fluid was removed. The patient had some mild chest tightness so no further fluid was removed at this time.

Marked decrease in shortness of breath. The patient tolerated the procedure well. Study was sent for cytology, chemistry, and micro.

Maurice Doater, MD

GODFREY REGIONAL HOSPITAL
123 Main Street • Aldon, FL 77714 • (407) 555-1234

EXERCISE 23

Level I

PROCEDURE NOTE

Patient information:

Patient name:	Date:
DOB:	Surgeon:
MR#:	Anesthetist:

Preoperative diagnosis:

HISTORY:
Ultrasound guidance

Postoperative diagnosis:

IMPRESSION:
Ultrasound guidance for placement of empyema drainage catheters in the right chest as described below

Procedure(s) performed:

U/S guide for thoracentesis and chest tube placement

Anesthesia:

Assistant surgeon:

Description of procedure:

ULTRASOUND GUIDANCE:
An area of loculated fluid collection was seen in the right posterior lower chest. An area was anesthetized appropriately using 9 cc of Xylocaine 2%. The area was punctured using an 18-gauge needle, and a guide wire was placed. This was done at 2 separate locations. Dilatation was performed using a 9 French dilator. An 8.5 French drainage catheter was inserted into the area of abnormality on each side with attempt at breaking up the loculations. The pus was withdrawn from both catheters. Approximately 100 cc of yellowish pus without odor was removed. Two mg of TPA was injected, 10 cc on each side. This was left in position for one hour, and a drain was placed. The patient is to return in 3 days for follow up.

Maurice Doater, MD

GODFREY REGIONAL HOSPITAL
123 Main Street • Aldon, FL 77714 • (407) 555-1234

EXERCISE 24

Level I

PROCEDURE NOTE

Patient information:	
Patient name: DOB: MR#:	Date: Surgeon: Anesthetist:

Preoperative diagnosis:

HISTORY:
Lung nodule

Postoperative diagnosis:

IMPRESSION:
CT guided lung biopsy

Procedure(s) performed:

CT guided lung biopsy

Anesthesia:

Assistant surgeon:

Description of procedure:

TECHNIQUE:
The patient was positioned prone on the table, and images were obtained, demonstrating the area of abnormality. An appropriate area of puncture was made. The skin was cleaned and the area anesthetized with 3 cc of 1% Xylocaine. A co-axial 18-gauge spring-loaded needle was inserted into the lesion; three cores of tissue were removed. No pneumothorax was seen after the procedure. The specimens were sent to the lab for appropriate analysis.

Maurice Doates, MD

GODFREY REGIONAL HOSPITAL
123 Main Street • Aldon, FL 77714 • (407) 555-1234

EXERCISE 25

Level I

EMERGENCY ROOM RECORD

Name:	Age:	ER physician:
	DOB:	Robert Rais

Allergies/type of reaction:	Usual medications/dosages:

Triage/presenting complaint:　　CC: Nosebleed on anticoagulants

Patient complains that immediately prior to arrival, she experienced a nosebleed, unable to stop.

Initial assessment:

ROS: Negative for chest pain, dyspnea, negative excessive bruising, fever, nausea, dizziness, syncope, vomiting
PMH/SH: Negative

Time	T	P	R	BP	Other:					

Medication orders:

Lab work:

X-ray:

Physician's report:

EXAM:
Vital signs are noted, patient appears well nourished, in mild distress

HEENT: Nose, dried blood right anterior nasal mucosa. Fresh clots right anterior nasal mucosa.
Pharynx: Unremarkable.
Chest: No visible signs of trauma
CV: All distal pulses are 2+
MS: Normal ROM, no swelling or deformities
Neuro: Alert, oriented to person, time, and place

TREATMENT:
Clots were cleared from nasal passages and oozing of flow continued. Both nares were treated with cauterization and the bleeding appeared to be well controlled at that time.

Diagnosis:	Physician sign/date
Anterior epistaxis	*Robert Rais MD*

Discharge	Transfer	Admit	Good	Satisfactory	Other:	

GODFREY REGIONAL HOSPITAL
123 Main Street • Aldon, FL 77714 • (407) 555-1234

CARDIOVASCULAR EXERCISES

EXERCISE 1

Level I

OPERATIVE REPORT

Patient information:	
Patient name: DOB: MR#:	Date: Surgeon: Anesthetist:

Preoperative diagnosis:

Metastatic colon cancer

Postoperative diagnosis:

Metastatic colon cancer

Procedure(s) performed:

1. Placement of a right internal jugular single chamber.
2. Infuse-A-Port placed onto the right anterior chest wall.

Anesthesia:

Assistant surgeon:

Description of procedure:

The patient is a very pleasant 65-year-old male who recently presented to my office with a history of colon cancer and is undergoing chemotherapy. He has very poor peripheral IV access and he presents for the above procedure.

OPERATIVE PROCEDURE:
The patient was taken to the operating room and placed in a supine position on the operating table. After adequate IV sedation was achieved, the patient's right neck and upper chest were prepped and draped in standard surgical fashion. Using 1% lidocaine, I carefully anesthetized an area over the anterior border, sternocleidomastoid muscle, as well as onto the anterior chest wall. Using a Seldinger technique, a guidewire was placed into the right internal jugular vein to the superior vena cava. This was verified using intraoperative fluoroscopy. I then made a pocket under the right anterior chest wall using the 15-blade and electric Bovie cautery, and created it so that the Infuse-A-Port would fit comfortably into the pocket. Then using the dilator introducer system, these were placed over the guidewire into the internal jugular vein. The guidewire and dilator were then removed, and the catheter itself was threaded into the superior vena cava. Again its position was verified using intraoperative fluoroscopy. I then used the tunneling device and tunneled the catheter onto the anterior chest wall, hooked it up to the Infuse-A-Port, placed the Infuse-A-Port into the pocket. I ensured that the Infuse-A-Port

GODFREY REGIONAL HOSPITAL
123 Main Street • Aldon, FL 77714 • (407) 555-1234

Continued

OPERATIVE REPORT

Patient information:	
Patient name: DOB: MR#:	Date: Surgeon: Anesthetist:

Preoperative diagnosis:

Postoperative diagnosis:

Procedure(s) performed:

Anesthesia:

Assistant surgeon:

Description of procedure:

worked properly using heparinized saline, both aspirating and then flushing. I then closed the pocket using a 3-0 Vicryl suture and the skin was closed with subcuticular 4-0 Monocryl. The neck incision was also closed with subcuticular 4-0 Monocryl. Benzoin and Steri-strips were placed over the incision.

The patient tolerated the procedure very well and returned to the recovery room in good condition.

Ruth Brady Mr

GODFREY REGIONAL HOSPITAL
123 Main Street • Aldon, FL 77714 • (407) 555-1234

EXERCISE 2

Level II

OPERATIVE REPORT

Patient information:

Patient name: Date:
DOB: Surgeon:
MR#:   Anesthetist:

Preoperative diagnosis:

End-stage renal disease, nonmaturation of left arm AV-fistula

CLINICAL HISTORY: The patient is status post left arm AV fistula. She has nonmaturation. Fistulogram shows one moderate size tributary just proximal anastomosis. She presents for elective ligation.

Postoperative diagnosis:

Same

Procedure(s) performed:

Ligation of AV-fistula tributaries

Anesthesia:

Assistant surgeon:

Description of procedure:

DESCRIPTION OF THE PROCEDURE:
The patient had three tributaries marked by ultrasound. One was close to the anastomosis; the other two were more proximal at the arm. We prepped and draped her left arm, anesthetized skin and subcu tissue with local. We dissected down and found the proximal tributary, ligated it, and stapled it. The fistula was still patent after we ligated the tributary. We could not find the more proximal tributary despite dissecting out the fistula for 2 cm. Rather than risk injuring the fistula, I did not proceed with attempts at finding a tributary. We did not attempt to locate the most proximal tributary either. We irrigated the two opened incisions and closed the skin with interrupted 4-0 Biosyn and placed sterile dressing.

The patient is to follow up in one month.

Ruth Brady Mr

GODFREY REGIONAL HOSPITAL
123 Main Street • Aldon, FL 77714 • (407) 555-1234

EXERCISE 3

Level II

OPERATIVE REPORT

Patient information:	
Patient name: DOB: MR#:	Date: Surgeon: Anesthetist:

Preoperative diagnosis:

Diatek cath

Postoperative diagnosis:

Procedure(s) performed:

Left Diatek catheter insertion

HISTORY: Malfunction of catheter

Anesthesia:

Assistant surgeon:

Description of procedure:

TECHNIQUE:
The examination was done through the existing tract of the left-sided catheter. A stiff guidewire was initially inserted through the catheter, but the catheter could not be withdrawn. A 0.035 angled Glidewire was inserted through the catheter, and again the indwelling catheter could not be withdrawn. Multiple attempts to release the catheter were unsuccessful. The skin between the exit incision and the internal jugular vein was entered and the catheter removed in its mid-portion and cut. The wire was then inserted through this area for better manipulation. After numerous attempts, the catheter was withdrawn over the wire. The Diatek catheter was then inserted over the wire to the appropriate position. The patient received 1 gram of Ancef intravenously at the start of the procedure, and the old and new tracks of the catheters were flushed with a solution of 1 gram of Ancef and 1 liter of normal saline. The position of the catheter was checked at the termination of the procedure by fluoroscopy. Less than one hour of fluoroscopy time was used for the procedure.

IMPRESSION: Insertion of left-sided Diatek tunneled catheter under fluoroscopic guidance.

Ruth Brady MD

GODFREY REGIONAL HOSPITAL
123 Main Street • Aldon, FL 77714 • (407) 555-1234

EXERCISE 4

Level II

OPERATIVE REPORT

Patient information:

Patient name: Date:
DOB: Surgeon:
MR#:   Anesthetist:

Preoperative diagnosis:

Left leg and thigh, symptomatic varicose veins

Postoperative diagnosis:

Same

Procedure(s) performed:

Varicose vein stripping and ligation of left leg and thigh—primarily lesser, but partial greater saphenous systems

Anesthesia:

Assistant surgeon:

Description of procedure:

The patient was placed in the sitting position for the spinal and then placed supine and in slight Trendelenburg, sterilely prepped and draped. The veins had been marked in the preoperative area. Each marked vein was approached in the following fashion: The skin was incised transversely with a number 11 blade. The vein was teased out. If there were perforator veins or terminal veins, these were ligated with 3-0 Vicryl; otherwise, they were sequentially dissected towards the next mark and then a counter incision was made to connect the dissections. In the lower leg, the veins were small and friable. In the upper thigh, the veins were quite sizable and thick. In this fashion veins were resected from the leg both anteriorly and posteriorly, as well as a significant system on the lateral aspect and on to the thigh initially, laterally, at the knee and extending medially on the more proximal thigh. Every mark had an identified vein that was resected. Skin was closed with 4-0 nylon in interrupted vertical mattress fashion. These were then dressed with Telfa, gauze, Kerlix, and Ace wrap.

She tolerated the procedure well.

[signature] Ruth Brady MD

GODFREY REGIONAL HOSPITAL
123 Main Street • Aldon, FL 77714 • (407) 555-1234

Level II

OPERATIVE REPORT

Patient information:	
Patient name: DOB: MR#:	Date: Surgeon: Anesthetist:

Preoperative diagnosis:

End-stage renal disease; infected Ash catheter

CLINICAL HISTORY: The patient is a 68-year-old white male who was undergoing dialysis. His Ash catheter became infected and required removal. He now presents for a Quinton catheter in his femoral vein.

Postoperative diagnosis:

End-stage renal disease; infected Ash catheter

Procedure(s) performed:

Left femoral Quinton catheter placement

Anesthesia:

Assistant surgeon:

Description of procedure:

The patient was brought to Ambulatory Care, placed in the supine position; right groin was prepped and draped in sterile fashion. We attempted to gain access to right femoral vein, but instead placed the needle into the femoral artery. We were using ultrasound, but the artery and vein were very close together. Patient had some edema from the prior catheter. We held pressure and aborted the procedure after one arterial stick. We then shaved and prepped the left groin and attempted to place the catheter in the left groin. Again, we incurred an arterial puncture. Patient developed a small hematoma. We aborted the left femoral approach. We then attempted the right IJ vein. We were able to gain access but could not thread the guidewire due to a thrombus in the vein. We aborted this procedure, then re-evaluated. The swelling in the left groin had diminished. We again did the ultrasound of the groin and we were able to see the vein with the ultrasound. We prepped and draped and were able to percutaneously enter the left femoral vein without puncturing the artery. We placed the guidewire dilator over the guidewire and then placed the catheter over the guidewire. We sutured it in place and flushed it. It flushed easily.

Plan is to get vancomycin again today, 1 gram. He had only gotten it one time, even though I ordered it with every dialysis; I told the dialysis tech that he needs it with every dialysis. I talked with his primary care physician and our long-term plan is to place a left forearm graft. I will look into the availability for immediate-use graft. If one is not available, we will use the Gore-Tex and wait two weeks to start accessing it.

The patient was transferred to the recovery room in good condition.

Ruth Brady MD

GODFREY REGIONAL HOSPITAL
123 Main Street • Aldon, FL 77714 • (407) 555-1234

EXERCISE 6

Level II

OPERATIVE REPORT

Patient information:	
Patient name:	Date:
DOB:	Surgeon:
MR#:	Anesthetist:

Preoperative diagnosis:

Renal failure, infected Ash catheter

CLINICAL HISTORY: The patient presented with swelling around his catheter several days ago. It was infected. We took it out. Today, he has some erythema around his site, but no pain. I could not expel anything from the tract. I tried several times, but nothing came out, so we did not need to open it. He presents now for right femoral in-and-out Quinton catheter, which we will do for a couple of weeks until we can replace either another Ash catheter or put some sort of arm graft into his arm.

Postoperative diagnosis:

Renal failure, infected Ash catheter

Procedure(s) performed:

Right femoral Quinton catheter placement, 20 cm

Anesthesia:

Assistant surgeon:

Description of procedure:

DESCRIPTION OF PROCEDURE:
The patient was placed in the supine position and his right groin was shaved, then prepped and draped in sterile fashion. We anesthetized the skin and subcu tissue with lidocaine, made a skin nick with the scalpel, and under ultrasound guidance, skin of the right femoral vein was located. We placed a guidewire through the needle, dilated over the guidewire, and then placed a 20-cm Quinton catheter over the guidewire. We flushed with saline and heparin and sutured it in place.

We placed a sterile dressing. Patient is to get dialysis today, then have the catheter removed and come back Wednesday for another catheter.

Ruth Brady MD

GODFREY REGIONAL HOSPITAL
123 Main Street • Aldon, FL 77714 • (407) 555-1234

EXERCISE 7

Level I

OPERATIVE REPORT

Patient information:

Patient name:
DOB:
MR#:

Date:
Surgeon:
Anesthetist:

Preoperative diagnosis:

1. End of life pacemaker
2. CVR

Postoperative diagnosis:

1. End of life pacemaker
2. CVR

Procedure(s) performed:

Insertion of permanent pacemaker; lead analysis and pulse generator placement

Anesthesia:

Assistant surgeon:

Description of procedure:

With the patient placed on the operating room table, the patient was prepped and draped in the usual fashion. A small incision was made over the previous scar, and we extruded the pulse generator and disimplanted the leads. Atrial lead is #4058, serial #02500; ventricular lead was model #4262, serial #060719. The threshold in the atrium impedance was 52 ohms; there was flutter. No other thresholds were obtained. The ventricular threshold was 0.7 volts, 1.2 MA and 630 ohms. R wave was 9.1.

The pacemaker was model Meridiem DR, Model #1276, serial number 415811. This was DDD mode, upper rate of 120, lower of 60. AV delay 150 milliseconds, amplitude 3.5 volts. Pulse width is 0.4 milliseconds, 0.75 millivolts. Atrial and ventricular, 2.5 millivolts. The pocket was irrigated and the closure was done in layers of Vicryl and nylon for the skin.

The patient was transferred to the recovery room in good condition.

GODFREY REGIONAL HOSPITAL
123 Main Street • Aldon, FL 77714 • (407) 555-1234

EXERCISE 8

Level I

OPERATIVE REPORT

Patient information:	
Patient name:	Date:
DOB:	Surgeon:
MR#:	Anesthetist:

Preoperative diagnosis:

Symptomatic left leg varicose veins

Postoperative diagnosis:

Left leg and thigh varicose veins involving the lesser and greater saphenous systems

Procedure(s) performed:

Left leg and thigh varicose vein stripping and ligation involving lesser saphenous systems

Anesthesia:

Assistant surgeon:

Description of procedure:

The patient was placed in the sitting position for placement of a spinal and then was placed supine and sterilely prepped and draped. Multiple testings were accomplished, and it did not appear that the spinal had any take. Therefore, general anesthesia was induced, and we proceeded. The veins had been marked in the preoperative area. At each marked site, a small incision was made with a No. 11 blade, and the vein was isolated with a hemostat or vein hook. The veins were then traced out distally and proximally. Segments that appeared to be perforating or went into unmarked areas of the leg were ligated with 2-0 Vicryl. In this way, sequential incisions were made up the veins to remove all the marked veins. She had enormous veins, particularly on the lateral aspect of the leg, knee, and anterior thigh. There were smaller veins on the medial thigh, posterior calf, and left lateral thigh. After all the marked veins were removed, the defects were closed with 3-0 nylon in interrupted vertical mattress fashion. These were then dressed with Telfa, gauze, Kerlix, and Ace wraps.

She tolerated the procedure well. All needle, sponge, and instrument counts were reported as correct.

Ruth Budy Mr

GODFREY REGIONAL HOSPITAL
123 Main Street • Aldon, FL 77714 • (407) 555-1234

GASTROINTESTINAL EXERCISES

EXERCISE 1

Level I

OPERATIVE REPORT

Patient information:	
Patient name: DOB: MR#:	CONSENT: Informed consent obtained from the patient after full disclosure of risks and indications to the patient.

Preoperative diagnosis:

Diarrhea. History of colon cancer.

Postoperative diagnosis:

See findings below.

Procedure(s) performed:

Colonoscopy with hot biopsies and cold biopsies

Anesthesia:

Assistant surgeon:

Description of procedure:

After obtaining an informed consent, the patient was brought to the OR and put in the left lateral position. IV line was maintained. IV sedation was given. Vitals were monitored throughout the procedure, which included pulse, pulse oximetry, blood pressure, level of consciousness, and EKG monitoring. Digital rectal examination was done, which showed normal anal tone, no tags, and no hemorrhoids. Scope was introduced and advanced all the way up to the cecum, identified by ileocecal valve and appendicular orifice and entering into the terminal ileum. Patient had lots of stool spread all over, some of this solid, especially in proximal colon. This was washed away repeatedly. Watched colonic mucosa carefully. However, small polyps could have been missed. There was a very small polyp at hepatic flexure, which was biopsied. Terminal ileum appeared normal. Cecum appeared normal. The distal colon area, rectosigmoid, and descending colon appeared a little inflamed. Multiple random biopsies were taken. Biopsy was also taken from the terminal ileum. She had very small to moderate-sized internal hemorrhoids. The rest of the examination revealed normal mucosa. No masses. No AV malformation. No other polyps seen.

FINDINGS:
1. Small polyp in hepatic flexure, hot biopsied and sent for histopathology with good fulguration of the base.
2. Biopsy from the terminal ileum.

GODFREY REGIONAL HOSPITAL
123 Main Street • Aldon, FL 77714 • (407) 555-1234

Continued

OPERATIVE REPORT

Patient information:

Patient name:
DOB:
MR#:

Preoperative diagnosis:

Postoperative diagnosis:

Procedure(s) performed:

Anesthesia:

Assistant surgeon:

Description of procedure:

3. Erythematous and inflamed-appearing mucosa in the distal colon, especially in the rectal area. Biopsies taken and sent for histopathology from both areas.
4. Poor prep. She had some solid stools spread all over, which were washed away. Mild small to moderate-sized internal hemorrhoids, non-bleeding and non-thrombosed.

PLAN:
Follow up with biopsy results.

Patk Adam MD

GODFREY REGIONAL HOSPITAL
123 Main Street • Aldon, FL 77714 • (407) 555-1234

EXERCISE 2

Level II

OPERATIVE REPORT

Patient information:
Patient name: DOB: MR#:

Preoperative diagnosis:
Left inguinal pain five years after left inguinal herniorrhaphy INDICATIONS: This is a 27-year-old male who has returned to my clinic multiple times complaining of left-sided inguinal pain. He'd had a bilateral inguinal herniorrhaphy five years ago, and then about 2 months or so ago, was lifting something heavy at work and felt

Postoperative diagnosis:
Same FINDINGS: Mesh is intact, negative groin exploration. Of note is that he had a previous McVay with mesh placed over the top. Even with the patient straining and coughing, I couldn't feel any defects or problem with the mesh.

Procedure(s) performed:
Left inguinal exploration

Anesthesia:

Assistant surgeon:

Description of procedure:
The patient was brought to the operating room and placed in a supine position on the operating room table. Anesthesia and some sedation were given. The patient's left groin was prepped and draped in the usual sterile fashion. After the administration of appropriate operative antibiotics, 1% lidocaine mixed with 0.25% Marcaine was used to anesthetize an area in the left groin. An ilioinguinal block was placed. The old incision was re-opened and the dissection was carried sharply down to the external oblique, which was, with some difficulty, dissected free along its anterior extent. The external ring was located and the external oblique opened in line with its fibers, beginning at the external ring. Spermatic cord was isolated, looped, and drawn up. The mesh was palpable beneath. It seemed to be solid; in fact, with patient coughing and straining, there was no defect in the mesh whatsoever. I did feel at both the neo-internal ring of the mesh and at the pubic tubercle as well as all the areas in between. Again, with the patient straining and coughing, there was no palpable hernia defect on direct palpation of his repair mesh. Hemostasis was achieved. The external oblique was closed in a running fashion with 2-0 Vicryl. The skin was closed in a running fashion with 4-0 Monocryl subcuticular stitch. Steri-Strips and a sterile dressing were applied. The patient was taken to the PACU in good condition.

GODFREY REGIONAL HOSPITAL
123 Main Street • Aldon, FL 77714 • (407) 555-1234

Continued

OPERATIVE REPORT

Patient information:

Patient name:
DOB:
MR#:

Preoperative diagnosis:

what he thought was some tearing and began to have pain in his left groin. Despite rest and nonsteroidal antiinflammatory drugs, he has not been able to resolve this pain. I have examined him multiple times in clinic and can feel no obvious hernia. He is tender in the area. I told him that although his exploration could possibly be negative, I thought that with his persistent pain we could go ahead and explore his left groin.

Postoperative diagnosis:

Procedure(s) performed:

Anesthesia:

Assistant surgeon:

Description of procedure:

[signature] Patk Adam MD

GODFREY REGIONAL HOSPITAL
123 Main Street • Aldon, FL 77714 • (407) 555-1234

EXERCISE 3

Level I

OPERATIVE REPORT

Patient information:

Patient name:
DOB:
MR#:

CONSENT:
Informed consent obtained from the patient after full
disclosure of risks and indications to the patient.

Preoperative diagnosis:

Colonic polyps seen on air contrast barium enema in the sigmoid colon

Postoperative diagnosis:

ASSESSMENT:
1. Abnormal appearing fold/area in the cecum with surface appearing as a cauliflower sessile
2. Two sigmoid polyps, one pedunculated and one sessile, both snared and sent for histopathology
3. Moderate sized internal hemorrhoids

Procedure(s) performed:

Colonoscopy with hot biopsy and polypectomy with snare

Anesthesia:

Assistant surgeon:

Description of procedure:

After obtaining informed consent, the patient was brought to the OR and put in the left lateral position. IV line was maintained.
IV sedation was given and vitals were monitored throughout the procedure that included pulse, pulse oximetry, blood
pressure, respiratory rate, level of consciousness, and ECG monitoring. Digital rectal examination was done first, and then
colonoscope Olympus GIF 140 was introduced and advanced all the way up to the cecum, identified by ileocecal valve and
appendicular orifice. Of note of importance, she does have a lot of twist, almost a 360° twist in the area of transverse and
descending colon, and also in the proximal ascending colon as well. Beyond the cecal valve was an area which appeared to
be flat with cauliflower-looking appearance on top of which was an almost flat lesion, no pedicle, spread over approximately
0.8 mm in size in cross-section. No ulceration observed. It was a little bit friable, and I took a few biopsies, hot and cold, from
that area. A minimum amount of blood oozing. The rest of the colon appeared normal. She had a few pockets of stools that
were washed away. In the area of the sigmoid region, two polyps were identified, which were seen on air contrast barium
enema. Both were in close approximation and were snared in toto and retrieved with suction. The rest of the colon was entirely
normal. She does have moderate sized internal hemorrhoids.

PLAN:
Follow up with Pathology. Follow up in clinic in one to two weeks.

Patrik Adam MD

GODFREY REGIONAL HOSPITAL
123 Main Street • Aldon, FL 77714 • (407) 555-1234

EXERCISE 4

Level I

OPERATIVE REPORT

Patient information:	
Patient name: DOB: MR#:	CONSENT: An informed consent was obtained from the patient and his father after explaining the risks, indications, and possible complications.

Preoperative diagnosis:

15-year-old with chronic pyrosis and now losing weight; diarrhea

Postoperative diagnosis:

See findings below.

Procedure(s) performed:

Esophagogastroduodenoscopy

Anesthesia:

Assistant surgeon:

Description of procedure:

After obtaining an informed consent, the patient was brought to the OR, put in the left lateral position. IV line was maintained and IV sedation was given. Vitals were monitored throughout the procedure, which included pulse, pulse oximetry, blood pressure, level of consciousness, and EKG monitoring. Mouth was sprayed with Cetacaine and then mouth block was applied. Esophagogastroduodenoscopy scope was passed in the mouth and easily intubated. Visually guided in the esophagus. The proximal esophagus showed longitudinal ulcer with clean margins at 16 cm. Scope was further advanced. No stricture or masses seen. The distal esophagus appeared normal. Scope was further advanced into the stomach. Rugae appeared normal, which flattened out normally on insufflation. The scope was advanced all the way to pylorus that appeared normal in size and shape. No distortion noticed. Scope was pushed into the duodenal bulb, which appeared normal, and scope was advanced beyond the 3rd part of the duodenum. A couple of biopsies were taken from the small bowel mucosa. Scope was withdrawn all the way back into the antrum. Retroflexion was done. Incisura appeared normal. The scope was dropped down into the fundus and body, both of which appear normal. The scope was straightened out, pulled back all the way up to the GE junction. Excess air was suctioned out. Then re-examined the esophageal ulcer at 16 cm, which extends from 16 to 17 cm, in a longitudinal fashion. One biopsy was taken. However, the patient had difficulty at this time with constant retching. Unable to do any more biopsies. This halted the procedure at this time and the scope was taken out.

GODFREY REGIONAL HOSPITAL
123 Main Street • Aldon, FL 77714 • (407) 555-1234

Continued

OPERATIVE REPORT

Patient information:
Patient name: DOB: MR#:

Preoperative diagnosis:

Postoperative diagnosis:

Procedure(s) performed:

Anesthesia:

Assistant surgeon:

Description of procedure:

FINDINGS:
1. Esophageal ulcer at 16 cm, extending all the way to 17 cm, longitudinal, non-bleeding with clear margins
2. Otherwise normal esophagogastroduodenoscopy with excessive reflux seen on endoscopy

PLAN:
Continue with Prevacid, follow up with biopsy results. Based on the biopsy results, may need another endoscopy after treating with PPI in the next couple of weeks.

Patk Adam MD

GODFREY REGIONAL HOSPITAL
123 Main Street • Aldon, FL 77714 • (407) 555-1234

EXERCISE 5

Level II

OPERATIVE REPORT

Patient information:

Patient name:
DOB:
MR#:

CONSENT:
Informed consent obtained from the patient after full disclosure of risks and indications to the patient.

Preoperative diagnosis:

Chronic pyrosis. Family history of colon cancer.

Postoperative diagnosis:

See impressions below.

Procedure(s) performed:

Colonoscopy with polypectomies and hot biopsies. Upper endoscopy with biopsy.

Anesthesia:

Assistant surgeon:

Description of procedure:

After obtaining an informed consent, patient was brought to the OR and placed in the left lateral position. Digital rectal examination was done. IV sedation was given. Vitals were monitored throughout the procedure, which included pulse, pulse oximetry, blood pressure, respiratory rate, level of consciousness, ECG monitoring. Colonoscope was introduced in advance all the way up to the cecum, in fact, by ileocecal valve and appendicular orifice. On the way up, had noticed in areas of the sigmoid and the rectum two polyps. Cecum was identified by ileocecal valve and appendicular orifice. Scope was carefully withdrawn. In the descending colon, two small polyps were identified, which were hot-biopsied and totally fulgurated. Good hemostasis and photo documentation obtained. The scope was withdrawn into the sigmoid colon, where there was a large pedunculated polyp. Photo documentation obtained. A small biopsy was taken from the tip of the polyp. Snare was put in. Polyp was snared in toto. Tissue retrieved. Scope was then pulled down into the rectal area. There were two polyps; both were snared. Tissue sent for histopathology. Retroflexion showed large internal hemorrhoids with some tags. No attempt to biopsy them. Scope was taken out. Prep was good. The rest of the examination was within normal limits. Examination was satisfactory.

Mouth was sprayed with Cetacaine. IV sedation was given, totaling the dose as described above. With some difficulty, was able to pass scope through the mouth, into esophagus and was advanced all the way into the antrum. He does have a long J-shaped stomach with antrum slightly distorted. However, easily entered into the duodenum. Showed severe duodenitis with lots of edema with at least two pseudo-polyps identified with a central ulceration. Biopsies were taken from the edges of the polyps. Then the scope was withdrawn into the antrum. The antrum looks a little bit deformed. Photo documentation obtained. CLOtest biopsy was taken in the antral area, which showed a few ulcerations as well. Retroflexion revealed two ulcers, healed, on the incisura. Biopsies were taken from one of the ulcers. They were small, non-bleeding. Then the scope was dropped into the body. This showed some atrophic gastritis, but no evidence of any inflammation or any ulcers. Scope was straightened out and

GODFREY REGIONAL HOSPITAL
123 Main Street • Aldon, FL 77714 • (407) 555-1234

Continued

OPERATIVE REPORT

Patient information:

Patient name:
DOB:
MR#:

Preoperative diagnosis:

Postoperative diagnosis:

Procedure(s) performed:

Anesthesia:

Assistant surgeon:

Description of procedure:

pulled up to the GE junction. He has a hiatal hernia approximately 43 cm to 39 cm. Mild distal esophagitis. No evidence of any salmon-colored mucosa seen. In the mid esophagus, he had a bleb appearing like a varix. This was surrounded by a little erythema. Biopsy not attempted, as could be a blood vessel. Scope was further withdrawn. A careful look at the vocal cords appeared normal. Scope was taken out.

FINDINGS:
COLONOSCOPY:
1. Two small polyps from the descending colon, both hot-biopsied and sent for histopathology.
2. A large polyp with thick pedicle from sigmoid colon, which was snared in toto and sent for histopathology.
3. Two rectal polyps, one medium sized and one small. Both were snared and sent for histopathology.
4. Large internal hemorrhoids. Small external hemorrhoids.
5. Prep was good. The rest of the examination was essentially normal.

UPPER ENDOSCOPY:
1. Severe duodenitis with edema and ulceration, non-bleeding, well healed with white formation (appears to look like two polyps). Biopsies were taken and sent for histopathology.
2. Antral gastritis with some deformity in the pylorus, CLO test biopsy taken.
3. Ulcers on the incisura are well-healed and non-bleeding. Small in size and two in number; biopsy taken.

GODFREY REGIONAL HOSPITAL
123 Main Street • Aldon, FL 77714 • (407) 555-1234

Continued

OPERATIVE REPORT

Patient information:
Patient name: DOB: MR#:

Preoperative diagnosis:

Postoperative diagnosis:

Procedure(s) performed:

Anesthesia:

Assistant surgeon:

Description of procedure:

4. The rest of the stomach showed atrophic mucosa.
5. Hiatal hernia approximately 3 cm in size, non-inflamed from 41 to 39 cm.
6. Mild distal esophagitis.
7. Varix-like vessel appearing cystic lesion in the mid esophagus with surrounding erythema. Biopsy not taken.

PLAN:
COLONOSCOPY:
Follow up with biopsy results. May need colonoscopy in 1 to 2 years for chronic pyrosis, most likely related to his peptic ulcer disease. He has duodenal ulcers. Will re-endoscope to look for duodenal polyps if they persist, even after treatment and on H2 blockers. May need to be snared.

UPPER ENDOSCOPY:
Also will get an esophagogram to delineate further the polyps/varix seen in the upper esophagus. That also needs further endoscopy in the next 4 to 8 weeks.

Patk Adam MD

GODFREY REGIONAL HOSPITAL
123 Main Street • Aldon, FL 77714 • (407) 555-1234

EXERCISE 6

Level I

OPERATIVE REPORT

Patient information:

Patient name:
DOB:
MR#:

CONSENT:
Informed consent obtained from the patient after full disclosure of risks and indications to the patient.

Preoperative diagnosis:

Hematochezia with weight loss

Postoperative diagnosis:

See findings below.

Procedure(s) performed:

Colonoscopy with biopsies

Anesthesia:

Assistant surgeon:

Description of procedure:

After obtaining informed consent, the patient was brought into the OR and put in the left lateral position. IV line maintained. IV sedation was given and vitals were monitored throughout the procedure, which included pulse, pulse oximetry, blood pressure, level of consciousness, and EKG monitoring. First digital rectal examination was done, and then Olympus 140 colonoscope was introduced into the rectum and advanced all the way up to the cecum, identified by the ileocecal valve and appendical orifice. There were lots of areas of pockets of stools, solid stools, which were washed away. Examination was fair; prep was fair. In the cecum there was an abnormal area of cecal fold that was biopsied; appeared to be inflamed, no polyps. The rest of the examination essentially was within normal limits. In the rectal area there was one abnormal-appearing fold with polypoid appearance to it, a flat lesion with shiny mucosa. It was hot-biopsied, and ulceration was seen. There are no masses, no tumors, and no AV malformation. She does have a moderate-sized internal hemorrhoid. Scope was taken out.

FINDINGS:
1. Abnormal cecal fold; biopsies taken to rule out IBD.
2. Normal-appearing rectal fold with some polypoid flat lesion on biopsies taken; sent for histopathology.
3. Moderate-sized internal hemorrhoid.

PLAN:
Follow up with biopsy results.

GODFREY REGIONAL HOSPITAL
123 Main Street • Aldon, FL 77714 • (407) 555-1234

EXERCISE 7

Level II

OPERATIVE REPORT

Patient information:

Patient name:
DOB:
MR#:

Preoperative diagnosis:

Recurrent squamous cell carcinoma of the oral cavity

CLINICAL NOTE:
The patient is an 82-year-old white female who several years ago underwent wide local resection of left anterior and lateral tongue and floor of mouth, squamous cell carcinoma. She had full-course radiation therapy postoperatively. She has been doing

Postoperative diagnosis:

Recurrent squamous cell carcinoma of the oral cavity

Procedure(s) performed:

Laser ablation of recurrent squamous cell carcinoma of the left anterior floor of mouth/mandibular alveolar mucosa/and left anterior tongue.

Anesthesia:

Assistant surgeon:

Description of procedure:

The patient was brought in the operating room and placed on the operating room table in a supine position. General anesthesia was administered endotracheally with a special laser tube. The left anterior tongue, floor of mouth, and alveolar area of tumor were seen and examined circumferentially. With margins this was marked with Bovie cautery prior to injecting with 1% lidocaine with 1:100,000 epinephrine. Using a hand-held laser set at 15 watts, super pulse power was utilized around the circumference of the lesion, and dysplasia was circumscribed with the laser as well. The central tumor and dysplastic tissue were then ablated and vaporized with the laser. Specimens were sent from the left anterior tongue, anterior and posterior alveolar mucosal margins, and left floor of mouth deep margins from the patient after ablation of the tumor. All these returned back negative for residual squamous cell carcinoma except the posterior alveolar margin that showed one small foci of carcinoma. This area was further ablated with the laser to destroy any residual tumor. There is adequate hemostasis obtained. There was meticulous hemostasis throughout the procedure.

The patient was then awakened from general anesthesia, extubated, and brought to the recovery room in stable condition, having tolerated the procedure well.

ESTIMATED BLOOD LOSS:
Less than 5 cc

GODFREY REGIONAL HOSPITAL
123 Main Street • Aldon, FL 77714 • (407) 555-1234

Continued

OPERATIVE REPORT

Patient information:
Patient name: DOB: MR#:

Preoperative diagnosis:
well, when on routine follow-up visit, was found to have recurrent squamous cell carcinoma that was biopsied in the office and confirmed the diagnosis. She is being brought to the operating room for resection/ablation.

Postoperative diagnosis:

Procedure(s) performed:

Anesthesia:

Assistant surgeon:

Description of procedure:

[signature] Patk Adam MD

GODFREY REGIONAL HOSPITAL
123 Main Street • Aldon, FL 77714 • (407) 555-1234

EXERCISE 8

Level II

OPERATIVE REPORT

Patient information:

Patient name:
DOB:
MR#:

Preoperative diagnosis:

Left parotid tumor

CLINICAL NOTE:
The patient is a 73-year-old white male with an enlarging left parotid mass. Frozen section intraoperatively showed this to be a benign Warthin's tumor. The mass was approximately 2.5 cm in diameter and was closely adherent to the upper facial nerve

Postoperative diagnosis:

Warthin's tumor, left parotid gland

Procedure(s) performed:

1. Left parotidectomy with facial nerve dissection
2. Left sternocleidomastoid muscle rotation flap

Anesthesia:

Assistant surgeon:

Description of procedure:

The patient was brought into the operating room and placed on the operating table in the supine position. General endotracheal anesthesia was performed. The left face was prepped and draped in sterile fashion and injected with saline with 1:100,000 parts epinephrine. A plane incision was injected subcutaneously with approximately 10 cc of the above. A modified Blair incision was made, extending along the preauricular crease around the earlobe and then on to the neck in curvilinear fashion. Incision was made with 15-blade scalpel and carried down through subcutaneous layer with Bovie cautery and meticulous dissection.

Using Metzenbaum scissors and meticulous dissection, with bipolar cautery, subcutaneous dissection just above the parotid fascia layer was performed and the facial flap was reflected anteriorly, exposing the parotid gland and tumor. The parotid tumor was in the preauricular area, just anterior to the tragal pointer of the ear cartilage, deep within the parotid gland.

Dissection was carried down along the preauricular region and tragal pointer tangentially to the anticipated course of the main trunk of the facial nerve. Hemostasis was obtained with bipolar cautery. Main trunk of the facial nerve was identified, and stylomastoid foramen was dissected out to the pes anserinus. Using cross-clamp technique, branches were followed that extended deep to the parotid tumor. Parotid tissue was cross-clamped and face observed for any facial movements, and then cut with 15-blade scalpel when clear. The parotid tumor was resected in a standard technique with the branches of the facial nerve visualized and preserved.

The mass was completely excised with several branches of the facial nerve, notably frontal and zygomatic branches dissected off the capsule of the tumor and preserved. Meticulous hemostasis was obtained with bipolar cautery and silk suture ties. Specimen was sent to Pathology for frozen and permanent section, and returned back showing Warthin's tumor.

GODFREY REGIONAL HOSPITAL
123 Main Street • Aldon, FL 77714 • (407) 555-1234

Continued

OPERATIVE REPORT

Patient information:

Patient name:
DOB:
MR#:

Preoperative diagnosis:

branch divisions. The frontal branch of the facial nerve had to be peeled off the capsule of the tumor and was left intact.

Postoperative diagnosis:

Procedure(s) performed:

Anesthesia:

Assistant surgeon:

Description of procedure:

The wound was irrigated copiously with normal saline and blotted dry. A superiorly based sternocleidomastoid muscle flap was made using the Bovie cautery and reflected up into the preauricular defect to cover the facial nerve to prevent scarring and Prey's syndrome. This was sutured with interrupted 3-0 chromic sutures to adjacent parotid fascia and preauricular soft tissue and fascia into position. A small diameter Jackson-Pratt drain was placed into the wound and brought out through a separate postauricular stab incision. It was sutured to the skin with 2-0 silk mattress sutures.

The wound was closed with inverted interrupted 3-0 chromic sutures for the deep subcutaneous layer and inverted interrupted 4-0 chromic sutures for the subcuticular layer. Skin was closed with running interlocking 5-0 nylon sutures with the exception of interrupted 5-0 nylon sutures around the earlobe. Bacitracin ointment was placed over the wound, followed by Telfa and light pressure dressing. The Jackson-Pratt was placed to self-suction.

The patient was awakened from general anesthesia, extubated, and brought to the recovery room in stable condition, having tolerated the procedure well.

Patk Adam MD

GODFREY REGIONAL HOSPITAL
123 Main Street • Aldon, FL 77714 • (407) 555-1234

EXERCISE 9

Level I

OPERATIVE REPORT

Patient information:

Patient name:
DOB:
MR#:

Preoperative diagnosis:

Esophageal food bolus

INDICATION:
This 77-year-old male came to the emergency room several hours after eating steak and felt it get stuck in his esophagus.
He has had this problem before and refuses to undergo dilatation because he thinks he will need it frequently after that.

Postoperative diagnosis:

Same

Procedure(s) performed:

EGD with removal of food bolus

Anesthesia:

Assistant surgeon:

Description of procedure:

The patient was taken to the operating room and put into the left lateral decubitus position on the operating room table. After the induction of anesthesia, the flexible fiberoptic scope was passed through the oropharynx and into the esophagus without difficulty. The scope was advanced through the esophagus. There was a large amount of what appeared to be meat in the esophagus. Upon reaching the lower portion of the esophagus, it was packed full, and we were unable to clearly identify a direction in which to push the food bolus through and it would not push through easily. Therefore the pelican forceps were used to remove large amounts of the meat so that the distal end of the esophagus and GE junction could be identified, and the remainder was pushed through. The patient tolerated the procedure well. The scope was removed. No apparent esophageal carcinoma was noted.

The patient was transferred to recovery in stable condition.

Patik Adam MD

GODFREY REGIONAL HOSPITAL
123 Main Street • Aldon, FL 77714 • (407) 555-1234

EXERCISE 10

Level II

OPERATIVE REPORT

Patient information:	
Patient name: DOB: MR#:	CONSENT: Signed and on chart

Preoperative diagnosis:

INDICATION:
Anemia, history of heme-positive stools, history of polyps

Postoperative diagnosis:

Colonic AVMs, polyps, diverticulosis coli, external hemorrhoids

Procedure(s) performed:

Colonoscopy with polypectomy and electrocoagulation with arteriovenous malformation

Anesthesia:

Assistant surgeon:

Description of procedure:

Prior to the procedure, the patient was consented. He was then taken to the endoscopy suite, placed in the left lateral decubitus position, and adequately sedated.

Next, digital rectal exam was performed revealing no mass, external hemorrhoids, good tone, and enlarged prostate.

Next, the Olympus CP-160L colonoscope was introduced into the patient's rectum and passed throughout the colon into the cecum. Free intubation of ileocecal valve and terminal ileum was not achieved. In the cecum, there were a couple of AVMs. These were treated with 7 French BICAP probe, 20 watt setting. Successful obliteration of AVMs. There was another one in the ascending colon that was also electrocoagulated. There were a few scattered diverticula noted in the right colon and ascending colon. There was a 5-mm polyp removed by hot snare polypectomy and placed in jar B. In the transverse colon, there were a few scattered diverticula, but no polyps, no AVMs. In the descending and sigmoid colon, there were scattered diverticula, but no polyps, no AVMs. The endoscope was brought back into the rectum. There were a couple of 2-mm polyps removed by fulguration polypectomy. On retroflexed view, he did not have enlarged internal hemorrhoids. The endoscope was straightened, reintroduced around the colon into the cecum. The patient was placed in the supine position. The endoscope was gradually withdrawn. The colon was deflated. No additional lesions were noted. The endoscope was then removed.

GODFREY REGIONAL HOSPITAL
123 Main Street • Aldon, FL 77714 • (407) 555-1234

Continued

OPERATIVE REPORT

Patient information:
Patient name: DOB: MR#:

Preoperative diagnosis:

Postoperative diagnosis:

Procedure(s) performed:

Anesthesia:

Assistant surgeon:

Description of procedure:

The patient tolerated the procedure well.

MEDICATIONS UTILIZED:
Versed 10 mg IV in increments; Demerol 130 mg IV in increments

IMPRESSION:
1. Colon polyps
2. AVMs
3. Diverticulosis coli
4. External hemorrhoids

PLAN:
At this time is to check biopsy results. Continue on iron supplements as previously mentioned. If he develops recurrent iron deficiency, we will need to place him on IV iron, as he has had previous antrectomy.

GODFREY REGIONAL HOSPITAL
123 Main Street • Aldon, FL 77714 • (407) 555-1234

EXERCISE 11

Level II

OPERATIVE REPORT

Patient information:
Patient name: DOB: MR#:

Preoperative diagnosis:
Abdominal pain, possible peptic ulcer disease INDICATIONS FOR SURGERY: This 66-year-old male has been having symptoms of reflux, also epigastric pain and bloating. Recent upper GI was performed, which showed irregularity in the duodenal bulb, and he is referred for upper endoscopy.

Postoperative diagnosis:
Duodenitis, gastritis, hiatal hernia, proximal gastric polyp FINDINGS: The esophagus does not appear acutely inflamed. The Z line is distinct 43 cm from the incisors. There is a small hiatal hernia but again no acute inflammation is seen. No evidence of stricturing or narrowing. The stomach shows some mild hyperemia in the

Procedure(s) performed:
Esophagogastroduodenoscopy with biopsy and removal of gastric polyp

Anesthesia:

Assistant surgeon:

Description of procedure:
The patient is taken to the operating room, given intravenous sedation, and the throat is topically anesthetized. The esophagus is intubated with the Olympus gastroscope and this is carefully advanced under direct visualization through the esophagus, stomach, and then the duodenum, where the first and second portions are carefully examined and the pyloric region is also carefully and clearly examined. Examination of the stomach is then performed, including retroflex examination of the fundus. Biopsies of the antrum are taken, and also a small polyp in the proximal stomach is removed with the biopsy forceps. There did not appear to be any excessive bleeding from the biopsy sites or polyp removal site. The gastroesophageal junction is carefully examined, and then the scope is fully withdrawn with the esophagus being again examined. The scope was removed and the patient was taken from the procedure room in satisfactory condition. Estimated blood loss is minimal. Complications none. Prognosis good. COMMENT: Operative findings were discussed with the patient. He will be notified when the pathology report returns. I suggested that he consider a two-week course of an acid-blocking medication in an effort to clear his duodenitis, and if biopsies show H. pylori, he may need additional medication.

GODFREY REGIONAL HOSPITAL
123 Main Street • Aldon, FL 77714 • (407) 555-1234

Continued

OPERATIVE REPORT

Patient information:

Patient name:
DOB:
MR#:

Preoperative diagnosis:

Postoperative diagnosis:

region of the antrum and pylorus but no definite ulcers. The duodenum demonstrates inflammation and some mild erosions of the mucosa. No definite ulceration is noted in the duodenal bulb. The second portion of the duodenum appears unremarkable. There is a 5-mm benign-appearing gastric polyp noted in the proximal stomach that was removed.

Procedure(s) performed:

Anesthesia:

Assistant surgeon:

Description of procedure:

Patk Adam MD

GODFREY REGIONAL HOSPITAL
123 Main Street • Aldon, FL 77714 • (407) 555-1234

EXERCISE 12

Level I

OPERATIVE REPORT

Patient information:

Patient name:
DOB:
MR#:

Preoperative diagnosis:

Foreign body (quarter) stuck in esophagus

Postoperative diagnosis:

Same

Procedure(s) performed:

Upper gastrointestinal endoscopy and foreign object removal

Anesthesia:

Assistant surgeon:

Description of procedure:

Patient is a 3-year-old who swallowed a quarter. X-ray confirms position in the high esophagus. The patient was brought to the endoscopy suite where continuous oximetry, blood pressure, and EKG monitoring were placed. Anesthesia administered (inhalation anesthesia—see their notes). Following this, oral airway was placed. The Olympus flexible fiberoptic endoscope was introduced through the pharynx without difficulty. Immediately upon entering the esophagus, the coin was noted. This was grasped with a tooth tenaculum and then pulled intact from the esophagus.

Patient tolerated the procedure well.

IMPRESSION:
Foreign object, 25-cent piece in esophagus, removed

GODFREY REGIONAL HOSPITAL
123 Main Street • Aldon, FL 77714 • (407) 555-1234

Level I

OPERATIVE REPORT

Patient information:

Patient name:
DOB:
MR#:

CONSENT:
An informed consent was obtained from the patient after full disclosure of risks and indications to the patient.

Preoperative diagnosis:

Hematochezia

Postoperative diagnosis:

See findings below.

Procedure(s) performed:

Colonoscopy

Anesthesia:

Assistant surgeon:

Description of procedure:

After obtaining an informed consent, the patient was brought to the OR and put in the lateral position. IV line was maintained. IV sedation was given. Vitals were monitored throughout the procedure that included pulse, pulse oximetry, blood pressure, level of consciousness, and ECG monitoring. Digital rectal examination was done, which revealed external hemorrhoids, non-bleeding and non-thrombosed. Non-tender digital exam. Normal anal tone. Endoscope was introduced and advanced all the way up to the cecum, identified by ileocecal valve, appendicular orifice, and light reflex transillumination. There was some difficulty in advancing the scope through the sigmoid and also from the ascending colon into the cecum. However, the scope was reached all the way down. Prep was good. A few pockets of liquid stools, which were washed away. Thorough examination was done. She has extensive diverticulosis with wide gaping mouths of diverticula all the way in left colon up to the transverse colon. No AV malformation noticed. No polyps or masses seen. She does have some moderate-sized internal hemorrhoids.

ASSESSMENT/FINDING:
Extensive diverticulosis involving left side of the colon with wide gaping mouths. Moderate-sized internal hemorrhoids. Moderate-sized external hemorrhoids, non-bleeding and non-thrombosed.

PLAN:
Her bleeding per rectum most likely was diverticular bleed, which resolved spontaneously. At this point, there is no evidence of any bleed, tumor, or any defect. She does have internal hemorrhoids and external hemorrhoids. If they become symptomatic, she may use Anusol plain or with AC as needed. Follow up with primary care physician.

GODFREY REGIONAL HOSPITAL
123 Main Street • Aldon, FL 77714 • (407) 555-1234

EXERCISE 14

Level I

OPERATIVE REPORT

Patient information:

Patient name:
DOB:
MR#:

CONSENT:
Informed consent was obtained from the patient after full disclosure of risks and indications to the patient.

Preoperative diagnosis:

History of polyps in the past

Postoperative diagnosis:

See assessment below.

Procedure(s) performed:

Colonoscopy with biopsies

Anesthesia:

Assistant surgeon:

Description of procedure:

After obtaining informed consent, the patient was brought to the OR and put in the left lateral position. IV line was maintained. IV sedation was given and vitals were monitored throughout the procedure that included pulse, pulse oximetry, blood pressure, and level of consciousness. Digital rectal examination was done, which revealed normal anal tone. No masses palpable. The scope was introduced and advanced all the way up to the cecum, identified by ileocecal valve and appendical orifice. The scope was withdrawn, watching all of the colonic mucosa. There were several pockets of liquid stools at various stages. Most of them were washed and cleaned away as much as possible, and a closer examination of the mucosa was performed. No AV malformation noticed, no masses, no polyps. Up until the sigmoid region there were two polyps adjacent to each other, one a little larger than the other, both of them less than 5 mm, which were hot-biopsied and sent for histopathology. In the rectum, retroflexion was done, which showed moderate-sized abdominal hemorrhoids non-bleeding, non-thrombosed, and the scope was straightened out and pulled out.

The patient tolerated the procedure well. Prep was fair. There were a few pockets of liquid stool that may have obscured the vision. Small polyps may have been missed. No gross abnormality was seen.

GODFREY REGIONAL HOSPITAL
123 Main Street • Aldon, FL 77714 • (407) 555-1234

Continued

OPERATIVE REPORT

Patient information:
Patient name: DOB: MR#:

Preoperative diagnosis:

Postoperative diagnosis:

Procedure(s) performed:

Anesthesia:

Assistant surgeon:

Description of procedure:

ASSESSMENT:
Two sigmoid polyps hot-biopsied, small in size, approximately less than 5 cm in size, sent for histopathology. Moderate-sized internal hemorrhoids. Otherwise normal exam.

PLAN:
Follow up with biopsy results.

Patk Adam MD

GODFREY REGIONAL HOSPITAL
123 Main Street • Aldon, FL 77714 • (407) 555-1234

EXERCISE 15

Level I

OPERATIVE REPORT

Patient information:
Patient name: DOB: MR#:

Preoperative diagnosis:

1) Recurrent tonsillitis. 2) Upper airway obstruction. 3) Hypertrophic tonsils and adenoids.

INDICATION:
4-year-old female with recurrent episodes of tonsillitis. She also has upper airway obstruction manifested by snoring and mouth breathing. Examination reveals hypertrophic tonsils and adenoids.

Postoperative diagnosis:

Same

Procedure(s) performed:

Tonsillectomy and adenoidectomy

Anesthesia:

Assistant surgeon:

Description of procedure:

After consent was obtained, the patient was taken to the operating room and placed on the operating table in supine position. After adequate level of general endotracheal anesthesia was obtained, the patient was turned and draped in appropriate manner for tonsillectomy and adenoidectomy. A McIver mouth gag was then placed to allow visualization of the tonsils. Attention was first focused on the left tonsil. The Allis clamps were placed in the superior pole and tonsils were retracted towards the midline. Then utilizing a needlepoint Bovie, the tonsil was removed in its entirety from superior to inferior direction. Hemostasis was achieved with electrocautery. Similar procedure was then performed on the right tonsil. A cath was then placed through the left nostril to elevate the soft palate. Examination of the nasopharynx showed hypertrophic adenoids. Utilizing suction cautery, the adenoids were removed. Hemostasis was achieved with suction cautery. Tonsillar fossae, as well as the nasopharynx, were then irrigated with saline. Neo-Synephrine spray was then placed in the nasopharynx. Subsequent re-inspection showed no active bleeding. The tension on the mouth gag and the catheter were then released. Re-inspection showed no active bleeding. The mouth gag and catheter were then removed. Prior to removal of mouth gag, 1% Xylocaine with 1:100,000 units of epinephrine was then infiltrated into the retromolar and soft palate areas bilaterally. Patient tolerated the procedure well. There was no break in technique.

The patient was extubated and taken to the post-anesthesia care unit in good condition.

Fluids administered: 1000 cc RL
Estimated blood loss: Less than 10 cc
Pre-operative medications: 4 mg Decadron and 500 mg ampicillin IV

Patik Adam MD

GODFREY REGIONAL HOSPITAL
123 Main Street • Aldon, FL 77714 • (407) 555-1234

EXERCISE 16

Level I

OPERATIVE REPORT

Patient information:

Patient name:
DOB:
MR#:

Preoperative diagnosis:

Cyst, right mucocele, right buccal mucosa

Postoperative diagnosis:

Same

Procedure(s) performed:

Wide excision mucocele, right buccal mucosa

Anesthesia:

This young lady was given IV sedation.

Assistant surgeon:

Description of procedure:

A mucocele measuring approximately 1.5 cm in diameter was noted on the mucosal surface of the right lower lip. The lesion was carefully outlined and infiltrated with Xylocaine 2% with epinephrine. The lesion was completely excised. The mucosa and submucosa were carefully closed with a 2-layer suture of 5-0 of Vicryl. She had no complications. We will see her back in follow-up.

Patk Adam MD

GODFREY REGIONAL HOSPITAL
123 Main Street • Aldon, FL 77714 • (407) 555-1234

EXERCISE 17

Level II

OPERATIVE REPORT

Patient information:

Patient name:
DOB:
MR#:

Preoperative diagnosis:

1. Bleeding per rectum
2. Increasing bowel movements

Postoperative diagnosis:

1. Spastic colon
2. Polyp in the colon
3. AV malformation
4. Minimal colitis
5. Minimal diverticulosis
6. Internal hemorrhoids

Procedure(s) performed:

Colonoscopy, polypectomy, cauterization of AV malformation and biopsy for colitis

Anesthesia:

RN sedation

Assistant surgeon:

Description of procedure:

The patient was brought to the endoscopy suite and placed in the left lateral position. After he was connected to the ECG, blood pressure and pulse oximeter were found to be within reasonable normal limits. IV sedation was given initially by IV Demerol and then IV Versed. After adequate sedation was obtained, Xylocaine cream was used in the perirectal area. Rectal examination was performed and was found to be normal.

The colonoscope was introduced and passed through all of the flexures into the cecum. Slight sigmoid pressure had to be exerted to go around the hepatic flexure. Then the scope was carefully withdrawn, visualizing all the sites of the colon. The patient did have very occasional diverticulosis. He had one polyp in the splenic flexure that was about 1 to 2 mm, was sessile, and was removed. He also had minimal AL malformation, solitary AV malformation. This was cauterized. The patient had minimal colitis. The patient did have a mild to moderate amount of spastic colon while I was intubating the scope, and required 1 mg of glucagon intravenous to be given slowly, which was done. The patient did, on retroflexion of the scope in the rectum, have minimal hemorrhoids. Then the scope was withdrawn.

The patient tolerated the procedure well and was transferred to the same-day surgery unit in a stable condition.

GODFREY REGIONAL HOSPITAL *Patk Adam MD*
123 Main Street • Aldon, FL 77714 • (407) 555-1234

EXERCISE 18

Level I

OPERATIVE REPORT

Patient information:

Patient name:
DOB:
MR#:

CONSENT:
Informed consent was obtained from the patient after full
disclosure of risks and indications to the patient.

Preoperative diagnosis:

Elevated liver enzymes

Postoperative diagnosis:

Same

Procedure(s) performed:

Subcutaneous liver biopsy

Anesthesia:

Assistant surgeon:

Description of procedure:

After obtaining informed consent, the patient was brought in the room and put in a left lateral position. IV line was maintained,
IV sedation was given with 2 mg Ativan prior to the procedure. Then the area of the liver span was mapped out by percussion,
confirmed with ultrasound during expiratory and inspiratory phases. The area of biopsy site was chosen and then the area was
cleaned. The patient was in the supine position. Patient was infiltrated with 2% Xylocaine in the skin and the deeper tissue all
the way up to the liver capsule. A small nick was made on the skin with a scalpel, 1 cm to 1/2 inch deep, and then the ASAP
gun was introduced and advanced all the way into the liver capsule. The patient was asked to hold her breath and then we
inserted the ASAP gun into the liver. We obtained core biopsy, which was immediately taken out and sent for histopathology.

Follow up with routine post-biopsy instructions.

Patk Adam MD

GODFREY REGIONAL HOSPITAL
123 Main Street • Aldon, FL 77714 • (407) 555-1234

EXERCISE 19

Level II

OPERATIVE REPORT

Patient information:
Patient name: DOB: MR#:

Preoperative diagnosis:
Right hydrocele, possible hernia

Postoperative diagnosis:
Same

Procedure(s) performed:
Right high ligation of hernia sac and hydrocelectomy

Anesthesia:

Assistant surgeon:

Description of procedure:
The patient was brought to the operating room, placed under general anesthesia. After prepping and draping was completed, incision was made in the lower abdominal skin-fold, through the skin with a scalpel, through the subcutaneous tissues with a Bovie exposing the external inguinal ring. The cord was dissected up along with the hernia sac. Circumferential dissection was carried out, and the hernia sac was then carefully dissected away from the cord structures and they were preserved. The sac was divided, rotated upon itself several revolutions, and suture-ligated with 3-0 silk. The hydrocele was then opened and imbricated back with two silk sutures. Hydrocele fluid was expressed. I then closed the subcutaneous tissues with Vicryl, the skin with undyed Vicryl, followed by Mastisol, Steri-Strips, and an OpSite dressing. The patient tolerated the procedure without any obvious abnormalities. *Patk Adam MD*

GODFREY REGIONAL HOSPITAL
123 Main Street • Aldon, FL 77714 • (407) 555-1234

EXERCISE 20

Level I

OPERATIVE REPORT

Patient information:

Patient name:
DOB:
MR#:

Preoperative diagnosis:

HISTORY:
Elevated ferritin

Postoperative diagnosis:

Procedure(s) performed:

Attempted transjugular liver biopsy

Anesthesia:

Assistant surgeon:

Description of procedure:

The examination was done through a right internal jugular approach using a #6 French micropuncture set. The right hepatic vein was cannulated using the catheter that was on the hepatic access tray with a Bentson wire. A very sharp angle is present at the takeoff. Cannulation by the catheter and the sheath could be performed, but the stiff metallic device could not be passed through this area due to the angle. Numerous attempts with numerous wires were made, and actually changing the angle of the distal metallic tip was attempted without success.

IMPRESSION:
Unsuccessful transjugular liver biopsy

Patk Adam MD

GODFREY REGIONAL HOSPITAL
123 Main Street • Aldon, FL 77714 • (407) 555-1234

EXERCISE 21

Level I

OPERATIVE REPORT

Patient information:

Patient name:
DOB:
MR#:

Preoperative diagnosis:

Umbilical hernia

Postoperative diagnosis:

Umbilical hernia

Procedure(s) performed:

Repair of umbilical hernia

Anesthesia:

Assistant surgeon:

Description of procedure:

Under spinal anesthesia, the patient was prepped and draped in the usual sterile manner. 0.5% Marcaine with epinephrine was injected along the incisional lines. An elliptical incision was made around the umbilicus. The incision was carried through subcutaneous tissue, basically all the way to the fascia level. The hernia sac was opened and excised along with the umbilicus. Limited exploration was done. The peritoneum was closed with #0 Vicryl sutures. The fascia was dissected above and below. The fascia was closed in imbricating fashion, pushing the lower edge under the upper part of the fascia. Mattress sutures were taken from above, a distance away from the edge, and the edge was then incorporated. Then on the way back, we took the suture from the edge to a distance away from the upper part of the fascia. This was tightened and tied so the lower edge would go underneath the upper part of the fascia. Eight of these interrupted sutures were made and they were tightened and tied. The upper edge was then sutured to the fascia below with a running suture of #1 Vicryl. There was good hemostasis. The subcutaneous tissue was closed with two layers of 2-0 Vicryl and skin was closed with 4-0 Dexon subcuticular sutures. The patient tolerated the procedure well and left the operating room in good condition.

INDICATIONS AND/OR FINDINGS:
This patient had a large umbilical hernia. The defect measured 3 cm.

Pattk Adam MD

GODFREY REGIONAL HOSPITAL
123 Main Street • Aldon, FL 77714 • (407) 555-1234

EXERCISE 22

Level II

OPERATIVE REPORT

Patient information:

Patient name:
DOB:
MR#:

Preoperative diagnosis:

Right parotid tumor versus postauricular cyst

CLINICAL NOTE:
The patient is a 62-year-old white male who has a 2-cm right postauricular mass that is soft with underlying deep parotid tissue surrounding it being much harder, measuring approximately 3.5 cm in diameter on palpation. The patient has no other palpable

Postoperative diagnosis:

Right parotid tumor, consistent with lipoma

Procedure(s) performed:

Right superficial parotidectomy with facial nerve preservation/dissection

Anesthesia:

Assistant surgeon:

Description of procedure:

The patient was brought to the operating room and placed on the operating table in supine position. General endotracheal anesthesia was performed. A modified Blair incision was made from the right preauricular region, around the earlobe, and onto the neck, two fingerbreadths below the inferior border of the mandible. This was injected subcutaneously with injectable saline with 1:100,000 parts epinephrine. The patient was prepped and draped in a sterile fashion. Using a 15-blade scalpel, incision was made through skin and subcutaneous tissue. Initially, dissection was performed around the cystic area, which appeared to be a lipoma, and it was found to involve the superficial portion of the parotid gland. The entire incision was opened, with hemostasis being obtained with bipolar cautery. A subcutaneous flap was elevated anteriorly and the flap was reflected anteriorly. Dissection was made along the pretracheal pointer, but not completely down to the stylomastoid foramen, using tangential dissection along the reposed pathway of the main trunk of the facial nerve. Using meticulous dissection and bipolar cautery, the entire area of the pretracheal pointer, down onto the anterior border of the sternocleidomastoid muscle, was dissected and exposed, exposing the tumor. The tumor easily peeled off the sternocleidomastoid muscle and levator scapulae muscle. Dissection was then carried through the superficial parotid fascia anteriorly, along the palpable margin of the tumor. Using standard cross-clamp technique, followed by sharp incision, stepwise dissection was performed circumferentially around the tumor. Along the deep portion of the tumor, the above standard technique was used. The tumor involved the superficial lobe of the parotid, just lateral to the branch of the facial nerve. Only the small branch of the marginal mandibular branch of the facial nerve was visualized, with the remainder of the facial nerve, including the main trunk and pes anserinus lying within the soft tissue deep to the plane of dissection. The tumor was removed and sent to Pathology for frozen and permanent section. Frozen section revealed this to be lipoma with no malignant cells seen. An adjacent parotid lymph node was dissected in the superior margin of the surgical field and sent for frozen and permanent section. This also came back benign.

GODFREY REGIONAL HOSPITAL
123 Main Street • Aldon, FL 77714 • (407) 555-1234

Continued

OPERATIVE REPORT

Patient information:

Patient name:
DOB:
MR#:

Preoperative diagnosis:

adenopathy in the neck. Operative findings, including frozen section, showed this to be consistent with benign lipoma. The lipoma involved the superficial portion of the parotid gland, comprising the inferior half of the parotid, from the earlobe down. It appeared to be herniating through the parotid fascia and superior region of the sternocleidomastoid muscle, causing the appearance of a postauricular cyst.

Postoperative diagnosis:

Procedure(s) performed:

Anesthesia:

Assistant surgeon:

Description of procedure:

No other masses were seen within the right parotid gland or neck.

Meticulous hemostasis was obtained with 3-0 silk sutures and bipolar cautery. The wound was copiously irrigated with normal saline and blotted dry. A 7-mm Jackson-Pratt drain was placed through a postauricular stab incision through the skin and sutured with 3-0 nylon purse-string sutures. This was placed just lateral to the area of dissection in the surgical field. The soft tissue of the parotid fascia was re-approximated to the anterior border of the sternocleidomastoid muscle. The deep soft tissue of the earlobe was re-approximated to the parotid fascia with interrupted 3-0 chromic sutures. The neck incision was closed with inverted interrupted 3-0 chromic sutures along the deep subcutaneous layer and around the region of the earlobe. Excess skin was excised posteriorly from the skin flap. The preauricular portion of the incision was closed in a similar fashion along the deep subcutaneous layer. Running interlocking 5-0 nylon sutures were used to close the skin in the preauricular and neck regions, followed by interrupted 5-0 nylon sutures around the earlobe. A Jackson-Pratt drain was placed to self-suction. The wound was dressed with Bacitracin ointment, followed by light Telfa occlusive dressing.

The patient was awakened from general anesthesia, extubated, and brought to the recovery room in stable condition, having tolerated the procedure well. In the recovery room, facial nerve function was intact bilaterally and symmetrically. No facial nerve function deficits were seen.

ESTIMATED BLOOD LOSS:
Less than 25 cc

GODFREY REGIONAL HOSPITAL
123 Main Street • Aldon, FL 77714 • (407) 555-1234

EXERCISE 23

Level II

OPERATIVE REPORT

Patient information:

Patient name:
DOB:
MR#:

Preoperative diagnosis:

Ranula, left floor of mouth

Postoperative diagnosis:

Same

Procedure(s) performed:

Excision of ranula and left sublingual glands

Anesthesia:

Assistant surgeon:

Description of procedure:

The patient was placed under IV sedation. Careful examination revealed a large swelling involving the left floor of mouth. This measured approximately 3 cm in length. It was along the submaxillary duct area. He had a previous excision of the submaxillary gland and also an excision of the submaxillary duct, followed by a cyst involving the anterior floor of mouth that I resected approximately 2 weeks ago. The cyst recurred. At this point it appears to be a significant ranula involving the floor of mouth. He was taken to the operating room and given IV sedation. Xylocaine 2% with epinephrine was used for infiltration anesthesia. Following this, an ellipse was made around the sac itself. This was carefully dissected, and following this, it was traced posteriorly. I inserted a dilator and indeed it extended into the area of the subungual gland. I isolated the gland by way of blunt dissection, carefully preserving the neurovascular bundle. The gland was excised. A small troublesome bleeder was found anteriorly along the mandible; however, this was controlled with a suture tie. At the termination of the procedure, a Penrose drain was inserted and anchored into the wound. The wound was then closed loosely with 3-0 chromic.

The patient had no complications and was taken to the recovery room in satisfactory condition.

Patk Adam MD

GODFREY REGIONAL HOSPITAL
123 Main Street • Aldon, FL 77714 • (407) 555-1234

EXERCISE 24

Level II

OPERATIVE REPORT

Patient information:
Patient name: DOB: MR#:

Preoperative diagnosis:
Rectal bleeding INDICATION FOR PROCEDURE: This 42-year-old male has significant episodes of rectal bleeding and pain. By examination, he only has one external skin tag, no evidence of hemorrhoids. By history, this patient has a fissure.

Postoperative diagnosis:
Same, plus anal fissure

Procedure(s) performed:
Examination under anesthesia with left lateral internal sphincterotomy

Anesthesia:

Assistant surgeon:

Description of procedure:
After adequate preparation, 1% Xylocaine plain was used to infiltrate a peri-anal block. Examination of the anal canal does not show significant internal hemorrhoids. He does have a posterior anal fissure. The left lateral mucosa over the internal sphincter was incised and hemostasis achieved. Under direct vision, the sphincter was completely divided. The mucous membrane was then oversewn in a running locking fashion with 3-0 Vicryl. The patient was taken to the recovery room in satisfactory condition.

Patrk Adam MD

GODFREY REGIONAL HOSPITAL
123 Main Street • Aldon, FL 77714 • (407) 555-1234

EXERCISE 25

Level II

OPERATIVE REPORT

Patient information:

Patient name:
DOB:
MR#:

Preoperative diagnosis:

Right hepatic cyst

INDICATIONS FOR OPERATION:
This is a 57-year-old male with a history of a GI bleed who for several months has had right upper quadrant abdominal pain. His studies are significant for a large hepatic cyst. His symptoms are not consistent with pain from gallbladder disease. An elective hepatic cystectomy is scheduled.

Postoperative diagnosis:

Right hepatic cyst

FINDINGS:
Large hepatic cyst adjacent to the abdominal wall. A large portion of this cyst wall is removed and the fluid aspirated away. It was slightly bile-tinged but not frankly bilious. Specimen in the hepatic cyst wall was sent for pathology.

Procedure(s) performed:

Laparoscopic hepatic cystectomy

Anesthesia:

Assistant surgeon:

Description of procedure:

The patient was brought to the operating room and placed in a supine position on the operating room table. General endotracheal anesthesia was induced and the patient's abdomen was prepped and draped in the usual sterile fashion. The patient was given IV cefotetan preoperatively. An infraumbilical incision was created, and the underlying tissue was dissected to the fascia, which was divided in the midline sharply. Stay sutures of 0 Vicryl were placed in the edges of the fascia. The laparoscope was then inserted into the abdomen via the balloon tip 10-mm port. The abdomen was insufflated with CO2 and laparoscope was inserted. Three additional 5-mm ports, two in the upper midline and one in the right lower quadrant, were placed. The liver was retracted to the left and superiorly. The large hepatic cyst was visualized. It seemed to be embedded in the abdominal wall. Its inferior portion was bluntly dissected free, as was its superior portion. The harmonic scalpel was then used to incise the cyst. The fluid was suctioned away. A large portion of this cyst wall, beginning at the anterior and superior portions and running inferiorly and posteriorly, created a large oval hole in this cyst. The oval hole was approximately 7 cm in diameter. This cyst was then removed through the infraumbilical port. Hemostasis was achieved. The abdomen was copiously irrigated, and all trocars were removed under direct visualization. The 10-mm port was closed with the previously placed stay sutures and an additional 0 Vicryl suture. All skin incisions were closed with 4-0 Monocryl subcuticular stitches. Sterile dressings were applied, and the patient was awakened and taken to the PACU in good condition.

Patk Adam MD

GODFREY REGIONAL HOSPITAL
123 Main Street • Aldon, FL 77714 • (407) 555-1234

EXERCISE 26

Level I

OPERATIVE REPORT

Patient information:
Patient name: DOB: MR#:

Preoperative diagnosis:

Postoperative diagnosis:

Procedure(s) performed:

Anesthesia:

Assistant surgeon:

Description of procedure:

The patient was taken to the OR and placed in a supine position. A vertical incision was made under the umbilicus and a 12-mm port inserted under direct visualization with the scope. The pneumoperitoneum was created. Two 5-mm ports were placed, and the appendix was grasped. The mesoappendix was clamped and cut using the Harmonic scalpel including the appendiceal artery. The Endo GIA was then placed across the base of the appendix and it was fired and the appendix released. It was then placed in the Endo bag and brought out through the umbilical incision. Irrigation was performed, hemostasis was noted. The ports were removed, the pneumoperitoneum was allowed to escape. The fascia was closed with 3-0 Vicryl as well as the skin.

The patient tolerated the procedure well and went to the recovery room in satisfactory condition.

Adam Westy MD

GODFREY REGIONAL HOSPITAL
123 Main Street • Aldon, FL 77714 • (407) 555-1234

EXERCISE 27

Level I

OPERATIVE REPORT

Patient information:
Patient name: DOB: MR#:

Preoperative diagnosis:
Chronic cholecystitis with cholelithiasis

Postoperative diagnosis:
Same

Procedure(s) performed:
Laparoscopic cholecystectomy

Anesthesia:

Assistant surgeon:

Description of procedure:
The abdomen was prepped and draped in a routine manner. An incision was made in the umbilicus, Veress needle placed and the abdomen insufflated with 3.2 liters of carbon dioxide. A 5-mm trocar was placed and a 10-mm trocar was also placed. It was then possible to grasp the gallbladder and push it laterally toward and above the liver. The cystic duct and cystic artery were identified. The gallbladder was removed in its entirity using cautery. The gallbladder was pulled out and multiple stones also pulled out. The area was irrigated well, the abdomen insufflated. The incisions were closed with figure of eight sutures of 2-0 Vicryl and Steri-strips applied.

Adm Westy MD

GODFREY REGIONAL HOSPITAL
123 Main Street • Aldon, FL 77714 • (407) 555-1234

GENITOURINARY EXERCISES

EXERCISE 1

Level I

OPERATIVE REPORT

Patient information:	
Patient name: DOB: MR#:	Date: Surgeon: Anesthetist:

Preoperative diagnosis:
Bladder neck infection

Postoperative diagnosis:
Same

Procedure(s) performed:
Incision of bladder neck infection

Anesthesia:
General

Assistant surgeon:

Description of procedure:
After the patient was prepped and draped in the lithotomy position, using the resectoscope, the urethra and bladder were inspected. He had about a ten French bladder neck contraction. Guidewire was inserted through the contraction, and then using the Collins knife cutting at the two, ten, seven, and five o'clock positions, the bladder neck was opened. Electrical cautery was used to obtain hemostasis. Patient tolerated procedure well. *Rachel Perez* MD

GODFREY REGIONAL HOSPITAL
123 Main Street • Aldon, FL 77714 • (407) 555-1234

EXERCISE 2

Level I

OPERATIVE REPORT

Patient information:	
Patient name: DOB: MR#:	Date: Surgeon: Anesthetist:

Preoperative diagnosis:

Postoperative diagnosis:

Procedure(s) performed:

OPERATIVE REPORTS:
This 1-day-old baby is brought into the hospital today for a circumcision. He also is to have his newborn screen blood draw done today. Mom was anxious to go home yesterday and went home in less than 24 hours and was asked to return today. Both mom and father desire to have a circumcision for Jakob. Risks and benefits are discussed, and the parents wish to proceed with the circumcision.

Anesthesia:

Assistant surgeon:

Description of procedure:

The patient was brought to the nursery and placed on the circumcision board. His legs were strapped down. The base of the penis was cleansed with alcohol, and 1% lidocaine without epinephrine was injected at the 10 and 2 o'clock positions. Less than 1 cc of 1% lidocaine was used. Good anesthetic effect. The patient was then prepped and draped in a sterile fashion. Hemostats were placed at the 9 and 3 o'clock positions to help with holding while adhesions were taken down from the glans. Adhesions were taken down, taking great care not to injure the glans. Hemostat was then placed at the dorsum sagittal line down to just distal to the corona. Hemostat was left in place for approximately 1 minute. After removal of the hemostat, an incision was made down to the apex. The foreskin was then retracted and further adhesions were removed. The foreskin was then brought back into place and the Mogen clamp was applied. While trying to bring the foreskin up through the Mogen clamp to the apex of the incision, the skin gave way and tore along the frenulum and along the apex. The Mogen clamp was never completely applied. The Mogen clamp was then removed.

Remainder of the foreskin attachment was then cross-clamped with hemostat for approximately 1 minute and then removed with scissors. Trying to maintain esthetics. Good hemostasis in this area. There was, however, oozing of blood along the volar aspect or frenulum part of the penis. Pressure was applied to this area. This was not enough to maintain hemostasis, so silver nitrate sticks were used with good results. The penis was then dressed with Vaseline gauze and patient was placed on observation status to

GODFREY REGIONAL HOSPITAL
123 Main Street • Aldon, FL 77714 • (407) 555-1234

Continued

OPERATIVE REPORT

| **Patient information:** | | |

Patient name: Date:
DOB: Surgeon:
MR#:   Anesthetist:

Preoperative diagnosis:

Postoperative diagnosis:

Procedure(s) performed:

Anesthesia:

Assistant surgeon:

Description of procedure:

watch for any signs of continued bleeding. Also to watch for urination. Patient was given some Tylenol during the procedure.

During the course of observation, blood began oozing on the dorsal aspect of the penis, and silver nitrate sticks were again used to stop the bleeding. No further bleeding throughout the stay. The patient tolerated diet well. He was given supplement as well as breast feeding while in the hospital. Incident of procedure was discussed with both mom and dad. Patient's pediatrician was contacted by telephone; he felt that all was done appropriately. His colleague was contacted as she was here in the clinic and she was brought to examine the patient. She observed good hemostasis and felt probable good outcome.

The baby was discharged to home approximately at 1:30 p.m. Care of circumcision was discussed with both Mom and Dad. They are strongly urged to come to the clinic with any signs of bleeding or infection. Okay to use Tylenol q4h in the first 24–48 hr. Return to clinic for recheck on Monday (3 days) and then follow up again at regular scheduled visit on Thursday, one week after delivery.

Upon discussion with Mom after she had taken baby home, he urinated shortly after getting home.

Adm Westy MD

GODFREY REGIONAL HOSPITAL
123 Main Street • Aldon, FL 77714 • (407) 555-1234

EXERCISE 3

Level I

OPERATIVE REPORT

Patient information:	
Patient name: DOB: MR#:	Date: Surgeon: Anesthetist:

Preoperative diagnosis:

Symptomatic uterine prolapse, declines pessary

CLINICAL NOTE: The patient is a very alert 93-year-old white female, para 0-0-1-0, with a long history of symptomatic uterine prolapse. In 1990, a pessary was placed with adequate relief. As she has gotten older, she has opted not to continue with the pessary and is now symptomatic with her prolapse. The cervix and anterior wall prolapse passed the introitus. She was counseled regarding the surgical procedure and was agreeable to proceed. She is not sexually active. She is aware of

Postoperative diagnosis:

Symptomatic uterine prolapse, declines pessary

Procedure(s) performed:

LeFort procedure

Anesthesia:

Spinal

Assistant surgeon:

Description of procedure:

OPERATIVE NOTE:
The patient was transferred to the operating room and onto the table where a spinal anesthetic was placed by the anesthesiologist. She was then positioned in the lithotomy position in the stirrups. The abdomen, vulva, and vagina were prepped with Betadine. A Foley catheter was placed to bag drainage. The cervix was extending outside the vagina. The cervix was grasped with a tenaculum. The anterior incision was made approximately 2 cm from the cervix and anteriorly up to approximately 5 cm from the urethral meatus. The denuded strip was approximately 2 to 3 cm in width. The denuded strip was grasped with a clamp. A posterior incision was made the same way. The procedure was then completed by suturing the anterior vaginal mucosa to the posterior vaginal mucosa and then by successive suturing to elevate the uterus and anterior bladder wall. The vaginal epithelium was then closed with a continuous suture of Vicryl. The procedure was terminated.

The patient was returned to the recovery room in satisfactory condition. Blood loss was about 30 cc. She did quite well. She will be maintained in the hospital for a 23-hour stay and then returned to the nursing home tomorrow.

GODFREY REGIONAL HOSPITAL
123 Main Street • Aldon, FL 77714 • (407) 555-1234

Rachel Perez MD

Continued

OPERATIVE REPORT

Patient information:

Patient name: Date:
DOB: Surgeon:
MR#:   Anesthetist:

Preoperative diagnosis:

potential surgical risks including blood loss, infection, and urinary dysfunction. Overall she has a good understanding. Medical clearance was obtained from hospitalist.

Her preop lab studies included a normal CHEM-7. CBC reported an H&H of 13 and 40, platelets 255,000, white count 7.4. Her ECG showed a sinus rhythm with a rate of 74, 1st-degree AV block, and left bundle branch block. X-ray showed no evidence of acute infiltrates. The lung spaces were clear. Osteoporosis was noted in the thoracic vertebrae. Pulmonary vasculature was normal. Some granulomatous type calcifications were seen bilaterally.

Postoperative diagnosis:

Procedure(s) performed:

Anesthesia:

Assistant surgeon:

Description of procedure:

GODFREY REGIONAL HOSPITAL
123 Main Street • Aldon, FL 77714 • (407) 555-1234

EXERCISE 4

Level II

OPERATIVE REPORT

Patient information:

Patient name: Date:
DOB: Surgeon:
MR#:   Anesthetist:

Preoperative diagnosis:

1. Right renal colic
2. Mild dilatation of the right collecting system, possible right distal ureteral calculus
3. Microscopic hematuria

Postoperative diagnosis:

1. Right renal colic
2. Mild dilatation of the right collecting system, possible right distal ureteral calculus
3. Microscopic hematuria
4. Possible spontaneously passed right ureteral calculus

Procedure(s) performed:

1. Cystourethroscopy
2. Right ureteroscopy
3. Right stent insertion

Anesthesia:

General

Assistant surgeon:

Description of procedure:

The patient was placed on the operating table in the lithotomy position after general anesthesia was given. External genitalia were prepped and draped in the usual manner. A #21 panendoscope was inserted transurethrally. Initial inspection of the bladder was not remarkable. Orifices were normal. Right retrograde pyelogram was performed using #8 acorn-tipped catheter, and the study revealed multiple filling defects, which were felt to represent air bubbles but no stones; however, because the patient's symptoms persisted (her microscopic hematuria and the dilatation of the collecting system on the right side, which persisted all the way down to the right UVJ), we elected to proceed with right ureteroscopy as follows:

Glidewire was inserted into the right orifice, advanced all the way to the right renal pelvis, following which the distal right ureter was dilated using a Microvasive balloon dilator, size 10 cm in length, 12 French in diameter. After the balloon was removed, a #9 rigid ureteroscope was introduced transurethrally and advanced in the dilated orifice, and ureter was dilated all the way to the right renal pelvis. No stones, tumors, or other abnormalities encountered.

Therefore we felt that the patient's symptoms and abnormal findings on the IVP could have been due to spontaneously passed stone and persistent edema of the right orifice.

GODFREY REGIONAL HOSPITAL
123 Main Street • Aldon, FL 77714 • (407) 555-1234

Continued

OPERATIVE REPORT

Patient information:	
Patient name:	Date:
DOB:	Surgeon:
MR#:	Anesthetist:

Preoperative diagnosis:

Postoperative diagnosis:

Procedure(s) performed:

Anesthesia:

Assistant surgeon:

Description of procedure:

Instrument removed. A #24 ureteral stent was inserted over the glidewire and left indwelling between the right renal pelvis and the bladder. The cystoscope was removed.

The patient tolerated the procedure well and was sent to the recovery room in satisfactory condition. She will be discharged home when discharge criteria are met. She will be given Cipro 500 mg bid for a week and she will be advised to continue taking Percocet 10 prn for pain. She will be scheduled for cysto and stent extraction in 5–7 days and further urological management as appropriate.

Rachel Perez, MD

GODFREY REGIONAL HOSPITAL
123 Main Street • Aldon, FL 77714 • (407) 555-1234

EXERCISE 5

Level I

OPERATIVE REPORT

Patient information:	
Patient name: DOB: MR#:	Date: Surgeon: Anesthetist:

Preoperative diagnosis:

Elevated prostatic specific antigen

Postoperative diagnosis:

Elevated prostatic specific antigen, benign prostatic hypertrophy

Procedure(s) performed:

Anesthesia:

Assistant surgeon:

Description of procedure:

The patient was placed on the operating table in the lithotomy position. He was sedated with anesthesia. 10 cc of Xylocaine was injected through the prostate via perineum and 10 cc of Xylocaine jelly was injected per urethra. Cystoscope was inserted. The urethra was unremarkable. The prostrate was trilobate and obstructing, quite large through the lumen, and a lot of anterior tissue was projecting into the bladder.

The bladder shows some trabeculation, but no mucosal lesions, no erythema, no stones. The bladder is emptied. Cystoscope is removed.

Finger was inserted into the rectum. His prostate is large. There is a hard, but not rock hard, ridge in the posterolateral prostate towards the apex. The rest of the prostate is just very large and firm. Needle was placed through the perineum, and finger-directed biopsies were taken from all four quadrants of the prostate.

Given the area of abnormality and palpation, he tolerated the procedure without difficulty.   *Rachel Perez MD*

GODFREY REGIONAL HOSPITAL
123 Main Street • Aldon, FL 77714 • (407) 555-1234

EXERCISE 6

Level I

EMERGENCY ROOM RECORD

Name:	Age:	ER physician:
	DOB:	

Allergies/type of reaction:	Usual medications/dosages:
	Flomax, baby aspirin, and saw palmetto

Triage/presenting complaint:

SUBJECTIVE: The patient presents complaining of urinary retention. The patient states that he woke this morning some time ago and was unable to void. States that he had a lot of pressure in the suprapubic area. About 12 years ago, he had a similar problem. They straight-cathed him and he was able to void without problems. After that, the patient has had multiple checks. Nothing ever developed. He has had biopsies done. No cancer noted. He has had an elevated

Initial assessment:

Time	T	P	R	BP	Other:					

Medication orders:

Lab work:

X-ray:

Physician's report:

OBJECTIVE:
The patient is a 74-year-old male in no acute distress. He is alert and oriented. Abdomen reveals bowel sounds in all four quadrants. There is definitely some suprapubic pressure and fullness felt there. There is no pain associated with this, just increased pressure. Rectal exam was deferred at this time. Catheter was placed and left indwelling until he drained completely. He had another 500 ml out. Sample was sent to the lab for a urinalysis. Those results are pending. The patient states immediate relief from the catheter, and this will be removed prior to his discharge.

PLAN:
Talked with primary care physician regarding this patient. She felt that as long as he is stating relief, we should be able to send him home, but he should follow up with his regular doctor within the next day or so. If he is unable to void after removal of the catheter, he should recheck with his physician today. Otherwise, he should increase his fluids, keep things flowing, and if there are any further problems, recheck.

Diagnosis:	Physician sign/date
IMPRESSION: Urinary retention with past history of enlarged prostate	*Adm Westy* MD

Discharge   **Transfer**   **Admit**   **Good**   **Satisfactory**   **Other:**

GODFREY REGIONAL HOSPITAL
123 Main Street • Aldon, FL 77714 • (407) 555-1234

Continued

EMERGENCY ROOM RECORD

Name:		Age:	ER physician:
		DOB:	

Allergies/type of reaction:	Usual medications/dosages:

Triage/presenting complaint: PSA in the past. He did have an episode after some shoulder surgery when he had some urinary retention as well. He had a catheter in for about a week, but after forcing lots of fluids, he was able to come out of that as well. He does have periods where sometimes he can't void, but he just lays down and relaxes and then he is able to void without problems. He increases his fluid intake and this seems to keep things flowing. He is here today to have this checked.

Initial assessment:

Time	T	P	R	BP	Other:					

Medication orders:

Lab work:

X-ray:

Physician's report:

Diagnosis:	Physician sign/date

Discharge   Transfer   Admit   Good   Satisfactory   Other:

GODFREY REGIONAL HOSPITAL
123 Main Street • Aldon, FL 77714 • (407) 555-1234

EXERCISE 7

Level I

OPERATIVE REPORT

Patient information:	
Patient name: DOB: MR#:	Date: Surgeon: Anesthetist:

Preoperative diagnosis:

Perimenopausal bleeding

Postoperative diagnosis:

Same

Procedure(s) performed:

D&C for control of perimenopausal bleeding. Patient had been seen in the office because of continued bleeding despite trial with hormonal manipulation. The impression was that this was probably related to perimenopausal status. Again, she was requesting to control bleeding and also afford a diagnosis. She was cleared medically by her family doctor who admitted her this morning for the same.

Anesthesia:

Assistant surgeon:

Description of procedure:

On admission an IV line was started. She was then brought to surgery. Procedure was to be done with local IV-monitored anesthesia. She was sedated IV-wise and then placed in the lithotomy position following perineal/vaginal prep. Operation was started. Weighted speculum was inserted into the posterior vagina. The anterior cervix was secured with tenaculum and weighted Hegar's dilators were utilized to size 10, and then a sharp curet was passed in, curetting generous amounts of endometrial tissue until nothing else could be felt except the firm, gritty sensation of myometrium. Operation was terminated at this point.

Patient was then taken from surgery to the recovery room in a satisfactory condition. She will be discharged today and will follow up with her primary care physician for continued care.

Adm Westy MD

GODFREY REGIONAL HOSPITAL
123 Main Street • Aldon, FL 77714 • (407) 555-1234

EXERCISE 8

Level II

OPERATIVE REPORT

Patient information:	
Patient name: DOB: MR#:	Date: Surgeon: Anesthetist:

Preoperative diagnosis:

1. Pelvic pain
2. Right ovarian cyst

Postoperative diagnosis:

1. Stage III endometriosis
2. Pelvic adhesions

Procedure(s) performed:

1. Exam under anesthesia
2. Laparoscopy
3. Lysis of adhesions

Anesthesia:

Assistant surgeon:

Description of procedure:

The patient was taken to the operating room and placed under adequate general anesthesia. She was then examined under anesthesia because prior ultrasound showed a 5 × 8 cm mass; however, on pelvic examination, the cystic lesion on the right side did not feel as big as what was seen on ultrasound. Therefore, repeat ultrasound was done under anesthesia. There was a 3-cm cyst noted on the right ovary. At that point, decision was made to perform a laparoscopy. Consent for the laparoscopy was obtained from the patient's husband.

The patient was placed in the lithotomy position and prepped and draped in the usual fashion. Foley catheter was placed in the bladder. Hulka tenaculum was then placed in the uterus for manipulation.

A small 5-mm infraumbilical incision was made, through which a Veress needle was passed without difficulty. After adequate insufflation with carbon dioxide gas, a 5-mm trocar was passed without difficulty. The laparoscope was passed through this and an intra-abdominal adhesion was noted. A suprapubic incision was made, 5 mm, in the midline, through which a 5-mm trocar was passed under direct visualization. The pelvis was inspected and the findings were as follows.

First, there were adhesions between the lower sigmoid colon and the posterior wall of the uterus with involved endometrial-type blebs. There were also deep black endometriotic implants along both uterosacral ligaments. Deeper in the cul-de-sac were red endometriotic implants. The right ovary was adhered to the right side of the uterine wall, and this was taken down bluntly. The cyst in the ovary opened up, and brown fluid could be seen coming from the cyst, which would be consistent with an endometrioma. It was opened completely and irrigated. The right

GODFREY REGIONAL HOSPITAL
123 Main Street • Aldon, FL 77714 • (407) 555-1234

Continued

OPERATIVE REPORT

Patient information:

Patient name:
DOB:
MR#:

Date:
Surgeon:
Anesthetist:

Preoperative diagnosis:

Postoperative diagnosis:

Procedure(s) performed:

Anesthesia:

Assistant surgeon:

Description of procedure:

adnexa was completely dissected off the uterus by blunt dissection. The lower sigmoid, upper rectal area was also dissected off the posterior wall of the uterus by blunt dissection. The sigmoid colon on the left, however, was adhered to a point just below the left ovary. This made it difficult to see the left ovary completely. However, the laparoscope was passed through the suprapubic cannula, and this allowed us to see the distal part of the tube. Both fimbriae appeared to be normal. There were some brown implants of endometriosis on the left ovary. The pelvis was extensively irrigated. At this point, there was no bleeding from the adhesiolysis.

A decision was made that the patient would benefit from a four- to six-month course of Lupron Depot to allow time for the pelvis to heal and some of the endometriosis to regress. At that point, a second-look laparoscopy will be performed with a laser to treat any residual endometriosis. Therefore, at this point, the procedure was terminated. The suprapubic cannula was removed under direct visualization without subsequent bleeding. CO_2 gas was released through the umbilical cannula, which was then removed. Both incisions were closed with Dermabond. Hulka tenaculum was removed from the cervix without subsequent bleeding. Needle and sponge counts were reported as correct by the circulating nurse.

General anesthesia was reversed and the patient was sent to the recovery room in stable condition.

Gunther Moss, MD

GODFREY REGIONAL HOSPITAL
123 Main Street • Aldon, FL 77714 • (407) 555-1234

EXERCISE 9

Level II

OPERATIVE REPORT

Patient information:

Patient name: Date:
DOB: Surgeon:
MR#:   Anesthetist:

Preoperative diagnosis:

Pelvic pain; dysmenorrhea; known endometriosis; failure of hormone therapy

Postoperative diagnosis:

Same with mild endometriosis; red, black, and clear (predominantly red) on both ovaries, both pelvic sidewalls (right greater than left), and a small amount in cul-de-sac

Procedure(s) performed:

Laser laparoscopy

Anesthesia:

Assistant surgeon:

Description of procedure:

The patient is brought to the operating room and placed under general anesthesia by endotracheal tube, prepped and draped in the usual sterile fashion, and placed in the lithotomy position. The bladder was drained with a small Foley, which was left in place. Hulka tenaculum was placed in the cervix. Examination under anesthesia revealed the uterus to be midline and midposition with no adnexal masses. Attention was turned to the upper abdomen after regowning and gloving.

Vertical incision was made through the patient's old laparoscopy incision and carried down through the subcu to the fascia. The fascia was delivered with hemostats and incised with a knife. The Veress needle was used in a modified procedure to inflate the abdomen. Then the Hasson cannula was placed. Next, the abdomen was inflated with CO_2. The laparoscope was introduced and upper abdomen was visualized and was normal. Lower abdomen showed the endometriosis.

Laser was used and the endometriosis was removed under direct visualization without subsequent bleeding. CO_2 gas was released through the umbilical cannula, which was then removed. Both incisions were closed with Dermabond. Hulka tenaculum was removed from the cervix without subsequent bleeding. Needle and sponge counts were reported as correct by the circulating nurse.

GODFREY REGIONAL HOSPITAL
123 Main Street • Aldon, FL 77714 • (407) 555-1234

Continued

OPERATIVE REPORT

Patient information:	
Patient name:	Date:
DOB:	Surgeon:
MR#:	Anesthetist:

Preoperative diagnosis:

Postoperative diagnosis:

Procedure(s) performed:

Anesthesia:

Assistant surgeon:

Description of procedure:

General anesthesia was reversed and the patient was sent to the recovery room in stable condition.

ESTIMATED BLOOD LOSS: Less than 10 cc

COMPLICATIONS: None

COUNTS: All counts correct

DISPOSITION: Patient to recovery room in stable condition

Rachel Perez, MD

GODFREY REGIONAL HOSPITAL
123 Main Street • Aldon, FL 77714 • (407) 555-1234

Level II

OPERATIVE REPORT

Patient information:	
Patient name:	Date:
DOB:	Surgeon:
MR#:	Anesthetist:

Preoperative diagnosis:

1. Weight loss
2. Elevated CA-125

Postoperative diagnosis:

Same

FINDINGS: As determined by exam under anesthesia, the patient has an essentially normal pelvic exam with possible fundal fibroid and retroverted uterus. On laparoscopy, she had a normal upper abdomen and pelvis except for some blebs or cysts at the distal end of each tube bilaterally. Additionally, there were several adhesions of the left ovary and these were

Procedure(s) performed:

Diagnostic scope with multiple biopsies

Anesthesia:

Assistant surgeon:

Description of procedure:

TECHNIQUE:
Following satisfactory and suitable anesthesia, she was placed in the lithotomy position and exam was performed. She was then prepped and draped in the usual fashion for this position. A dilator was used as a manipulator, and the uterus was sounded to 9 cm. Surgeon changed gloves, and laparoscopic portion was commenced. Initially, a Veress needle was used, but I could not maintain appropriate pressure, so the 12-mm trocar was then inserted and the scope passed to ensure proper location and lack of injury. CO_2 was then insufflated to a pressure of 12 mm, and an additional 5-mm suprapubic puncture was made. Examination of the upper abdomen and pelvis was performed and biopsies of both tubal cyst areas were performed. These were multiple little blebs of approximately 3–4 mm at the greatest dimension. The left ovary was then biopsied and the adhesions cut and a specimen taken as well. The peritoneal discolorations were documented on film and then biopsied in typical area. The upper abdomen biopsy was taken under the diaphragm as mentioned above. Irrigation was used, and a specimen was sent for cytology. Following this, hemostasis was noted and the CO_2 gas was allowed to escape after initial frozen-section reports came back as negative. The instruments were removed and the incision sewn with 4-0 undyed Vicryl in a subcuticular fashion with a deep stitch being placed in the 12-mm site. An additional right-

GODFREY REGIONAL HOSPITAL
123 Main Street • Aldon, FL 77714 • (407) 555-1234

Continued

OPERATIVE REPORT

Patient information:	
Patient name:	Date:
DOB:	Surgeon:
MR#:	Anesthetist:

Preoperative diagnosis:

Postoperative diagnosis:

cut and biopsied. There was some brownish discoloration of the anterior peritoneum in typical area of biopsy. Additionally, up under the diaphragm near the liver were some fatty deposits, and these were biopsied and felt to be benign. Frozen-section report on all specimens was benign and peritoneal fluid was also sent. A small left functional cyst was biopsied and also reported as benign.

Procedure(s) performed:

Anesthesia:

Assistant surgeon:

Description of procedure:

sided 5-mm mid-abdominal puncture had been made to allow us to get the subdiaphragmatic biopsy. This was also closed with 4-0 undyed Vicryl. Vaginal instruments were removed after sterile dressings were placed.

The patient was transferred to the recovery room in good condition.

Rachel Perez MD

GODFREY REGIONAL HOSPITAL
123 Main Street • Aldon, FL 77714 • (407) 555-1234

EXERCISE 11

Level II

OPERATIVE REPORT

Patient information:

Patient name:
DOB:
MR#:

Date:
Surgeon:
Anesthetist:

Preoperative diagnosis:

Infertility

Postoperative diagnosis:

1. Infertility
2. Tubo-ovarian adhesions

Procedure(s) performed:

1. Diagnostic laparoscopy
2. Lysis of adhesions
3. Fimbriectomy

Anesthesia:

Assistant surgeon:

Description of procedure:

The patient was taken to the operating room in the supine position. After general endotracheal anesthesia was induced, she was prepped and draped in a sterile fashion. A vertical incision was made in the umbilicus and taken down bluntly to the fascia. The abdomen was extended with the operator's hand and a Veress needle was inserted and directed toward the pelvis. Hanging drop test was performed. Pneumoperitoneum was created with 2 1/2 liters of CO_2 gas, with pressure being maintained below 12 mm of mercury. Once pneumoperitoneum was created, the Veress needle was removed. 12-mm trocar was inserted directly toward the pelvis. Visualization of the abdomen and pelvis revealed the above-noted findings, and photographs were taken. There was no evidence of trauma due to entry.

An accessory trocar was placed in the left lower quadrant lateral to the inferior epigastric vessels. It was placed under direct visualization. Sharp and blunt dissection was used to free up the adhesions of the ovaries to the sidewall. It was also used to free up the adhesions of the right fallopian tube distally to expose more of the fimbria. The areas were hemostatic. Once this was performed, the ovaries were wrapped in Interceed. The pneumoperitoneum was then allowed to escape. Trocar was removed. Fascial incision to the umbilicus was closed with a figure-of-eight stitch of 0 Vicryl. The skin was closed with subcuticular stitch of 3-0 Vicryl. The accessory trocar site was closed with a single stitch of 3-0 nylon.

GODFREY REGIONAL HOSPITAL
123 Main Street • Aldon, FL 77714 • (407) 555-1234

Continued

OPERATIVE REPORT

Patient information:

Patient name:
DOB:
MR#:

Date:
Surgeon:
Anesthetist:

Preoperative diagnosis:

Postoperative diagnosis:

FINDINGS: Filmy adhesions of the ovary and tube down to the pelvic sidewall bilaterally. The left fallopian tube was completely clubbed and no fimbria were visualized. The right fallopian tube was visualized and slightly clubbed; however, fimbria were visualized slightly. The bowel, liver, and gallbladder appeared normal.

Procedure(s) performed:

Anesthesia:

Assistant surgeon:

Description of procedure:

The patient tolerated the procedure well and went to the recovery room in stable condition. All needle, sponge, and instrument counts were correct.

ESTIMATED BLOOD LOSS: Minimal

COMPLICATIONS: None

SPECIMENS: None

Adm Westg MD

GODFREY REGIONAL HOSPITAL
123 Main Street • Aldon, FL 77714 • (407) 555-1234

EXERCISE 12

Level II

OPERATIVE REPORT

Patient information:	

Patient name:	Date:
DOB:	Surgeon:
MR#:	Anesthetist:

Preoperative diagnosis:

Acute left testicular torsion with nonviable right testicle secondary to previous traumatic scrotal injury

INDICATIONS: This is a 16-year-old male who presented to the ED earlier this morning secondary to acute onset of left testicular pain, beginning at approximately 2:30 a.m. this morning with associated nausea and emesis. Urologic history is significant for nonviable right testicle secondary to traumatic scrotal injury for which the patient and his family deferred scrotal exploration to assess viability of the right testicle. A scrotal ultrasound performed this morning demonstrates heterogeneous right testicle with absent vascular flow, most consistent with nonviable right testicle. Homogeneous echotexture is noted within the left testicle in the absence of solid testicular mass and associated decreased

Postoperative diagnosis:

Acute left testicular torsion with nonviable right testicle secondary to previous traumatic scrotal injury with subsequent salvage of viable left testicle

OPERATIVE FINDINGS: Physical exam performed in the ED demonstrated findings consistent with acute left testicular torsion with marked left testicular discomfort and foreshortening of the left spermatic cord with associated left spermatic cord thickening. Right testicle is significantly enlarged with associated induration and firmness throughout with radiographic imaging, most consistent with nonviable right testicle. On exploration of the left hemiscrotal contents, a small reactive left hydrocele is present with straw-colored fluid for which the testicle

Procedure(s) performed:

OPERATION PERFORMED:
Scrotal exploration; manual detorsion of left testicle with left orchiopexy; right scrotal orchiectomy

Anesthesia:

Assistant surgeon:

Description of procedure:

After informed consent was obtained from the patient's mother, the patient was taken to the operating room, placed in the supine position, and given general endotracheal anesthesia per protocol. The anterior scrotum was shaved and the lower abdomen and genitalia subsequently prepped with Betadine solution and draped in the usual sterile fashion. The left testicle was grasped between the thumb and index finger and raised to the anterior surface of the scrotum where a vertical midline scrotal incision was made within the median raphe. Sharp dissection was carried through the subcutaneous tissues to the tunica vaginalis. A small rent was made within the tunica vaginalis with drainage of hydrocele fluid, straw-colored in nature. The left testicle was then delivered into the surgical field where it was dusky in appearance. Application of warm sterile gauze was performed, and after approximately 20 minutes, viability was evident.

Attention was then directed toward the right hemiscrotum where planned orchiectomy was performed secondary to nonviable right testicle. Significant desmoplastic reaction was present as well as chronic inflammation and fibrosis for which the right testicle was sharply dissected from the underlying dartos tissue using Metzenbaum scissors in an avascular plane. After adequate mobilization of the nonviable right testicle had been obtained, the vascular pedicle and vas deferens were separated and subsequently transected over Kelly clamps where the right testicle was removed from the surgical field and

GODFREY REGIONAL HOSPITAL
123 Main Street • Aldon, FL 77714 • (407) 555-1234

Continued

OPERATIVE REPORT

Patient information:	
Patient name:	Date:
DOB:	Surgeon:
MR#:	Anesthetist:

Preoperative diagnosis:

vascular flow. Small left reactive hydrocele is present in addition to small left varicocele. Physical exam confirmed radiographic findings, most consistent with acute left testicular torsion for which the patient is being taken emergently to the operating room for scrotal exploration with manual detorsion of left testicle and left orchiopexy in addition to right scrotal orchiectomy secondary to nonviable right testicle. Further reference is made to the previously dictated admission history and physical exam. The risks and benefits of the surgery procedure were discussed preoperatively with both the patient and his mother; the specific risks include bleeding, infection, scrotal hematoma, chronic testicular pain, injury to the testicular vascular supply resulting in testicular atrophy, recurrent testicular torsion, injury to the vas deferens/

Postoperative diagnosis:

is dusky in nature and most consistent with acute left testicular torsion. The left testicle was twisted approximately 1 1/2 to 2 rotations where subsequent manual testicular detorsion was performed. Application of warm compresses resulted in gradual return of testicular viability with resolution of dusky color and sluggish red arterial bleeding with small incision made within the left tunica albuginea. No palpable left testicular mass or evidence of torsion of the appendix testis involving the left testicle. Exploration of the right hemiscrotal contents reveals large right testicle, firm and indurated throughout, with associated desmoplastic reaction secondary to right testicular nonviability.

Procedure(s) performed:

Anesthesia:

Assistant surgeon:

Description of procedure:

submitted for pathologic evaluation. Double ligatures consisting of 0 chromic stick ties were created to encompass both vascular pedicles, for which appropriate hemostasis was obtained. Absent right hemiscrotum was thoroughly irrigated with sterile saline, and hemostasis of small perforating vasculature was obtained with electrocautery.

Prior to returning the left testicle to its appropriate location within the left hemiscrotum, the left testicle was affixed in three points in order to prevent future left testicular torsion. 3-0 Prolene sutures were individually placed within the tunica albuginea and the midline of the scrotal septum. The testicle was then returned to the left hemiscrotum where each suture was tied to affix the left testicle within the left hemiscrotum. The wound was again thoroughly irrigated and appropriate hemostasis noted. Viability of the left testicle was sluggish in nature. The left hemiscrotum was closed in a single layer to include the dartos layer with a running 2-0 chromic sutures in locking fashion. Similarly, the right hemiscrotum was closed with care taken to obliterate dead space, as a right hemiscrotal drain was not placed. The skin edges of the scrotal sac were re-approximated with a 2-0 chromic suture in horizontal mattress fashion.

Application of antibiotic ointment to the incisional site was performed with sterile gauze and fluffs placed along with a jockstrap for adequate scrotal support and elevation. Final needle, sponge, and instrument counts were correct. The left

GODFREY REGIONAL HOSPITAL
123 Main Street • Aldon, FL 77714 • (407) 555-1234

Continued

OPERATIVE REPORT

Patient information:	
Patient name:	Date:
DOB:	Surgeon:
MR#:	Anesthetist:

Preoperative diagnosis:

epididymis resulting in future infertility, possible nonsalvageable left testicle resulting in potential removal with the specific risks including infertility, impotence, and dependency upon external testosterone replacement. Surgical consent was obtained after review of the informed consent document.

Postoperative diagnosis:

Procedure(s) performed:

Anesthesia:

Assistant surgeon:

Description of procedure:

testicle was descended within the dependent portion of the left hemiscrotum at completion of the surgical procedure. Estimated blood loss was less than 10 cc. The patient tolerated the procedure well without complications. He was subsequently transferred to the recovery room, extubated, and in stable condition.

Rachel Perez MD

GODFREY REGIONAL HOSPITAL
123 Main Street • Aldon, FL 77714 • (407) 555-1234

EXERCISE 13

Level II

OPERATIVE REPORT

Patient information:	
Patient name: DOB: MR#:	Date: Surgeon: Anesthetist:

Preoperative diagnosis:

Menorrhagia

Postoperative diagnosis:

Menorrhagia

Procedure(s) performed:

Evaluation under anesthesia, hysteroscopy, dilatation and curettage, endometrial ablation

Anesthesia:

General endotracheal

Assistant surgeon:

Description of procedure:

The patient was taken to the operating room. After an adequate level of general endotracheal anesthesia, the patient was placed in a modified lithotomy position in Allen stirrups. Evaluation under anesthesia revealed the uterus upper limits of normal, a multiparous cervix. No adnexal masses. A weighted vaginal speculum was placed in the vagina. Cervix was grasped with single-tooth tenaculum and dilated to a #6 Hegar dilator. Using a Stortz hysteroscope of 30 degrees and D5W, a hysteroscopy was performed, which revealed a fluffy appearance to the uterus consistent with menorrhagia and a proliferative endometrium. The ostia were noted to be normal. There were no submucous myomata. At this time the hysteroscope was removed. A dilation and curettage was performed with moderate amount of tissue. Then using an Ethicon endometrial ablation apparatus, the catheter was primed to 2150 mm Hg and placed into the uterus that had been sounded to 8 cm. Using D5W, the catheter was then primed to 180 mm Hg and the cycle was turned on. There was an endometrial ablation of the cavity of 8 minutes at 87 degrees Celsius. After this, it was removed after it had cooled down. The uterus took approximately 10 cc of D5W to fill. Single-tooth tenaculum was removed, as was the weighted vaginal speculum.

Using a medium-sized sharp curet, the endometrial cavity was curetted and curettings were sent to Pathology.

GODFREY REGIONAL HOSPITAL
123 Main Street • Aldon, FL 77714 • (407) 555-1234

Continued

OPERATIVE REPORT

Patient information:

Patient name: Date:
DOB: Surgeon:
MR#:   Anesthetist:

Preoperative diagnosis:

Postoperative diagnosis:

Procedure(s) performed:

Anesthesia:

Assistant surgeon:

Description of procedure:

Hysteroscope was reintroduced. The appearance of the cavity was much smoother.

At this point the procedure was terminated. A single-tooth tenaculum and bivalve speculum were removed from the cervix and vagina, respectively.

The patient tolerated the procedure well and was sent to the recovery room in stable condition.

Adm Westg MD

GODFREY REGIONAL HOSPITAL
123 Main Street • Aldon, FL 77714 • (407) 555-1234

EXERCISE 14

Level II

OPERATIVE REPORT

Patient information:	
Patient name: DOB: MR#:	Date: Surgeon: Anesthetist:

Preoperative diagnosis:

Pelvic pain, ovarian cyst

Postoperative diagnosis:

Pelvic pain with adhesions and right ovarian cyst

Procedure(s) performed:

Laparoscopy, lysis of adhesions, and right ovarian cystectomy

Anesthesia:

Assistant surgeon:

Description of procedure:

The patient was taken to the operating room here after an adequate level of general endotracheal anesthesia, and placed in a modified lithotomy position in Allen stirrups. A Foley was placed, and the patient was draped and prepped in the usual sterile fashion. A 45-degree side-open vaginal speculum was placed in the vagina. The cervix was grasped with a single-tooth tenaculum and a Hulka uterine manipulator. A subumbilical incision was made with a 15-blade, taken down through the subcutaneous tissue to the fascia, and the fascia was scored and taken transversely. Rectus muscle split. Peritoneum opened. Stay sutures of 2-0 Vicryl on a UR6 placed in the fascia. A blunt origin cannula was placed through which a 9.9 flow demand of CO_2 with a maximum pressure of 15 mm Hg was inserted. A second suprapubic port, as well as a left lateral port, was placed. It should be noted that there are adhesions from the omentum to the anterior abdominal wall as well as to the uterus. Also on the left-hand side, the sigmoid colon was adhered to the sidewall. This was taken down by blunt dissection and also with a laparoscopic cutting shears 5 mm. The previous tubal was noted, and at this point, the adhesions were freed up and the left ovary was noted to be normal. The right ovary had two ovarian cysts and the cyst walls were opened and marsupialized. Thus at the end of the procedure, there was no endometriosis. There were no adhesions left. All the adhesions had been freed up. The previous tubal ligation had been noted to be normal. And all adhesions had been

GODFREY REGIONAL HOSPITAL
123 Main Street • Aldon, FL 77714 • (407) 555-1234

Continued

OPERATIVE REPORT

Patient information:	
Patient name: DOB: MR#:	Date: Surgeon: Anesthetist:

Preoperative diagnosis:

Postoperative diagnosis:

Procedure(s) performed:

Anesthesia:

Assistant surgeon:

Description of procedure:

taken down from the omentum to the anterior abdominal wall as well as to the left lateral pelvic sidewall, and the two ovarian cysts on the right side had been marsupialized. All scopes were taken out under direct visualization. The previous subumbilical incision was closed with 2-0 Vicryl. The subcu was injected with 0.5% Marcaine and the skin was re-approximated with 3-0 Monocryl.

Estimated blood loss: Scant
Fluid received: Ringer's lactate
Pathology: None

The patient tolerated the procedure well and left for the recovery room in satisfactory condition.

Adm Westg MD

GODFREY REGIONAL HOSPITAL
123 Main Street • Aldon, FL 77714 • (407) 555-1234

EXERCISE 15

Level I

OPERATIVE REPORT

Patient information:	
Patient name: DOB: MR#:	Date: Surgeon: Anesthetist:

Preoperative diagnosis:

Postmenopausal bleeding, cervical polyp

Postoperative diagnosis:

Postmenopausal bleeding, cervical polyp

Procedure(s) performed:

Evaluation under anesthesia, removal of cervical polyp, dilation and curettage

Anesthesia:

General endotracheal

Assistant surgeon:

Description of procedure:

Patient was taken to the operating room. After adequate level of general endotracheal anesthesia, the patient was placed in a modified lithotomy position. Patient was draped and prepped in usual sterile fashion. Evaluation under anesthesia revealed a normal uterus. No adnexal masses. Weighted vaginal speculum was placed in the vagina. Cervix was grasped with single-tooth tenaculum. There was a small polyp or redundant cervix, which was removed. Cervix had been dilated to a #21 French Bratt dilator, and an endometrial curettage revealed scant tissue. The single-tooth tenaculum was removed, as was the weighted vaginal speculum.

The patient tolerated the procedure well and was sent to recovery room in satisfactory condition.

ESTIMATED BLOOD LOSS: 10 cc

PATHOLOGY: Endocervical polyp, endometrial curetting

Adm Westg MD

GODFREY REGIONAL HOSPITAL
123 Main Street • Aldon, FL 77714 • (407) 555-1234

EXERCISE 16

Level II

OPERATIVE REPORT

Patient information:	
Patient name:	Date:
DOB:	Surgeon:
MR#:	Anesthetist:

Preoperative diagnosis:

1. Endometriosis
2. Chronic pelvic pain secondary to possible pelvic adhesions

Postoperative diagnosis:

Same with no evidence of pelvic adhesions. Endometriosis is noted in cul-de-sac and on right salpinx. One small area of endometriosis on right ovary. Stage IV endometriosis noted. Patent tubes documented bilaterally.

Procedure(s) performed:

1. Examination under anesthesia
2. Operative laser laparoscopy
3. Laser ablation of endometriotic implants
4. Chromotubation

Anesthesia:

Assistant surgeon:

Description of procedure:

With the patient prepped and draped in the usual fashion for a laparoscopy and under adequate general anesthesia, an examination was performed. Cervix was closed, thick. Uterus was midline, nongravid, anteflexed. No adnexal masses appreciated.

An Auvard weighted speculum was used for retraction in the posterior vault. Sims retractor was used for retraction in the anterior vault, and the anterior lip of the cervix was grasped with a single-tooth tenaculum. An acorn tenaculum was then placed, and the urinary bladder was emptied with a Foley catheter.

Attention was then turned to the umbilicus in which an approximately 2-cm infraumbilical incision was performed, through which a Veress needle was introduced. The peritoneum was insufflated with approximately 3.5 liters of CO_2. The Veress needle was removed. The disposable trocar was introduced without difficulty, and the scope was introduced under direct vision. There was no evidence of trauma at the insertion site. The liver surface was grossly normal. The bowels were grossly normal. The appendix was grossly normal. The bladder surface was grossly normal. The uterus was grossly normal. The cul-de-sac showed evidence of endometriosis, primarily on the left uterosacral area. The right salpinx showed evidence of endometriosis. The right ovary showed evidence of endometriosis. The left salpinx and left ovary were grossly normal.

GODFREY REGIONAL HOSPITAL
123 Main Street • Aldon, FL 77714 • (407) 555-1234

Continued

OPERATIVE REPORT

Patient information:

Patient name: Date:
DOB: Surgeon:
MR#:   Anesthetist:

Preoperative diagnosis:

Postoperative diagnosis:

Procedure(s) performed:

Anesthesia:

Assistant surgeon:

Description of procedure:

There were multiple cysts on the left ovary, consistent with benign follicular cysts. The laser apparatus was used to ablate the endometriotic implants on the left uterosacral and cul-de-sac area as well as on the right salpinx and the right ovary. Care was taken to avoid laser injuries to contiguous structures. Hemostasis was adequate.

Chromotubation was then performed and bilateral tubal patency was documented. The scope was removed. The peritoneum was deflated. The trocar was removed. The intraumbilical incision was re-approximated using 4-0 Vicryl in a subcuticular stitch. The acorn tenaculum was removed as well as the single-tooth tenaculum and also the Foley catheter.

The patient tolerated the procedure well and left the operating room in good condition, breathing spontaneously, and with vital signs stable. All sponge, instrument, and needle counts were correct at the end of the procedure.

Adm Westg MD

GODFREY REGIONAL HOSPITAL
123 Main Street • Aldon, FL 77714 • (407) 555-1234

EXERCISE 17

Level I

OPERATIVE REPORT

Patient information:

Patient name: Date:
DOB: Surgeon:
MR#:   Anesthetist:

Preoperative diagnosis:

Recurrent interstitial cystitis with history of gross hematuria

INDICATIONS: This is a 21-year-old female previously referred secondary to recurrent cystitis with associated gross hematuria. Previous antibiotic therapy has included both oral Cipro and Tequin with prior urine culture negative for growth. IVP recently obtained, from which the upper urinary tract was found to be within normal limits with the ureters seen in their entirety and the urinary bladder distended in the absence of intraluminal filling defect. She presents for cystoscopy with

Postoperative diagnosis:

Recurrent cystitis with history of gross hematuria; bladder mucosal lesions consistent with inflammatory bladder disease

OPERATIVE FINDINGS: The urethra is within normal limits except for a few inflammatory pseudopolyps present at the anterior bladder neck, which are nonfriable. The bladder neck is open and patent. Careful systematic survey of the bladder demonstrates no evidence of tumor, foreign body, calculus, or mucosal ulceration. Both ureteral orifices are visualized in their normal anatomic positions with clear efflux of urine noted bilaterally. No significant bladder trabeculation is noted with

Procedure(s) performed:

OPERATIVE PROCEDURE: Cystoscopy; hydrodilation of the bladder

Anesthesia:

Assistant surgeon:

Description of procedure:

After informed consent was obtained, the patient was taken to the cystoscopy room, given laryngeal mask anesthesia per protocol, and placed in the lithotomy position. The external genitalia were prepped with Betadine solution and draped in the usual sterile fashion. An umbilical ring was present. The patient did receive one dose of oral antibiotic consisting of Levaquin prior to initiation of the surgical procedure. The 22 French endo sheath and obturator were passed transurethrally to the bladder without difficulty. The obturator was removed and the bladder drained of a scant volume of clear yellow urine in the absence of gross hematuria. Careful systematic survey of the bladder was performed using both the 70-degree and 30-degree lenses, with the findings dictated above. The bladder was then cycled on three consecutive occasions with sterile irrigant, with final bladder capacity under anesthesia being 900 cc. Fine submucosal petechial hemorrhages were noted at completion of the second bladder cycling, most consistent with inflammatory bladder disease suggestive of interstitial cystitis. The bladder was then emptied and the cystoscope slowly retracted to the level of the bladder neck where the entire urethra was visualized using the 12-degree lens. The cystoscope was then removed, as there was no significant postoperative hematuria noted, and the procedure terminated.

GODFREY REGIONAL HOSPITAL
123 Main Street • Aldon, FL 77714 • (407) 555-1234

Continued

OPERATIVE REPORT

Patient information:	
Patient name:	Date:
DOB:	Surgeon:
MR#:	Anesthetist:

Preoperative diagnosis:

hydrodilation of the bladder to complete the lower urinary tract evaluation regarding hematuria, and in addition, to rule out inflammatory bladder disease most consistent with interstitial cystitis. The risks and benefits of the surgical procedure were reviewed preoperatively and include bleeding, infection, urethral injury resulting in stricture formation, bladder perforation, ureteral injury resulting in stricture formation and/or obstruction of the renal unit, postoperative hematuria, and persistent postoperative irritative voiding symptoms and pelvic pain. Full surgical consent was obtained after review of the informed consent document.

Postoperative diagnosis:

bladder filling or evidence of diverticulum formation. Mucosal changes overlying the trigone consistent with trigonitis present. The bladder was cycled on three consecutive occasions, with final capacity under anesthesia being 650 cc, 800 cc, and 900 cc, respectively. After completion of the second bladder cycle, fine submucosal petechial hemorrhages were present, originating from the left and right lateral bladder walls in addition to posterior bladder wall and bladder dome. Although the degree of erythema was not typical of the usual inflammatory bladder disease, these findings were suggestive of interstitial cystitis where a light terminal hematuria was noted with each completion of bladder cycling.

Procedure(s) performed:

Anesthesia:

Assistant surgeon:

Description of procedure:

The patient tolerated the procedure well without complications and was subsequently transferred to the recovery room, extubated, and in stable condition.

Adm Westg MD

GODFREY REGIONAL HOSPITAL
123 Main Street • Aldon, FL 77714 • (407) 555-1234

EXERCISE 18

Level I

OPERATIVE REPORT

Patient information:	
Patient name:	Date:
DOB:	Surgeon:
MR#:	Anesthetist:

Preoperative diagnosis:

Incomplete abortion at eight weeks' gestation, twin gestation noted

Postoperative diagnosis:

Same

Procedure(s) performed:

Suction D&C under ultrasound guidance

Anesthesia:

Assistant surgeon:

Description of procedure:

The patient was prepped and draped in the usual fashion for suction D&C. Under adequate general anesthesia, and with ultrasound guidance, the cervix was dilated and a #10 suction cannula was introduced. The anterior, posterior, and lateral walls of the endometrial cavity were curetted, yielding a moderate amount of products of conception. No endometrial defects were encountered. A medium-sized sharp curette was then introduced. The anterior, posterior, and lateral walls of the endometrial cavity were gently curetted, yielding a scant amount of additional tissue. Again, no endometrial defects were encountered. No injury to the uterus was noted. A Foley catheter was used to fill the bladder for proper visualization during the procedure. IV oxytocin was infused as well as Methergine 0.2 mg IM, and after the procedure, two 100 mg tablets of Cytotec were placed intrarectally.

The patient tolerated the procedure well, left the operating room in good condition, breathing spontaneously, vital signs stable. All sponge, instrument, and needle counts were correct at the end of the procedure.

Rachel Perez, MD

GODFREY REGIONAL HOSPITAL
123 Main Street • Aldon, FL 77714 • (407) 555-1234

EXERCISE 19

Level I

OPERATIVE REPORT

Patient information:	
Patient name: DOB: MR#:	Date: Surgeon: Anesthetist:

Preoperative diagnosis:

Multiparity

Postoperative diagnosis:

Multiparity with chronic pelvic inflammatory disease

Procedure(s) performed:

1. Examination under anesthesia
2. Operative laparoscopy with lysis of adhesions
3. Bilateral fulguration of the salpinges for elective voluntary permanent tubal sterilization
4. Intraoperative administration of Rocephin, 2 grams

Anesthesia:

Assistant surgeon:

Description of procedure:

With the patient prepped and draped in the usual fashion for laparoscopic tubal ligation, and under adequate general anesthesia, an examination was performed. The cervix was closed, thick, uterus midline, nongravid, anteflexed; no adnexal masses were appreciated. An Auvard weighted speculum was used for retraction in the posterior vault. Sims retractor was used for retraction in the anterior vault, and the anterior lip of the cervix was grasped with a single-tooth tenaculum. A Hulka tenaculum was placed without difficulty and the other instruments were removed. The urinary bladder was then emptied with a straight catheter and a very strong odor was noted to the urine. At this time, it was discussed that nitrites were present in the urine and the decision was made to treat the patient for a urinary tract infection. Attention was then directed to the umbilicus, in which an approximately 2-cm infraumbilical incision was performed through which a Veress needle was introduced. The peritoneum was insufflated with approximately 3.5 liters of CO_2. The trocar was introduced without difficulty and the scope was introduced under direct vision. There was no evidence of trauma at the insertion site. The liver surface was grossly normal. The gallbladder was grossly normal. There was some old blood noted in the cul-de-sac. There was a mosaic pattern noted on the surface of the uterus, consistent with inflammation. The right salpinx and right tube showed evidence of inflammation. The left salpinx and left tube showed evidence of chronic inflammation with an adhesion involving

GODFREY REGIONAL HOSPITAL
123 Main Street • Aldon, FL 77714 • (407) 555-1234

Continued

OPERATIVE REPORT

Patient information:	
Patient name: DOB: MR#:	Date: Surgeon: Anesthetist:

Preoperative diagnosis:

Postoperative diagnosis:

Procedure(s) performed:

Anesthesia:

Assistant surgeon:

Description of procedure:

the left salpinx and the posterior wall of the uterus. No active infection was noted. There was no purulent material. The decision was made to proceed with adhesiolysis for further evaluation of the pelvic organs. This was performed with the bipolar cautery device used for electrocauterization and the endoscopic scissors used for excision of the pelvic adhesions. Once there was restoration of near normal anatomy, the pelvic organs were again re-evaluated.

The decision was made to proceed with the tubal sterilization, since this appeared like a chronic process and the patient was not recently symptomatic. The right salpinx was grasped with a bipolar cautery device and it was cauterized, with care being taken to ensure blanching into approximately 1 cm of the mesosalpinx and to ensure that the resistance needle reverted back to its original position. This was performed the second time on the right, with care being taken to avoid thermal or mechanical injuries to contiguous structures. The same procedure was performed on the left with the same precautions used.

The scope was removed under direct vision. The peritoneum was deflated. The infraumbilical incision was re-approximated using 4-0 Vicryl in a subcuticular stitch. Hulka tenaculum was removed.

Once inflammation was noted, IV Rocephin 2 grams was infused. The patient will be discharged with doxycycline 100 bid for 14 days.

Adam Westy, MD

GODFREY REGIONAL HOSPITAL
123 Main Street • Aldon, FL 77714 • (407) 555-1234

EXERCISE 20

Level II

OPERATIVE REPORT

Patient information:	
Patient name: DOB: MR#:	Date: Surgeon: Anesthetist:

Preoperative diagnosis:

1. Endometrial hyperplasia treated with Provera; this is a re-evaluation
2. Stenotic cervix

Postoperative diagnosis:

FINDINGS:
1. Uterus six weeks size, severe retroversion
2. Severe scarring of the cervical os, impenetrable with Pratt dilator and lacrimal duct. Ultrasound guidance was used to aid in the dilatation but was unable to be done secondary to scarring.
3. Ultrasound findings as above

Procedure(s) performed:

Attempted cervical dilatation and curettage that could not be done; scar tissue was far too thick; lacrimal ducts were used; surgeon unable to safely develop a canal into the endocervical canal; ultrasound guidance was used, endometrium was found to be 1.2 mm thick, retroverted uterus, simple cyst on the right ovary, 2 × 1 cm, no change times one year. Attempt to dilate with guidance still failed secondary to severe scarring and distortion of the endocervical canal. The procedure was not able to be adequately done at this time.

Anesthesia:

Light mask anesthesia

Assistant surgeon:

Description of procedure:

After obtaining informed consent, the patient was taken to the operating room and placed in the dorsal supine position, and placed under light mask anesthesia. The patient was prepped and draped in the usual sterile fashion. She was placed in the lithotomy position with Allen stirrups. Weighted speculum was placed in her introitus after being prepped and draped. Single-tooth tenaculum was placed in the 12 o'clock position of the cervix. She was attempted to be dilated with Pratt dilators but an adequate cervical opening could not be found. Lacrimal ducts were used from the smallest size to the medium size; unable to penetrate the external os through various attempts at cervical opening. Ultrasound was called in for ultrasound guidance. The uterus was found to be retroverted, and a 1.2-mm simple cyst was noted on the right ovary, unchanged from previous evaluation. Again, attempts were made to dilate under ultrasound guidance, and again, no tract could be made from the external os at all through several attempts secondary to the thin endometrial lining. As the result of the difficulty and inability to properly dilate, the procedure was deemed completed at this time.

The patient was taken to the recovery room in stable condition. Instrument counts and sponge counts were correct times two.

COMPLICATIONS: Severe scarring

GODFREY REGIONAL HOSPITAL
123 Main Street • Aldon, FL 77714 • (407) 555-1234

Continued

OPERATIVE REPORT

Patient information:	
Patient name: DOB: MR#:	Date: Surgeon: Anesthetist:

Preoperative diagnosis:

Postoperative diagnosis:

Procedure(s) performed:

Anesthesia:

Assistant surgeon:

Description of procedure:

ESTIMATED BLOOD LOSS: Zero
IV FLUIDS: 400 cc
URINE OUTPUT: Not available

Rachel Perez MD

GODFREY REGIONAL HOSPITAL
123 Main Street • Aldon, FL 77714 • (407) 555-1234

EXERCISE 21

Level I

OPERATIVE REPORT

Patient information:	
Patient name:	Date:
DOB:	Surgeon:
MR#:	Anesthetist:

Preoperative diagnosis:

Extrauterine IUD

Postoperative diagnosis:

Extrauterine IUD

Procedure(s) performed:

Laparoscopic removal of extrauterine Lippes Loop

Anesthesia:

Assistant surgeon:

Description of procedure:

The patient was taken to the OR, placed in the lithotomy position, and prepped and draped in the usual fashion. A weighted speculum was inserted, and the anterior and posterior lips of the cervix were grasped with a tenaculum. A French catheter was then inserted into the bladder and taped to the traction handle. The patient was then turned for the laparoscopic procedure.

For traction, #2 silk sutures were placed lateral to the umbilicus and grasped with Kelly clamps. A small infraumbilical incision was made in the area of the previous laparoscopic scar. The Veress needle was inserted. Normal saline was injected and not aspirated. A good pneumoperitoneum was obtained after insufflating approximately 3 1/2 liters of CO_2. The large trocar was inserted, followed by insertion of a laparoscope. The uterus, tubes, and ovaries appeared to be normal. There was no evidence of where the IUD had perforated the uterus. Upon inspection, the IUD was noted to be embedded in the omental pad anteriorly. Using the grasper through the laparoscope, it was freed up and pulled out in toto through the portal of the infra-abdominal incision. The laparoscope was reinserted and the area where the IUD had been embedded was re-inspected, and no bleeding was noted. It was removed intact, being a Lippes Loop-type IUD. The laparoscope was removed. CO_2 was allowed to escape through the trocar sleeve. Incision was then closed using an interrupted suture of 3-0

GODFREY REGIONAL HOSPITAL
123 Main Street • Aldon, FL 77714 • (407) 555-1234

Continued

OPERATIVE REPORT

Patient information:	
Patient name:	Date:
DOB:	Surgeon:
MR#:	Anesthetist:

Preoperative diagnosis:

Postoperative diagnosis:

Procedure(s) performed:

Anesthesia:

Assistant surgeon:

Description of procedure:

Dexon. The cervical tenaculum and French catheter were then removed intact.

The patient tolerated the procedure well. Estimated blood loss was less than 10 cc. She was sent to the recovery room in stable post-op condition.

Adm Westy MD

GODFREY REGIONAL HOSPITAL
123 Main Street • Aldon, FL 77714 • (407) 555-1234

EXERCISE 22

Level I

OPERATIVE REPORT

Patient information:	
Patient name: DOB: MR#:	Date: Surgeon: Anesthetist:

Preoperative diagnosis:

1) Chronic pelvic pain; 2) Abnormal uterine bleeding

Postoperative diagnosis:

Same plus bilateral ovarian cyst

FINDINGS: Normal-appearing endometrial cavity, normal-appearing uterus. Adhesions of omentum to anterior abdominal wall at the umbilicus and right lower abdominal wall. There is a simple-appearing 2-cm cyst on the right ovary and approximately 4–5 cm simple cyst on the left ovary. The EBL is 100 cc.

Procedure(s) performed:

Hysteroscopy, D&C, laser laparoscopy with bilateral ovarian cystotomies, and fulguration of the right fallopian tube

Anesthesia:

Assistant surgeon:

Description of procedure:

The patient was taken to the operating room and placed in the supine position. After general endotracheal anesthesia was induced, she was placed in Allen stirrups and prepped and draped in a sterile fashion. A Foley catheter was placed. Speculum was placed in the vagina. Anterior lip of the cervix is grasped with single-tooth tenaculum. The cervix was serially dilated to accommodate the hysteroscope. The scope was inserted using normal saline as distending medium. The above findings were documented with photographs.

Sharp curettage was performed of all four quadrants and the endocervical canal. Instruments had been removed and Hulka tenaculum applied to the cervix.

The operator then changed gloves. The abdominal portion of the case was then performed.

A transverse incision was made in the lower aspect of the umbilicus and taken down bluntly to fascia. The fascia was incised with Mayo scissors, and stay sutures were placed in the fascia bilaterally. The Hasson cannula was introduced into the peritoneal cavity and scope was inserted, with intra-abdominal placement confirmed. Pneumoperitoneum was created with CO_2 gas. The patient was placed in Trendelenburg, and the above-noted findings were documented with photographs.

Accessory ports were also placed. They were placed under direct visualization with no evidence of trauma. The laser was then connected, and using 10 watts of power, the cysts were lysed bilaterally. Attempt was then made, using blunt dissection and hydrodissection, to remove the cyst wall of the left ovarian cyst. However, only a portion of the cyst wall was removed. The interior of the ovarian cavity was irrigated with

GODFREY REGIONAL HOSPITAL
123 Main Street • Aldon, FL 77714 • (407) 555-1234

Continued

OPERATIVE REPORT

Patient information:

Patient name: Date:
DOB: Surgeon:
MR#:   Anesthetist:

Preoperative diagnosis:

Postoperative diagnosis:

Procedure(s) performed:

Anesthesia:

Assistant surgeon:

Description of procedure:

normal saline and noted to be hemostatic. The remainder of the pelvis was irrigated. The right fallopian tube, which had tubal ligation three months ago, did not appear to be interrupted despite the fact that the pathology report revealed a portion of the fallopian tube had been removed. For this reason, fulguration with bipolar cautery was used to pulverize a 2-cm portion of the tube, approximately 3 cm from the fundus. Again, irrigation was performed.

The accessory trocar was then removed. The pneumoperitoneum was allowed to escape. The umbilical port was removed. The fascia at the umbilical incision was closed with figure-of-eight stitch of #0 Vicryl. The skin was closed with 3-0 Vicryl. The accessory port sites were closed with horizontal mattress stitches of 3-0 nylon. Hulka tenaculum and Foley catheter were removed.

The patient went to the recovery room in stable condition. All needle, sponge, and instrument counts were correct.

COMPLICATIONS: None

DRAINS: None

SPECIMENS: Endometrial curettings and portions of left ovarian cyst wall

Adm Westg, MD

GODFREY REGIONAL HOSPITAL
123 Main Street • Aldon, FL 77714 • (407) 555-1234

EXERCISE 23

Level I

OPERATIVE REPORT

Patient information:	
Patient name:	Date:
DOB:	Surgeon:
MR#:	Anesthetist:

Preoperative diagnosis:

Bladder symptoms; ureteral colic

Postoperative diagnosis:

Bladder symptoms; ureteral colic

Procedure(s) performed:

Cystoscopy and retrograde stent placement

Anesthesia:

Assistant surgeon:

Description of procedure:

The patient was placed on the operating table in the lithotomy position. She was prepped and draped sterilely. She was sedated with conscious sedation.

Cystoscope was inserted into the bladder. The bladder shows diffuse erythema throughout.

The orifices were in normal placement and configuration. No specific lesions in the bladder. 5 French stent was advanced into the right ureteral orifice. Foley catheter was in place. After removing the Foley, the stent was left in the orifice and tied to the Foley. We are going to do a retrograde film through the stent that was left in place.

Adm Westg MD

GODFREY REGIONAL HOSPITAL
123 Main Street • Aldon, FL 77714 • (407) 555-1234

Level II

OPERATIVE REPORT

Patient information:

Patient name:
DOB:
MR#:

Date:
Surgeon:
Anesthetist:

Preoperative diagnosis:

1. Recurrent urinary retention
2. Enlarged prostate with bladder outlet obstruction
3. Generalized debilitation due to pancreatitis

Postoperative diagnosis:

1. Recurrent urinary retention
2. Enlarged prostate with bladder outlet obstruction
3. Generalized debilitation due to pancreatitis

FINDINGS: The anterior urethra was normal. Membranous urethra was normal. The prostatic urethra revealed enlargement of the prostate causing bladder outlet obstruction.

Procedure(s) performed:

1. Flexible cystourethroscopy   2. Percutaneous cystostomy insertion

Anesthesia:

Assistant surgeon:

Description of procedure:

With the patient in the supine position, the lower midline abdomen and the penis and genitalia were prepped and draped in sterile fashion. The lower midline abdomen, two fingerbreadths above the symphysis pubis, was the site for this cystostomy catheter insertion. This area was infiltrated subcutaneously with 1% plain Xylocaine and infiltration continued inward to the level of the rectus fascia.

A small stab incision was made in this site with an 11-blade knife. Flexible cystourethroscopy was then performed, with the above findings noted. The bladder was distended with the irrigation fluid until the bladder was palpable in the suprapubic area. The cystostomy trocar was then advanced through the stab incision just above the symphysis pubis and passed in all the way through the anterior bladder wall and into the lumen of the bladder under direct vision with the cystoscope in place. The 12 French cystostomy catheter was advanced through the sheath after removing the trocar, and the sheath was then removed, leaving the catheter in place. The balloon of the catheter was inflated with 10 cc of sterile water.

The cystostomy catheter was then attached to a sterile drainage bag. A single stitch of 3-0 nylon was used to tighten the stab incision at the site of the cystostomy catheter. The cystoscope was removed.

The patient tolerated the procedure well and was taken to the day surgery unit in satisfactory condition.

GODFREY REGIONAL HOSPITAL
123 Main Street • Aldon, FL 77714 • (407) 555-1234

Rachel Perez MD

Continued

OPERATIVE REPORT

Patient information:	
Patient name: DOB: MR#:	Date: Surgeon: Anesthetist:

Preoperative diagnosis:

Postoperative diagnosis:

Examination of the bladder revealed some areas of acute cystitis secondary to recent Foley catheterization, and there were some changes of chronic bladder outlet obstruction with trabeculation of the bladder, but there were no stones, tumors, diverticula, or ulcerations seen.

Procedure(s) performed:

Anesthesia:

Assistant surgeon:

Description of procedure:

GODFREY REGIONAL HOSPITAL
123 Main Street • Aldon, FL 77714 • (407) 555-1234

EXERCISE 25

Level II

OPERATIVE REPORT

Patient information:

Patient name: Date:
DOB: Surgeon:
MR#:   Anesthetist:

Preoperative diagnosis:

Chronic pelvic pain with irritative voiding symptoms; history of endometriosis

INDICATIONS: This is a 43-year-old female previously referred secondary to chronic pelvic pain with associated irritative voiding symptoms including urinary dysuria. Previous gynecological history has included diagnostic laparoscopy with aspiration of left ovarian cyst, negative for malignant cells, in addition to a total abdominal hysterectomy with bilateral salpingo-oophorectomy, absent of malignancy. Her specific complaint is urinary dysuria with difficulty with urination for which an indwelling Foley catheter was placed. Subsequent radiographic imaging consisting of CT scan of the abdomen/pelvis was performed, showing no upper tract urinary pathology for which the bladder is contracted

Postoperative diagnosis:

Chronic pelvic pain with irritative voiding symptoms; history of endometriosis; reduced total bladder capacity under anesthesia

OPERATIVE FINDINGS: The urethra is within normal limits without evidence of inflammatory lesion or mass. Multiple pseudopolyps are seen at the anterior bladder neck and are nonfriable in nature. Systematic survey of the bladder demonstrates a solitary erythematous patch posterior to the right ureteral orifice, felt to be most consistent with Foley catheter irritation. Despite indwelling Foley catheter present, significant bullous edema involving the bladder mucosa is not noted. No evidence of tumor, foreign body, calculus, or mucosal ulceration is noted within the urinary bladder. Both ureteral orifices are visualized in their normal anatomic positions with clear efflux of urine noted

Procedure(s) performed:

Cystoscopy; hydrodilation of bladder; superficial bladder biopsies × 3

Anesthesia:

Assistant surgeon:

Description of procedure:

After informed consent was obtained, the patient was taken to the cystoscopy room, given laryngeal mask anesthesia per protocol, and placed in the lithotomy position. The present indwelling Foley catheter was removed. The external genitalia were prepped with Betadine solution and draped in the usual sterile fashion. The patient did receive one dose of oral prophylactic antibiotic consisting of Levaquin prior to initiation of the surgical procedure. The 22 French endo sheath and obturator were passed transurethrally to the bladder without difficulty. The obturator was removed, and no significant return was obtained as the bladder had been decompressed with current indwelling Foley catheter. Careful systematic survey of the bladder was then performed using both the 70-degree and 30-degree lenses, with the findings dictated above. Consecutive cycling of the bladder under anesthesia with instillation of sterile saline showed consistent bladder capacity of 300 cc under anesthesia, for which the typical cystoscopic findings of interstitial cystitis were not present as dictated above. Significant reduction in overall bladder capacity is present and is felt to be most consistent with inflammatory bladder disease. Due to the irritative nature of voiding symptoms in the absence of true cystoscopic findings consistent with interstitial cystitis, superficial random bladder biopsies were then performed. The flexible cold-cup biopsy forceps were passed through the working channel where biopsy specimens were taken from the right posterior bladder wall, midline posterior bladder wall, and left posterior bladder wall. Each biopsy site was cauterized using the Bugbee electrode where

GODFREY REGIONAL HOSPITAL
123 Main Street • Aldon, FL 77714 • (407) 555-1234

Continued

OPERATIVE REPORT

Patient information:

Patient name: Date:
DOB: Surgeon:
MR#:   Anesthetist:

Preoperative diagnosis:

secondary to current indwelling Foley catheter. Removal of the Foley catheter to further evaluate for cystoscopic changes consistent with inflammatory bladder disease was discussed preoperatively. The patient deferred catheter removal until the surgical procedure secondary to concern with voiding dysfunction for which she does realize the potential limitation of the planned procedure.

The risks and benefits of the surgical procedure were reviewed preoperatively and include bleeding, infection, urethral injury resulting in stricture formation, bladder perforation requiring surgical repair, ureteral injury resulting in stricture formation and/or obstruction of renal unit, postoperative hematuria, postoperative urinary retention, and persistent postoperative chronic pelvic pain with irritative voiding symptoms. Full surgical consent was obtained after review of the informed consent document.

Postoperative diagnosis:

bilaterally. No significant bladder trabeculation is evident with bladder filling or evidence of diverticulum formation present. Consecutive bladder cycling with instillation of sterile saline shows decreased bladder capacity, with final bladder capacity under anesthesia being 300 cc. The findings are most consistent with inflammatory bladder disease; however, typical submucosal petechial hemorrhages and glomerulations are not present as diagnostic for interstitial cystitis. A solitary small cellule is seen along the right posterolateral bladder wall above the right ureteral orifice. Significant terminal hematuria after each consecutive bladder cycling is not present.

Procedure(s) performed:

Anesthesia:

Assistant surgeon:

Description of procedure:

adequate hemostasis was obtained. All specimens were submitted in one container and labeled "random bladder biopsy" for further pathologic evaluation. No significant terminal hematuria was noted with each consecutive bladder cycling. The bladder was then emptied and the cystoscope slowly retracted, visualizing the urethra in its entirety. Multiple pseudopolyps were present at the bladder neck. However, no specific inflammatory urethral mass or lesion was noted. The 22 French endo sheath was then re-inserted, with the obturator removed and the bladder drained at the completion of cystoscopic evaluation. The patient tolerated the procedure well without complications.

She was subsequently transferred to the recovery room, extubated, and in stable condition.

Adm Westy MD

GODFREY REGIONAL HOSPITAL
123 Main Street • Aldon, FL 77714 • (407) 555-1234

EXERCISE 26

Level II

OPERATIVE REPORT

Patient information:	
Patient name:	Date:
DOB:	Surgeon:
MR#:	Anesthetist:

Preoperative diagnosis:

1) Right labial mass; 2) Vulvar and vaginal condyloma; 3) HIV positive

Postoperative diagnosis:

Same

FINDINGS: A 2-3-2 cm firm mass involving the right labia. Upon removal of this, it appeared as a large condyloma. Multiple condylomata of the vulvar, perianal, and vaginal areas are noted.

SPECIMENS: Right labial mass

Procedure(s) performed:

Incision of vaginal mass and laser vaporization of condyloma

Anesthesia:

Assistant surgeon:

Description of procedure:

The patient was taken to the operating room and placed in the supine position. Her legs were placed in candy-cane stirrups, and she was prepped and draped in a sterile fashion. Spinal anesthesia was found to be adequate.

The knife was used to make an incision over the right labial mass, which was excised using Metzenbaum scissors and Bovie. The deep tissues were closed with interrupted figure-of-eight sutures of #3 Vicryl and a subcuticular stitch of 3-0 Vicryl was used to close the epithelium. The laser was then used to vaporize the condyloma; it was set on 15 watts of power and test-fired. Vaporization was then performed at the various vulvar and intravaginal regions. Silvadene cream was then applied to the areas.

The patient tolerated the procedure well and went to the recovery room.

She was given a prescription for Vicodin 5/500 #40 to take one po q4h prn for pain, Silvadene cream to use twice a day, and EMLA cream to use prn for vulvar pain. She is to follow up in the office in one week.

Rachel Perez, MD

GODFREY REGIONAL HOSPITAL
123 Main Street • Aldon, FL 77714 • (407) 555-1234

EXERCISE 27

Level I

OPERATIVE REPORT

Patient information:	
Patient name: DOB: MR#:	Date: Surgeon: Anesthetist:

Preoperative diagnosis:

Vaginal bleeding from granulation tissue at area of colonic vaginal fistula repair

Postoperative diagnosis:

Vaginal bleeding from granulation tissue at area of colonic vaginal fistula repair

Procedure(s) performed:

Exam under anesthesia, curettage of granulation tissue with biopsy and cauterization of vaginal vault granulation tissue

Anesthesia:

Assistant surgeon:

Description of procedure:

The patient was brought to the operating room, placed under general anesthesia by oral airway, and prepped and draped in usual sterile fashion. Anti-embolism pumps were running on the leg. Exam under anesthesia revealed granulation tissue we had previously seen. Small, sharp curette of approximately 1-cm width was used to curette the granulation tissue area under direct visualization with removal of a small permanent suture, apparently some Ethibond. The granulation tissue area was curetted out until clean.

Next, the Bovie was set at 20 watts cautery and tissue was gently cauterized with ball electrode. At this point, all the tissue had been freshened. Cauterization had been carried out. Rectovaginal exam was negative.

Patient tolerated the procedure well and went to the recovery room in stable condition.

COMPLICATIONS: None. All counts correct 3 3. Patient taken to recovery room in stable condition.

Rachel Perez MD

GODFREY REGIONAL HOSPITAL
123 Main Street • Aldon, FL 77714 • (407) 555-1234

Level I

OPERATIVE REPORT

Patient information:	
Patient name: DOB: MR#:	Date: Surgeon: Anesthetist:

Preoperative diagnosis:

Pelvic pain

Postoperative diagnosis:

Pelvic pain with adhesions, right ovarian cyst, and pelvic congestion syndrome or pelvic varicosities

Procedure(s) performed:

Laparoscopy, lysis of adhesions, and right ovarian cystectomy

Anesthesia:

General endotracheal

Assistant surgeon:

Description of procedure:

Patient was taken to operating room here. After an adequate level of general endotracheal anesthesia, patient was placed in a modified lithotomy position in Allen stirrups. Foley was placed; patient was draped and prepped in usual sterile fashion. A 45-degree side-open vaginal speculum was placed in the vagina. Cervix was grasped with single-tooth tenaculum and a Hulka uterine manipulator was placed. A subumbilical incision was made, taken down through the subcutaneous tissue to fascia. Fascia was picked up and incised. Peritoneum was opened. Stay sutures of 2-0 Vicryl on UR6 were placed. A blunt origin cannula was placed, through which a 9.9 flow demand of CO_2 with maximum pressure of 15 mm Hg was inserted. A second suprapubic port was made. It should be noted that the appendix was normal, the liver was normal, and the bowel was run and noted to be normal. There were no signs of any endometriosis. The patient's previous tubal ligation was noted. On the patient's right side in the sigmoid, there were a few adhesions to the side wall, which were taken down by sharp dissection. No cautery. The left ovary was noted to be normal. On the right ovary there was a 5-cm cyst, which was marsupialized with scissors and allowed to drain with clear fluid. Also, it should be noted that there were large varicosities of the pelvic wall bilaterally. It should be noted that we put the patient in and out of Trendelenburg to try to reduce or increase them. Even at maximum reverse Trendelenburg and increasing the pressure of the abdomen, there were still large pelvic

GODFREY REGIONAL HOSPITAL
123 Main Street • Aldon, FL 77714 • (407) 555-1234

Continued

OPERATIVE REPORT

Patient information:	
Patient name: DOB: MR#:	Date: Surgeon: Anesthetist:

Preoperative diagnosis:

Postoperative diagnosis:

Procedure(s) performed:

Anesthesia:

Assistant surgeon:

Description of procedure:

varicosities. Thus we had to remove the adhesions, and we opened up the ovarian cyst and marsupialized and noted the pelvic varicosities. All scopes were taken out under direct visualization. The previous subumbilical incision was closed with 2-0 Vicryl. Subcu was injected with 0.5% Marcaine with epinephrine, and the skin was re-approximated with 3-0 Monocryl.

ESTIMATED BLOOD LOSS: Scant

FLUID RECEIVED: Ringer's lactate

PATHOLOGY: None

The patient tolerated the procedure well and went to the recovery room in satisfactory condition.

Rachel Perez MD

GODFREY REGIONAL HOSPITAL
123 Main Street • Aldon, FL 77714 • (407) 555-1234

EXERCISE 29

Level II

OPERATIVE REPORT

Patient information:	
Patient name:	Date:
DOB:	Surgeon:
MR#:	Anesthetist:

Preoperative diagnosis:

Status post bladder neck suspension with vesical sling with erosion

Postoperative diagnosis:

Erosion of vesical sling

Procedure(s) performed:

Removal of eroded bladder neck vesical sling

Anesthesia:

General

Assistant surgeon:

Description of procedure:

The patient was placed on the operating table in the lithotomy position after general anesthesia was given. External genitalia and vagina were prepped and draped in the usual sterile manner. Foley catheter was inserted in the bladder and left indwelling throughout the procedure. The labia were retracted laterally. The weighted speculum was placed on the posterior vaginal wall.

A small incision on the anterior vaginal wall was performed with the cautery over the eroded sling. The synthetic sling was grasped at a right angle and pulled, and the lateral sutures were cut and the sling removed. We were able to pull the suture on the left side completely; however, we were able to pull it partially on the right side. Surgical field was irrigated thoroughly with large amount of antibiotic solution.

The small vaginal incision was left open in order to let it granulate, since the opening was very small and because of infection evidence.

The patient tolerated the procedure well. She was sent to the recovery room in satisfactory condition, and she will be discharged home when discharge criteria are met and after her Foley catheter is removed.

DISCHARGE MEDICATIONS: Levaquin 500 mg one tablet daily for 10 days. She will be advised to have follow-up in the office in 4–6 weeks or as needed.

GODFREY REGIONAL HOSPITAL
123 Main Street • Aldon, FL 77714 • (407) 555-1234

Rachel Perez MD

EXERCISE 30

Level I

OPERATIVE REPORT

Patient information:	
Patient name: DOB: MR#:	Date: Surgeon: Anesthetist:

Preoperative diagnosis:

Urinary retention

Postoperative diagnosis:

Urinary retention

Procedure(s) performed:

Cystoscopy and percutaneous placement of suprapubic catheter

Anesthesia:

Assistant surgeon:

Description of procedure:

The patient was placed on the operating table in the lithotomy position. His perineum was prepped and draped sterilely. 10 cc of Xylocaine jelly was injected per urethra. The scope was inserted. His urethra is unremarkable. Prostate is very large with trilobated hypertrophy and a big median bar that you have to go up and over.

The bladder shows a lot of catheter cystitis and a lot of trabeculation, just diffusely inflamed. The bladder was filled under vision with the cystoscope. I then approached him two fingerbreadths suprapubically infiltrated with Xylocaine through the skin and fascia until I accessed the bladder and could aspirate bladder. I looked in the bladder and I could see the needle coming in the dome of the bladder. I then made a stab incision, and using the Amplatz dilator, dilated to 28 French, leaving the sheath, and placed a 24 French Foley catheter. This was sewn in place. The cystoscope was removed.

He tolerated the procedure without difficulty.

Rachel Perez MD

GODFREY REGIONAL HOSPITAL
123 Main Street • Aldon, FL 77714 • (407) 555-1234

EXERCISE 31

Level II

OPERATIVE REPORT

Patient information:	
Patient name: DOB: MR#:	Date: Surgeon: Anesthetist:

Preoperative diagnosis:

Cancer of the prostate, status post seed implant for prostate cancer, and hematuria

INDICATION FOR PROCEDURE: This patient had a seed implant for prostate cancer in 1997. Recently, the patient has been having blood in the urine. Sometimes it is significant. IVP is negative. The patient also has urgency and urgency incontinence.

Postoperative diagnosis:

Cancer of the prostate, status post seed implant and prostatic urethral stone and bladder stones

Procedure(s) performed:

Cystoscopy, stone extraction, and bilateral retrograde pyelogram

Anesthesia:

Assistant surgeon:

Description of procedure:

The patient was brought to the operating room and spinal anesthesia was given. The patient was placed in lithotomy position. Genitalia were prepped and draped. The cystoscope was introduced. Anterior urethra was normal. Posterior urethra was found to be nonobstructive. But there is evidence of bleeding from this area, especially in the posterior aspect of the prostatic urethra. The prostatic urethra had been resected before. There is no significant obstruction of the prostatic urethra. Bladder neck was found to be open. There are stones stuck in the prostatic urethra. I pushed it back with the cystoscope into the bladder. There were three stones. One of the stones was in the bladder. The stones measure about 1/2 cm. The stones were removed by irrigation. The bladder was examined with a right-angle lens as well as the regular lens. Both ureteric orifices were normal. There is no stone or tumor in the bladder. Then the retrograde was performed by inserting a catheter bilaterally; retrograde is negative. Then the scope was removed, a Foley catheter was inserted, and the patient was sent to the recovery room in good condition.

The patient tolerated the procedure and there was no change in vital signs.

The patient will go home today and we will be removing the catheter tomorrow morning at the office.

GODFREY REGIONAL HOSPITAL
123 Main Street • Aldon, FL 77714 • (407) 555-1234

Rachel Perez MD

NERVOUS SYSTEM EXERCISES

EXERCISE 1

Level II

OPERATIVE REPORT

Patient information:	
Patient name: DOB: MR#:	Date: Surgeon: Anesthetist:

Preoperative diagnosis:

Postoperative diagnosis:

Procedure(s) performed:

Spinal cord stimulator trial; intraoperative spinal cord stimulator screening

Anesthesia:

Assistant surgeon:

Description of procedure:

After an IV was started, the patient was taken to the operating room and placed prone on the operating table. A couple of pillows were placed under the abdomen to straighten out the spinal flexion. The lumbar area was prepped and draped in the usual sterile fashion using DuraPrep, and under direct fluoroscopy the T10 to L2 spinous processes were identified and marked. The skin overlying the L1-2 interspace was infiltrated with 5–6 cc of a mixture of 1% lidocaine and 0.5% bupivacaine.

A small stab wound was made in the L1-2 interspace just above the spinous process. A 15-gauge Tuohy needle was inserted under direct fluoroscopy control through the stab wound and guided into the L1-2 interspace. Under direct fluoroscopy control, the needle was then advanced further until the epidural space was identified using the loss-of-resistance technique. After negative aspiration for blood or CSF was confirmed, a guidewire was inserted through the Tuohy needle and advanced up into the epidural space without any problems. The system was then inserted through the Tuohy needle, and under direct fluoroscopy control, was gradually advanced up into the epidural space in the midline. The final positioning of the tip of the lead was noted to be at the mid body of the T10 vertebra.

The stylet inside the quad lead was removed and a shorter lead connector was inserted into the lead system. This

GODFREY REGIONAL HOSPITAL
123 Main Street • Aldon, FL 77714 • (407) 555-1234

Continued

OPERATIVE REPORT

Patient information:

Patient name: Date:
DOB: Surgeon:
MR#:   Anesthetist:

Preoperative diagnosis:

Postoperative diagnosis:

Procedure(s) performed:

Anesthesia:

Assistant surgeon:

Description of procedure:

connector was then attached to the screening cable and locked into place. The patient was allowed to wake up at this time in preparation for the intraoperative screening. Various combinations were tried intraoperatively, and the final settings of the screener were noted before the lead was disconnected from the screening cable. The Tuohy needle was then withdrawn into the subcutaneous tissue very carefully, and the positioning of the lead was confirmed after the needle was withdrawn. The lead was basically noted to be intact after the needle was withdrawn and removed. The lead was then fixed in place using Steri-Strips, and an extension lead was connected to the quad lead system. Sterile dressing was applied over the lead system, and the patient was transported to the recovery area where she was observed for a few minutes before being discharged home.

POSTOPERATIVE SCREENING:
In the recovery area the patient was educated in detail about the use of the screener and the final settings were as follows: Lead 0 was negative, lead 1 was positive, 2 was off, and 3 was off. Pulse width was 390, rate was at 40, and aptitude was 4.1. The patient was shown how to use the machine and was discharged home on Keflex 500 mg po q8h for seven days and was told to come back for follow-up in one week, at which time we will consider further options, depending on her

GODFREY REGIONAL HOSPITAL
123 Main Street • Aldon, FL 77714 • (407) 555-1234

Continued

OPERATIVE REPORT

Patient information:	
Patient name: DOB: MR#:	Date: Surgeon: Anesthetist:

Preoperative diagnosis:

Postoperative diagnosis:

Procedure(s) performed:

Anesthesia:

Assistant surgeon:

Description of procedure:

response to this modality of treatment. Until such time the patient will continue her OxyContin and baclofen and will also continue her physical therapy exercises. At the time of discharge, the patient reported excellent pain relief as far as her burning neuropathic pain is concerned; however, she continued to have some dull aching, spasmodic pain in the hip joint and in the muscles of the leg.

The patient reported good coverage in both her lower extremities with a slight predominance on the left side.

Rachel Perez MD

GODFREY REGIONAL HOSPITAL
123 Main Street • Aldon, FL 77714 • (407) 555-1234

EXERCISE 2

Level II

OPERATIVE REPORT

Patient information:

Patient name: Date:
DOB: Surgeon:
MR#:   Anesthetist:

Preoperative diagnosis:

Cervical radiculopathy; dystrophy, right upper extremity; headaches

Postoperative diagnosis:

Cervical radiculopathy; dystrophy, right upper extremity; headaches

Procedure(s) performed:

Cervical epidural steroid injections under fluoroscopy and sedation, trigger point injection to right paravertebral neck and suprascapular region on the right side

Anesthesia:

Assistant surgeon:

Description of procedure:

The patient was taken to the operating room. IV fluids given, 200 cc lactated Ringer's preoperatively as prehydration. Monitors placed. IV with sedation given.

Surgical scrub to lower neck under fluoroscopic guidance. C7-C8 intervertebral space was identified. The skin was infiltrated with 1% lidocaine 2 cc. Epidural needle #17 Tuohy, loss-of-resistance technique; loss of resistance positive. Needle position confirmed by fluoroscopy, and 2 cc of 0.25% bupivacaine injected as a test dose. Test dose was negative. No CSF, no heme on aspiration. Then 5 cc of normal saline preservative-free with 40 mg of Depo-Medrol was injected though the epidural space and the needle was removed. Two trigger points were done on the right side, one at the right paravertebral neck and the second at the right suprascapular region. Each trigger point was injected with 2.5 cc of 0.25% bupivacaine and 20 mg of Depo-Medrol to each side.

OPERATIVE REPORT: The patient tolerated the procedure well. Vital signs are stable. The patient was taken to PACU.

POSTOPERATIVE PLAN: Discharge home, ice packs to lower back, follow-up in the office in seven days.

COMPLICATIONS: Nil

Adm Westg MD

GODFREY REGIONAL HOSPITAL
123 Main Street • Aldon, FL 77714 • (407) 555-1234

E X E R C I S E 3

Level II

OPERATIVE REPORT

Patient information:	
Patient name: DOB: MR#:	Date: Surgeon: Anesthetist:

Preoperative diagnosis:

Postoperative diagnosis:

Procedure(s) performed:

Spinal cord stimulator trial; intraoperative screening of the cord lead placement

Anesthesia:

Assistant surgeon:

Description of procedure:

The patient had an IV started and received 1 gram of Ancef IV prior to the procedure. The patient was taken to the operating room and placed prone on the spinal table with a couple of pillows under her hips. The lumbar area was prepped and draped in the usual sterile fashion, and the L2-3 interspace was identified and marked under fluoroscopy. The T9-10 vertebrae were also identified and marked, and a temporary plan to place the tip of the needle around the T9-10 level was made before proceeding with the procedure. The L2-3 interspace was infiltrated with about 6 to 8 cc of 1% lidocaine on the right side. A 17-gauge Tuohy needle was inserted under direct fluoroscopic control into the interspace and advanced gradually until the epidural space was identified using a loss-of-resistance technique. Once the epidural space was identified, an introducer was passed through the needle and advanced a few cm into the epidural space without any resistance. The cord lead was then inserted through the needle and advanced under direct fluoroscopic control gradually into the epidural space and advanced gradually until the tip of the needle was at the T9-10 interspace level. Positioning of the lead was confirmed, both in the AP and the oblique views, and the positioning of the needle was confirmed to be in the posterior epidural space just to the right side of the midline.

The cord lead was then connected to the screener and a trial screening was conducted using various lead settings. The patient had a good coverage of the lower back as well as the right lower extremity and was very satisfied with the type of pain relief that she received with this screening.

The epidural needle was then gradually withdrawn into the subcutaneous tissues, and positioning of the lead was once again confirmed to be

GODFREY REGIONAL HOSPITAL
123 Main Street • Aldon, FL 77714 • (407) 555-1234

Continued

OPERATIVE REPORT

Patient information:	
Patient name: DOB: MR#:	Date: Surgeon: Anesthetist:

Preoperative diagnosis:

Postoperative diagnosis:

Procedure(s) performed:

Anesthesia:

Assistant surgeon:

Description of procedure:

in the T9-10 level. The lead was then taped in place using Steri-Strips, and the stylet was then removed. The cord lead was then connected to extension lead, and gauze dressing was then placed over the leads.

The patient was then taken to the recovery area and final stimulator settings were then performed in the recovery area.

The patient had a good response to the stimulation and had good coverage over the area of her pain.

The patient tolerated the procedure well and had very minimal blood loss. The patient was given her discharge instructions and discharged home after the usual discharge criteria were met.

FOLLOW-UP PLAN: The patient will follow up in the pain clinic in two weeks or so, at which time we will evaluate the patient further, and if she has good control of her pain with this modality, we will go ahead and implant the lead and the generator. Until such time, the patient will take Keflex 500 mg po q8h along with methadone 2.5 mg po q4 to 6 hours prn for breakthrough pain. Patient will also take Soma to treat any muscle spasms.

Adm Westy MD

GODFREY REGIONAL HOSPITAL
123 Main Street • Aldon, FL 77714 • (407) 555-1234

EXERCISE 4

Level I

OPERATIVE REPORT

Patient information:	
Patient name: DOB: MR#:	Date: Surgeon: Anesthetist:

Preoperative diagnosis:

Ulnar neuropathy, right elbow; carpal tunnel syndrome, right wrist

Postoperative diagnosis:

Same

Procedure(s) performed:

Transposition of the ulnar nerve, right elbow, and release of carpal tunnel, right wrist and hand

Anesthesia:

Assistant surgeon:

Description of procedure:

After induction of general anesthesia by CRNA, the patient's right arm was prepped and draped in the usual fashion with a high brachial tourniquet. The arm was elevated and exsanguinated with an Esmarch bandage, and the tourniquet was inflated for a little over an hour during the procedure. The medial right elbow was approached through a curving posteromedial incision. The ulnar nerve was identified proximally. A Penrose drain was placed around it, and it was followed to the cubital tunnel and freed from the tunnel and dissected distally to the flexor carpi ulnaris. Hemostasis was obtained, and the nerve was freed along its course until it could easily be positioned medially anterior to the epicondyle. The subcutaneous pocket was fashioned in this location and 2-0 Vicryl was used to close the pocket over the ulnar nerve in its new position. There was no undue tension. Flexion and extension of the elbow showed no bow stringing or snapping of the ulnar nerve. The wound was copiously irrigated, and subcutaneous layer was closed over the subcutaneous pocket with interrupted 2-0 Vicryl sutures.

Attention was turned to the right hand, which was placed on the hand table, and a palmar incision was made in line with the 4th ray, extending from the distal flexion crease of the wrist distally to the proximal flexion crease of the palm. The palmar aponeurosis was divided. The superficial arterial arch was protected ulnarly, and the flexor tendons were identified and followed to the carpal ligament, which was cleared on both its superficial and deep surfaces, so that it could be divided under direct vision. The ligament was divided well into the distal forearm to ensure complete incision of the transverse carpal ligament. Copious irrigation of the wound was carried out. The median nerve lay radial in the carpal tunnel. External neurolysis was performed. The tenosynovium appeared to be somewhat thickened, but not overtly diseased. Limited synovectomy was carried out to de-bulk the carpal tunnel, and the skin alone was closed with interrupted 4-0 nylon sutures.

GODFREY REGIONAL HOSPITAL
123 Main Street • Aldon, FL 77714 • (407) 555-1234

Continued

OPERATIVE REPORT

Patient information:	
Patient name:	Date:
DOB:	Surgeon:
MR#:	Anesthetist:

Preoperative diagnosis:

Postoperative diagnosis:

Procedure(s) performed:

Anesthesia:

Assistant surgeon:

Description of procedure:

Staples were then used to close the elbow incision and a sterile bulky Robert Jones dressing was applied with the Bunnell hand dressing. The wrist was held in dorsiflexion with a splint and a posterior splint was applied to hold the elbow in 90 degrees of flexion.

The tourniquet was deflated and the patient was sent to the recovery room in satisfactory condition. There were no complications.

Adm Westg MD

GODFREY REGIONAL HOSPITAL
123 Main Street • Aldon, FL 77714 • (407) 555-1234

EXERCISE 5

Level I

PAIN MANAGEMENT REPORT

Patient information:

Patient name: Date:
DOB: Surgeon:
MR#:   Anesthetist:

Preoperative diagnosis:

Postoperative diagnosis:

Procedure(s) performed:

Anesthesia:

Assistant surgeon:

Description of procedure:

INTRATHECAL PUMP INCREASE:
82-year-old gentleman comes to our clinic for increase in pump refill. This patient comes to our clinic due to geographical proximity to his home.

Patient has intrathecal pump, and his PCP asked us to increase the patient's dose by 10%. Concentration of the medication in the pump is morphine 25 mg per cc and bupivacaine 7.5 mg per cc.

The patient was placed supine on the examination table. Telemetry was performed, and patient has current reserve volume of 13.4 cc until continuous rate of 0.45 mg per hour or 10.80 mg per day.

His pump was increased to provide a continuous rate of 0.495 mg per hour to a total of 11.882 mg per day.

The patient tolerated the procedure well. Patient left the clinic in stable condition.

GODFREY REGIONAL HOSPITAL
123 Main Street • Aldon, FL 77714 • (407) 555-1234

Continued

PAIN MANAGEMENT REPORT

Patient information:

Patient name: Date:
DOB: Surgeon:
MR#:   Anesthetist:

Preoperative diagnosis:

Postoperative diagnosis:

Procedure(s) performed:

Anesthesia:

Assistant surgeon:

Description of procedure:

ASSESSMENT/PLAN:
This is an 82-year-old gentleman with chronic low back pain who is status-post laminectomy and failed back syndrome. He has the intrathecal pump in place, which delivers both morphine and bupivacaine. He comes into our clinic for pump reprogramming. His PCP requested increase by 10% and that was done today.

Thank you for letting us participate in this patient's care.

Rachel Perez MD

GODFREY REGIONAL HOSPITAL
123 Main Street • Aldon, FL 77714 • (407) 555-1234

Level I

PAIN MANAGEMENT REPORT

Patient information:	
Patient name:	Date:
DOB:	Surgeon:
MR#:	Anesthetist:

Preoperative diagnosis:

Postoperative diagnosis:

Procedure(s) performed:

Trigger point injections

Anesthesia:

Assistant surgeon:

Description of procedure:

Mary Smythe is a 58-year-old lady who has myofascial pain syndrome. She was doing better after the last set of trigger point injections; however, she went to a funeral out of town, and from riding that distance, she states that her back pain had increased.

PROCEDURE: Risks, benefits, and options discussed. Written consent was obtained. Vital signs stable, afebrile. The patient is placed in the sitting position. Palpation of the longissimus muscle and also the multifidus muscle reveals eight total trigger points. These trigger points were marked, skin prepped with alcohol, aseptic technique. 26-gauge needle and Marcaine 0.25% 1 cc was injected into each trigger point. The patient tolerated the procedure well and left the clinic in stable condition.

ASSESSMENT AND PLAN:
Myofascial pain syndrome in the lower lumbar and upper sacral areas. The patient received trigger point injections as above. The patient will return to clinic in one week for repeat trigger point injections. Will consider MRI of the lumbar spine if series of trigger point injections does not improve her low back. The patient is to continue physical therapy.

Thank you for letting us participate in this patient's care.

Rachel Perez MD

GODFREY REGIONAL HOSPITAL
123 Main Street • Aldon, FL 77714 • (407) 555-1234

Continued

EXERCISE 7

Level I

PAIN MANAGEMENT REPORT

Patient information:	
Patient name:	Date:
DOB:	Surgeon:
MR#:	Anesthetist:

Preoperative diagnosis:

Postoperative diagnosis:

Procedure(s) performed:

Trigger point injections

Anesthesia:

Assistant surgeon:

Description of procedure:

The patient is a 59-year-old lady who comes in for trigger point injections for treatment of myofascial pain syndrome. She states that she is having some increased pain in the right side of her lower lumbar upper sacral area. She has been to the tanning bed and she is sunburned on the back.

PROCEDURE: Risks, benefits, and options were discussed, and written consent was obtained. Vital signs stable, afebrile. The patient is placed sitting on the examination table. Palpation of the right longissimus muscles in the lumbar area and also the multifidus muscle reveals a total of eight trigger points. These trigger points were marked, skin prepped with alcohol. 1 cc of 0.25% Marcaine with 3 mg of Kenalog was injected into each trigger point. The patient tolerated the procedure well and left the clinic in stable condition.

ASSESSMENT AND PLAN:
1. Chronic low back pain, status post back surgery, failed back syndrome
2. Patient is status post three caudal epidural injections. The patient is on medications for chronic pain. She is currently taking MS Contin 15 mg q12 hours.
3. Myofascial pain syndrome. The patient received trigger point injections as above. The patient will return to the clinic in approximately one or two weeks for possible repeat trigger point injections.

Thank you for allowing us to participate in this patient's care.

Adm Westy MD

GODFREY REGIONAL HOSPITAL
123 Main Street • Aldon, FL 77714 • (407) 555-1234

EXERCISE 8

Level I

PAIN MANAGEMENT REPORT

Patient information:	
Patient name: DOB: MR#:	Date: Surgeon: Anesthetist:

Preoperative diagnosis:

Postoperative diagnosis:

Procedure(s) performed:

Bilateral injections of steroids into the wrists

Anesthesia:

Assistant surgeon:

Description of procedure:

A 24-year-old lady has bilateral wrist pain with occasional radiation of the pain into the arms and elbows. She was involved in a motor vehicle accident. The patient states that she continues to have bilateral wrist pain and it has not improved. I talked to her about possibly injecting some steroids between the articular processes in her wrists bilaterally. The risks, benefits, and options were discussed. She understood and accepted.

After oral and written consent, sterile prep with Betadine and alcohol, a 22-gauge needle was used to inject 0.125% bupivacaine plain along with Kenalog, approximately 6 mg per cc. The patient's wrists were injected on the dorsal side. She received an injection near the articular fossa of the ulna and the pisiform bone; 1 cc was injected in a fanlike manner in that area. Then another 1 cc was injected between the lunate and the radius in a fanlike manner and this was again done at the radius and the scaphoid bone. This was done on both wrists.

The patient tolerated the procedure well. She stated relief prior to leaving the clinic.

GODFREY REGIONAL HOSPITAL
123 Main Street • Aldon, FL 77714 • (407) 555-1234

Continued

PAIN MANAGEMENT REPORT

Patient information:

Patient name:	Date:
DOB:	Surgeon:
MR#:	Anesthetist:

Preoperative diagnosis:

Postoperative diagnosis:

Procedure(s) performed:

Anesthesia:

Assistant surgeon:

Description of procedure:

ASSESSMENT/PLAN:

Patient was involved in a motor vehicle accident in January 2002. Most of her aches and pains have been getting gradually better except for her wrists bilaterally. She did not have wrist pain before the accident. She has wrist pain after the accident.

Patient was unable to be seen by orthopedic service due to her current lawsuit situation.

Patient received injection of steroids at the wrists to decrease possible inflammation in the dorsal wrist area of bone and ligaments.

Patient will return to the clinic in 1 to 2 weeks for possible repeat injection.

Thank you for letting us participate in the patient's care.

Adm Westy MD

GODFREY REGIONAL HOSPITAL
123 Main Street • Aldon, FL 77714 • (407) 555-1234

EXERCISE 9

Level II

PAIN MANAGEMENT REPORT

Patient information:

Patient name: Date:
DOB: Surgeon:
MR#:   Anesthetist:

Preoperative diagnosis:

Postoperative diagnosis:

Procedure(s) performed:

Left lumbar facet denervation with pulse radiofrequency

Anesthesia:

Assistant surgeon:

Description of procedure:

The patient follows up at the pain clinic for radiofrequency pulse denervation of her left lumbar facet nerve. All risks and benefits of the procedure are explained to the patient and the patient wishes to proceed.

After sterile prep and drape and localization of the skin using a 20-gauge SMK spinal needle, the needle was advanced down into the medial portion of the left L2 transverse process, corresponding to the left L1-L2 facet nerve after a stimulation test that was positive for pain but negative for radiculopathy, was performed. This area was pulsed for a total of 120 seconds at 42–44 degrees Celsius heat and the patient tolerated the procedure well.

The exact same procedure was carried out at the left L2-L3 facet nerve.

The exact same procedure was carried out at the left L3-L4 facet nerve.

The exact same procedure was carried out at the left L4-L5 facet nerve.

The exact same procedure was carried out at the left L5-S1 facet nerve. A negative motor stimulation test was performed.

ASSESSMENT: Lumbar facet disease with chronic low back pain.

GODFREY REGIONAL HOSPITAL
123 Main Street • Aldon, FL 77714 • (407) 555-1234

Continued

PAIN MANAGEMENT REPORT

Patient information:		
Patient name: DOB: MR#:		Date: Surgeon: Anesthetist:

Preoperative diagnosis:

Postoperative diagnosis:

Procedure(s) performed:

Anesthesia:

Assistant surgeon:

Description of procedure:

PLAN: The plan will be for the patient to follow up in the pain clinic in one week, and we will see how she is doing after the completion of her lumbar facet pulse denervation. She is to continue with all her current medications.

Rachel Perez MD

GODFREY REGIONAL HOSPITAL
123 Main Street • Aldon, FL 77714 • (407) 555-1234

EXERCISE 10

Level I

PROGRESS NOTE

Patient information:

Patient name: Date:
DOB: Surgeon:
MR#:   Anesthetist:

Preoperative diagnosis:

Postoperative diagnosis:

Procedure(s) performed:

Anesthesia:

Assistant surgeon:

Description of procedure:

The patient follows up to the pain clinic for investigation of facet nerve with discogram. The patient understands all the risks and benefits of the procedure and she wishes to proceed.

After sterile prep and drape and localization of the skin using a discogram needle set, the introducer needle was passed into the right L4-L5 disk and the discogram needle was passed into the right L4-L5 disk, and this area was pressurized with 1/2 cc of Isovue-M 300, which was mixed with Ancef. The patient tolerated the injection well and there was no pain during the injection.

The exact same procedure was carried out at the L5-S1 disk. At this level during pressurization of the L5-S1 disk with 1/2 cc of Isovue-M 300, the patient noted concordant pain that was 80–90% reproduction of her usual low back pain. Therefore, this is a positive provocative discogram. We are going to go ahead and send her to CT scanner today.

ASSESSMENT: Status post discogram with chronic low back pain

PLAN: We are going to go ahead and have the patient follow up in one week and we will discuss with her the findings of the discogram, as well as the findings of the CAT scan.

Adm Westy MD

GODFREY REGIONAL HOSPITAL
123 Main Street • Aldon, FL 77714 • (407) 555-1234

EXERCISE 11

Level II

OPERATIVE REPORT

Patient information:	
Patient name:	Date:
DOB:	Surgeon:
MR#:	Anesthetist:

Preoperative diagnosis:

Internal disk disruption at L4-L5 and lumbar disk bulge at L3-L4

Postoperative diagnosis:

Internal disk disruption at L4-L5 and lumbar disk bulge at L3-L4

Procedure(s) performed:

Nucleoplasty at L3-L4 and right L4-L5 IDET

Anesthesia:

Assistant surgeon:

Description of procedure:

PREOPERATIVE INFORMATION: All risks and benefits of the procedure were explained to the patient to include paralysis, nerve injury, worsening of the symptoms, failure of the procedure, bleeding, and infection. The patient understands all of these risks and the patient wishes to proceed. The patient is given 1 gram of vancomycin IV piggyback prior to taking him into the operating room.

DESCRIPTION OF PROCEDURE:
The patient is placed prone on the spinal table in the operative suite, and the patient is sterilely prepped and draped. After localization of the skin at the L3-L4 level, coming in from the right side, a 17-gauge introducer needle is passed into the L3-L4 disk and confirmed on two planes by fluoroscopy, after which the Per-D catheter is passed into the L3-L4 disk, and at this level a total of 8 channels are created at the 2, 4, 6, 8, and 10 o'clock positions along with two additional channels. At each of these channels, coblation is performed during entry into the disk and coagulation is performed during exit from the disk.

The patient experienced muscle spasms during creation of several of these channels, and during the muscle spasm episodes, the coblation was discontinued. Each of the muscle spasms was during coblation and not coagulation. At each time that the patient had muscle spasms, the tip of the needle was confirmed on fluoroscopy. The patient tolerated this procedure well without complications.

The IDET procedure was then set up at the L4-L5 level and initial attempt was made from the right side after entering into the L4-L5 disk with a 17-gauge needle that is part of the IDET kit. The IDET catheter kinked during passage into the L4-L5 disk from the right side, and therefore,

GODFREY REGIONAL HOSPITAL
123 Main Street • Aldon, FL 77714 • (407) 555-1234

Continued

OPERATIVE REPORT

Patient information:	
Patient name:	Date:
DOB:	Surgeon:
MR#:	Anesthetist:

Preoperative diagnosis:

Postoperative diagnosis:

Procedure(s) performed:

Anesthesia:

Assistant surgeon:

Description of procedure:

the needle and the catheter were removed and the L4-L5 disk was entered from the left side. After the disk was entered with 17-gauge needle, the intradiskal catheter was passed into the L4-L5 disk without complications and was seen to wrap completely around the posterior lateral aspect of the right L4-L5 disk without paresthesias and without complications.

At this level, the catheter tip temperature was set at 65 degrees centigrade, after which it was increased by 1 degree centigrade to a total of 90 degrees centigrade where it was maintained for 4 minutes. There were no paresthesias and there was no radiculopathy during this procedure.

The patient tolerated this without complications.

POSTOPERATIVE DISCUSSION: The patient is given 40 tablets of Lortab 10/650 for postop pain control. The patient states that he must travel tonight and states that he is going to go ahead and put a bed in the back of his car and he will go in the supine position. The patient states that he needs to go because there is no one to take care of him here, and therefore, I have cautioned him against this trip. But he is determined to go, and therefore, I have given him his pain medication that he can take on an as-needed basis. Instructions for him I have given to him on two separate sheets—one for recovery from nucleoplasty and one for recovery from IDET. The patient is to wear a back brace for the first week during recovery in which he is to not perform any strenuous exercises. He is to slowly increase his activity over the next 2 to 3 weeks after his recovery. The patient is to call the pain clinic if he has any problems at all or any signs of an infection. The patient will start his physical therapy sometime around 3 to 4 weeks, depending on his recovery process.

Adm Westg MD

GODFREY REGIONAL HOSPITAL
123 Main Street • Aldon, FL 77714 • (407) 555-1234

EXERCISE 12

Level II

OPERATIVE REPORT

Patient information:	
Patient name:	Date:
DOB:	Surgeon:
MR#:	Anesthetist:

Preoperative diagnosis:

Lumbar disk bulge with chronic low back pain with radiculopathy at L5-S1

Postoperative diagnosis:

Same

Procedure(s) performed:

Nucleoplasty at right L4-L5

Anesthesia:

Assistant surgeon:

Description of procedure:

PREOPERATIVE INFORMATION:
The patient is seen in the preop holding area where all risks and benefits of the procedure are explained to the patient once again to include failure of the procedure, increased paresthesia, increased back pain, bleeding, infection, nerve injury, and paralysis. The patient understands all of these risks and she wishes to proceed.

The patient is given IV antibiotics, that is Ancef IV piggyback for 1 gram, and the patient is taken into the operating suite.

DESCRIPTION OF PROCEDURE: In the operating suite in the prone position, the patient's back is prepped with DuraPrep, and after finding the L4-L5 interspace with fluoroscopic guidance, using the 17-gauge introducer needle, the needle is advanced into the L4-L5 disk from the right side and confirmed on two planes by fluoroscopy. After the needle is slightly retracted to the outer edge of the annulus, the Per-D catheter is advanced to the anterior annulus and then retracted back into the 17-gauge discogram needle. Then the procedure is started where coblation is started during advancement of the Per-D catheter at the 12 o'clock position, and then the catheter is slightly retracted at increments of 0.5 cm per second with coagulation performed during retraction of the needle. These procedures are carried out at the 2, 4, 6, 8, and 10 o'clock positions of the disk along with two other positions, totaling eight channels created within the right side of the L4-L5 disk.

GODFREY REGIONAL HOSPITAL
123 Main Street • Aldon, FL 77714 • (407) 555-1234

Continued

OPERATIVE REPORT

Patient information:	
Patient name:	Date:
DOB:	Surgeon:
MR#:	Anesthetist:

Preoperative diagnosis:

Postoperative diagnosis:

Procedure(s) performed:

Anesthesia:

Assistant surgeon:

Description of procedure:

The patient tolerated the procedure well. The patient was awake during most of the procedure and lightly sedated, and experienced no paresthesias and no complications.

POSTOP DISCUSSION: The nucleoplasty at the right L4-L5 was done without complications. The plan will be for the patient to be on antibiotics for ten days and I have given her a prescription for Cipro at 500 mg to take twice a day for the next ten days. The patient is to undergo rest and I have given her a sheet that describes the rest period and what she can and cannot do. She is going to go ahead and undergo rest for a week and then slowly increase her activity, and then we are going to go ahead and follow her up back at the pain clinic in about two weeks. The patient will be given a prescription for Darvocet for a total of 40 tablets, 100 mg, that she can take on an as-needed basis for pain.

Adm Westg MD

GODFREY REGIONAL HOSPITAL
123 Main Street • Aldon, FL 77714 • (407) 555-1234

EXERCISE 13

Level I

OPERATIVE REPORT

Patient information:

Patient name: Date:
DOB: Surgeon:
MR#:   Anesthetist:

Preoperative diagnosis:

Postoperative diagnosis:

Procedure(s) performed:

Caudal epidural steroid injection

Anesthesia:

Assistant surgeon:

Description of procedure:

In the prone position, after sterile prep and drape and localization of the skin using a 22-gauge 3.5-inch spinal needle, the tip of the needle is placed into the epidural space caudally and confirmed with 2 cc of Isovue M-300, which is seen to spread into the sacral space. After a negative aspiration, 15 cc of 1/8% bupivacaine with a total of 80 mg of Depo-Medrol was injected without difficulty.

The patient tolerated the injection well. There were no complications.

ASSESSMENT: Chronic low back pain with radiculopathy.

PLAN: The patient received his second epidural steroid injection today via the caudal route without complications. The patient states that the first epidural steroid injection did not help him with his low back pain. Therefore we decided to go ahead and deliver the epidural steroid injection from the caudal route to see if this could give us any benefit in his chronic pain. Will go ahead and have him follow up in ten days, and if he does not notice any benefit from the second epidural steroid injection, then will go ahead and proceed with diagnostic lumbar facet blocks, since some of his low back pain may be secondary to facet disease. The patient was given a prescription for hydrocodone last year, but the patient states that

GODFREY REGIONAL HOSPITAL
123 Main Street • Aldon, FL 77714 • (407) 555-1234

Continued

OPERATIVE REPORT

Patient information:		

Patient name: Date:
DOB: Surgeon:
MR#: Anesthetist:

Preoperative diagnosis:

Postoperative diagnosis:

Procedure(s) performed:

Anesthesia:

Assistant surgeon:

Description of procedure:

the hydrocodone made him feel sick. Therefore he was given a prescription for Dilaudid, but he states that he did not feel as though the Dilaudid was helping him very much. So therefore he has discontinued his current medications. He is still taking Mobic without complications.

Rachel Perez MD

GODFREY REGIONAL HOSPITAL
123 Main Street • Aldon, FL 77714 • (407) 555-1234

EXERCISE 14

Level II

OPERATIVE REPORT

Patient information:

Patient name:
DOB:
MR#:

Date:
Surgeon:
Anesthetist:

Preoperative diagnosis:

Post lumbar laminectomy pain syndrome

Postoperative diagnosis:

Post lumbar laminectomy pain syndrome

Procedure(s) performed:

1. Implantation of constant flow aero pump. The pump chosen is a 50 cc pump with a 1 cc per day delivery rate.
2. Implantation of intrathecal aero catheter with tunneling
3. Intrathecal myelogram with interpretation
4. Intraoperative use of fluoroscopy
5. Pump refill with total of 50 cc of morphine sulfate, concentration 0.5 mg/cc to deliver 0.5 mg of morphine per day
6. Pump re-bolus with 0.5 mg of morphine sulfate using a special aero type of intrathecal bolus injection needle

Anesthesia:

General endotracheal

Assistant surgeon:

Description of procedure:

COMPLICATIONS: None
BLOOD LOSS: Less than 25 cc
DESCRIPTION OF PROCEDURE:
After informed consent, and after detailed description of the procedure and its rationale, including complications, benefits, alternatives, and risks, the patient understands and wishes to proceed. The patient was placed on standard monitors with oxygen supplementation and positioned prone on the fluoro table. Mid to lower back area was then prepped with Betadine and draped in the usual sterile fashion. After general anesthesia was administered, he was positioned in the left lateral decubitus, and the right lower back, right flank, and right lower abdominal area were prepped with Betadine and draped in the usual sterile fashion.

Initially, incision was made in the lower lumbar region, along the previous scar. Dissection was carried down to the fascia plane under continuous fluoroscopy, and the 17-gauge intra-thecal needle was used to access the intra-thecal space. At the level of L3, L4, the intra-thecal space was identified and brisk CSF backflow was noted. Under continuous fluoroscopy, the titanium alloy catheter was threaded in a cephalad direction to the lower border of T11. At this time, the distal end of the catheter was accessed and approximately 5 cc of Isovue 200 was injected with visualization of the intrathecal myelographic effect, which was seen to extend from the upper border of T9 to the lower border of L4. A picture was saved for the records. Subsequently, the intrathecal needle was removed and the catheter was secured with

GODFREY REGIONAL HOSPITAL
123 Main Street • Aldon, FL 77714 • (407) 555-1234

Continued

OPERATIVE REPORT

Patient information:

Patient name:
DOB:
MR#:

Date:
Surgeon:
Anesthetist:

Preoperative diagnosis:

Postoperative diagnosis:

Procedure(s) performed:

Anesthesia:

Assistant surgeon:

Description of procedure:

pursestring sutures using 4-0 Prolene, and the catheter was secured to the underlying catheter using 2-0 silk at three different points. Subsequently, attention was directed to the right lower abdominal area where a transverse incision was made about the level of the umbilicus, and the tissues were dissected down to the fascia where a pocket was created to accommodate the pump reservoir. The catheter was tunneled from the lumbar region to the site of the pump reservoir. The pump was secured to the underlying fascia using three different points with 0 Prolene sutures. The intrathecal catheter was connected to the pump catheter in the usual manner and a test flow was carried out to verify adequate CSF backflow without any obstruction or leak. The pump was then filled with a total of 50 ccs first delivery of morphine sulfate, concentration 0.5 mg/cc. A special bolus injection needle was introduced and the position appropriately verified, and a total of 0.5 mg of morphine was given as a direct intrathecal bolus.

Both wounds were thoroughly irrigated with Bacitracin-containing irrigant. Verifying adequate hemostasis, the wounds were closed in two layers using 3-0 Vicryl sutures for subcutaneous closure, interrupted. Staples were used for the skin. The patient tolerated the procedure well without complication and was transferred to the recovery room in stable condition. The patient received 2 grams of Ancef preoperatively and will be continued on Ancef IV throughout his hospitalization. He will be admitted to the observation suite. Postoperatively, he was examined and he was found to be hemodynamically and neurologically stable.

PLAN:
1. Admit to the observation suite.
2. Follow up and re-assess.

Adam Westy MD

GODFREY REGIONAL HOSPITAL
123 Main Street • Aldon, FL 77714 • (407) 555-1234

EXERCISE 15

Level II

OPERATIVE REPORT

Patient information:

Patient name: Date:
DOB: Surgeon:
MR#:   Anesthetist:

Preoperative diagnosis:

1. Status post implantation of programmable Medtronic pump
2. End of battery life

Postoperative diagnosis:

1. Status post implantation of programmable Medtronic pump
2. End of battery life

Procedure(s) performed:

1. Explantation of Medtronic pump
2. Revision of the implant pocket
3. Implantation of constant-flow aeropump type of pump implanted with 30 cc reservoir with 0.5 cc per day delivery rate
4. Pump refill with a total of 18 cc, the first delivery of morphine sulfate concentration, 10 mg per cc with clonidine concentration 100 micrograms per cc, a total of only 18 cc was used to fill the pump reservoir.
5. Pump bolus with 0.5 mg of morphine sulfate as a direct intrathecal bolus by the implanted catheter for anesthesia/pain management.

Anesthesia:

Endotracheal anesthesia

Assistant surgeon:

Description of procedure:

BLOOD LOSS: Less than 10 cc

COMPLICATIONS: None

INSTRUMENT AND LAP COUNT: Correct

DESCRIPTION OF PROCEDURE:
Following informed consent, and after detailed description of the procedure, complications, and risks, the patient understands and accepts the risks and complications and wishes to proceed. The patient was cleared by primary care physician. The patient was taken to the operating suite and positioned supine on the fluoroscopy table. The existing Medtronic pump was prepped with Betadine and draped in the usual sterile fashion. Incision was made along the previous scar and the tissues were dissected down to the fascial plane. The anchoring sutures of the existing pump were released. It was evident at that point that the previous Medtronic pump was implanted subcutaneously and it was not anchored to the underlying fascia. We then proceeded to dissect the capsule out. The floor of the capsule was completely removed. Subsequently, the subcutaneous tissues were dissected down to the fascial plane. The fascia was exposed. At this point, three 0-Proline sutures were used to anchor the aeropump to the underlying fascia at three different rings. The aeropump catheter was then connected to the existing intrathecal catheter using a special metallic connector. A test flow was then carried out using a special aero intrathecal bolus injection needle with visualization of CSF backflow without any obstruction or leakage. Subsequently, a total of 0.5 mg of morphine sulfate was given

GODFREY REGIONAL HOSPITAL
123 Main Street • Aldon, FL 77714 • (407) 555-1234

Continued

OPERATIVE REPORT

Patient information:

Patient name: Date:
DOB: Surgeon:
MR#:   Anesthetist:

Preoperative diagnosis:

Postoperative diagnosis:

Procedure(s) performed:

Anesthesia:

Assistant surgeon:

Description of procedure:

as a direct intrathecal bolus. The pump reservoir was then filled with a total of 18 cc of morphine sulfate, concentration at 10 mg per cc, with clonidine concentration 100 mcg per cc. The wound was thoroughly irrigated. Adequate hemostasis was then achieved. Wound was then closed in two layers using 3-0 Vicryl interrupted subcutaneous closure and staples of the skin. Betadine ointment, Telfa, and sterile dressing were applied.

The patient was taken to the recovery room in stable condition. The patient received antibiotic prophylaxis preoperatively and will be continued on oral antibiotics as an outpatient. He will be released today once he is assessed to be hemodynamically and neurologically stable, which he is at this time. The patient will be seen in follow-up in the office for further care.

Adm Westy MD

GODFREY REGIONAL HOSPITAL
123 Main Street • Aldon, FL 77714 • (407) 555-1234

EXERCISE 16

Level II

OPERATIVE REPORT

Patient information:

Patient name: Date:
DOB: Surgeon:
MR#:   Anesthetist:

Preoperative diagnosis:

Postoperative diagnosis:

DIAGNOSES:
1. Chronic, intractable, excruciating low back pain with lower extremity pain, which resists treatment. The patient had a successful trial of morphine pump to control the pain using a continuous morphine drip.
2. Post hemilaminectomy pain syndrome associated with neuropathic pain in the bilateral lower extremities

Procedure(s) performed:

1. Placement of intrathecal subarachnoid implantable non-programmable catheter
2. Thoracic myelogram
3. Placement of non-programmable Arrow implantable morphine pump

Anesthesia:

Using MAC/fentanyl and propofol drip accompanied with local infiltration of the wounds with bupivacaine 0.25% with epinephrine and spinal anesthesia for the rest of the case with MAC

Assistant surgeon:

Description of procedure:

ESTIMATED BLOOD LOSS: Minimal, 5 to 10 ml blood

DESCRIPTION OF THE PROCEDURE:
The patient signed an informed consent after full discussion and explanation with the patient and his friend about the procedure, rationale, side effects, complications, limitations, risks, and alternatives. The patient received 2 mg Ancef intraoperatively intravenously, and he will receive another 1 mg in the PACU.

The patient was brought to the operating room and positioned in the left lateral decubitus. The sites of the wound incisions in the back and in the right lower abdominal wall were marked. The patient was then prepped and draped in sterile technique, which was maintained all through. The back and the right side of the abdomen were prepared in routine sterile fashion. The L2-L3 vertebral spine was identified and infiltrated using bupivacaine 0.25% with epinephrine. The percutaneous 17-gauge Tuohy needle was inserted at the level of L2/3. The bevel was cephalad. The dura was punctured at about 5 cm deep from the skin. After free flow, an intrathecal special catheter was threaded through the needle with bevel directed cephalad. The tip of the catheter was placed around T12 and was threaded up in the subarachnoid space, about 10 to 12 cm. A C-arm fluoroscope with a TV monitor was used. The contrast material, Isovue 266 about 1.25 ml, was injected and was given a good intrathecal spread with myelogram picture without any pathological findings. A midline skin incision was made and carried out through subcutaneous tissue to the dorsal fascia. A clear flow was tested again. No blood but clear cerebral spinal fluid. With the needle in place,

GODFREY REGIONAL HOSPITAL
123 Main Street • Aldon, FL 77714 • (407) 555-1234

Continued

OPERATIVE REPORT

Patient information:	
Patient name: DOB: MR#:	Date: Surgeon: Anesthetist:

Preoperative diagnosis:

Postoperative diagnosis:

Procedure(s) performed:

Anesthesia:

Assistant surgeon:

Description of procedure:

purse-string stitches were placed using 3-0 Prolene. The catheter stylet was removed. Then 3-0 Prolene ties sutured the anchor to the underlying fascia using 3-0 Prolene and secured the catheter.

At the same time, another physician, at the other side of the table, created a pocket in the lower part of the right abdominal quadrant of the abdominal wall to hold the Arrow pump, and a transverse skin incision about 3 to 4 inches was made through the subcutaneous tissue to the external oblique fascia. The other surgeon used the previously marked pocket site, which was in between the costal margin and the iliac crest region, using cautery to desiccate down through the subcutaneous tissue to the level about the fascia and the pocket, adequate to accommodate the pump. The other physician created a pocket there. Meticulous hemostasis was used on the abdominal wall and back where the catheter was placed. Using the tunneling device provided, a subcutaneous tunnel was created between the posterior incision and the abdominal incision. The tubing that connected to the catheter with reservoir was brought through the tunnel. Of course, we provided titanium connector to connect them. Sutures secured the connection. The Arrow pump with capacity of 30 ml and 0.5 ml per day perfusion rate was prepped at the back table by emptying its water content and was refilled with 18 ml of the preservative-free Duramorph 1 mg/ml concentration. The extension tubing was connected as mentioned above to the Arrow pump after tying the catheter. The morphine pump was secured in place. Subcutaneously, the Arrow pump was placed into the pocket and secured to the underlying fascia using an 0 Prolene suture. Hemostasis was adequately achieved throughout the procedure using electrocautery. Hemostasis was meticulously performed. At this

GODFREY REGIONAL HOSPITAL
123 Main Street • Aldon, FL 77714 • (407) 555-1234

Continued

OPERATIVE REPORT

Patient information:

Patient name:
DOB:
MR#:

Date:
Surgeon:
Anesthetist:

Preoperative diagnosis:

Postoperative diagnosis:

Procedure(s) performed:

Anesthesia:

Assistant surgeon:

Description of procedure:

time, using a special needle to prime the catheter, 0.5 ml and another 0.5 ml which equals 0.5 ml Duramorph were used to prime the catheter and to give bolus intrathecally to the patient. The wounds were copiously irrigated with Bacitracin solution and closed in layers in routine fashion using 3-0 Vicryl for the subcutaneous tissue. The skin was closed using 2-0 nylon sutures with continuous stitches. After the sterile dressing was applied, the instrument, needle, and sponge counts were correct after being counted by scrub nurse and both surgeons.

The patient is transferred to the PACU in stable condition with no complications and absolute pain-free status. The patient will remain in the recovery room or in the same-day surgery unit for a few hours and will be discharged home per criteria to follow as outpatient with the surgeon.

Rachel Perez MD

GODFREY REGIONAL HOSPITAL
123 Main Street • Aldon, FL 77714 • (407) 555-1234

EXERCISE 17

Level II

OPERATIVE REPORT

Patient information:	
Patient name: DOB: MR#:	Date: Surgeon: Anesthetist:

Preoperative diagnosis:

Chronic back pain, status post back injury and multiple herniated disks and back surgery

Postoperative diagnosis:

Chronic back pain, status post back injury and multiple herniated disks and back surgery

Procedure(s) performed:

Insertion of morphine pump in conjunction with another surgeon

Anesthesia:

Assistant surgeon:

Description of procedure:

After the patient was given sedation by anesthesiologist, he was put with his left side down, and the abdomen and back were prepped with Betadine and then sterile towel-draped. After the other surgeon did his incision in the back and inserted the epidural catheter, I did an incision in the left upper outer quadrant area, about 3.5 inches, and then I dissected down and created a pocket about 5 inches below that and then subcutaneous over the fascia, and hemostasis was done with cautery. I flushed the wound with Kantrex antibiotics. Then I inserted the pump and sutured it in four places with nylon 0 to the deep fascia to keep it in place. Then we ran a tunnel between this wound and the spine wound, and we tied the spinal catheter to the abdominal wound. Then we connected the catheter from the pump and spinal catheter together with a special device. We made a loop of them, about 3 inches to 4 inches, to be lying without tension, and the loop of the catheter behind the pump, and the pump was filled first before with morphine, and after we inserted the catheters together, we inserted 1 cc of morphine to the pump as requested by the representative of the pump. Then the wound was again irrigated with Kantrex antibiotics; we closed the subcutaneous tissue with chromic 3-0 and silk with nylon 3-0 as well, and the patient lost maybe 4–5 cc of blood and tolerated the procedure.

The other surgeon finished his wound and the patient tolerated the procedure and went to the recovery room. The patient received Ancef before and during the procedure by IV.

Rachel Perez MD

GODFREY REGIONAL HOSPITAL
123 Main Street • Aldon, FL 77714 • (407) 555-1234

EXERCISE 18

Level I

OPERATIVE REPORT

Patient information:	
Patient name: DOB: MR#:	Date: Surgeon: Anesthetist:

Preoperative diagnosis:

Carpal tunnel syndrome, left wrist

Postoperative diagnosis:

Carpal tunnel syndrome, left wrist

Procedure(s) performed:

Left carpal tunnel release

Anesthesia:

Assistant surgeon:

Description of procedure:

SURGICAL TECHNIQUE: The patient was brought to the operating room and placed in the supine position. After adequate block, the arm was prepped with DuraPrep and sterilely draped in the usual manner. We made a small incision directly over the carpal ligament and deep and via careful scissors dissection to the ligament itself. The ligament was then sharply incised. Once we accessed tunnel, the ligament was released under direct visualization, both proximally and distally at its entire length. The nerve was initially quite pale and then turned purple. We made sure the nerve was free and we irrigated the wound and closed the skin with 4-0 nylon. The patient tolerated the procedure well and was placed in a splint and taken to the recovery room in good condition.

Adm Westy MD

GODFREY REGIONAL HOSPITAL
123 Main Street • Aldon, FL 77714 • (407) 555-1234

EXERCISE 19

Level II

PAIN CONSULTATION PROCEDURE NOTE

Patient information:	
Patient name: DOB: MR#:	Date: Surgeon: Anesthetist:

Preoperative diagnosis:

PROVISIONAL DIAGNOSIS:
1. Low back pain with left radicular symptoms
2. Probable significant degenerative arthritis, lumbar disk disease and L5 or S1 neuropathy

Postoperative diagnosis:

Procedure(s) performed:

Anesthesia:

Assistant surgeon:

Description of procedure:

HISTORY:
Kathy is a frail 82-year-old woman who presents today for an empiric epidural steroid injection because of persistent and worsening low back pain with left leg pain. She reports that she has had back and neck pain on and off now for years. She has had several superficial injections done by another physician in the office, but none in the last 6 months. Since the early part of the summer, the back pain and the left leg pain have become quite significant and pronounced. There really are no inciting factors or any history of injury. She has pain not only when she is walking, but also when she is lying or sitting, and the pain extends all the way down into her foot. She does state though that it seems to be a little bit more pronounced and frequent when she is upright and active doing any type of activity.

Her past medical history is significant for multiple medical problems. She has had long-standing coronary artery disease and had CABG times two both in '82 and '87. She is on multiple medications for her heart and has had frequent admissions for angina and chest pain. She also has a history of not only frequent pneumonias but also obstructive pulmonary disease. Osteoarthritis of almost all the major joints in her body. She also states that she has had problems since childhood with scoliosis. Her current medication list includes Cardizem, nitroglycerin patch, Darvocet, Premarin, trazodone, alprazolam, Micro-K, enalapril, Lasix, Miacalcin, Prilosec, Coreg, Arthrotec, Plavix, albuterol nebulizers, and Azmacort. She has been off her Plavix since last Wednesday; this would make this 9 days off her Plavix, which should be more than sufficient for the anti-platelet affect to have receded. The medications she can't take include aspirin, alcohol, caffeine, sulfa, Bentyl, Pepcid, Zantac, and multiple antibiotics including Augmentin, erythromycin, oxacillin, monacoliln, and Bactrim. None of these medications have caused

GODFREY REGIONAL HOSPITAL
123 Main Street • Aldon, FL 77714 • (407) 555-1234

Continued

PAIN CONSULTATION PROCEDURE NOTE

Patient information:	
Patient name: DOB: MR#:	Date: Surgeon: Anesthetist:

Preoperative diagnosis:

Postoperative diagnosis:

Procedure(s) performed:

Anesthesia:

Assistant surgeon:

Description of procedure:

anaphylaxis but most of them do have side effects she can't tolerate, usually GI in nature.

There were no imaging studies to review or recent x-rays of her lumbar spine.

Limited physical exam was done. The patient walks with a very guarded gait, although it is not antalgic in nature. Surprisingly, the sensory exam of the lower extremities is well preserved. She does have both decreased dorsal and plantar flexion in the left foot, as there is decreased left lower leg extension. Hip flexors are normal and symmetric bilaterally. Deep tendon reflexes at the knees are 21 symmetric and absent at the ankles. There is a positive straight leg raise sign at 50 degrees, with pain going down into the left calf. Contralateral on the right side was negative. Examination of her lower back revealed no overt trigger points or evidence of significant SI joint dysfunction. She does have a leftward tilting scoliosis that extends from about T-12 into the L4-5 region. Further questioning of the patient revealed that she has not had any increase or evidence of bowel or bladder dysfunction.

After a lengthy discussion with the patient and her husband, we went ahead and did an empiric L4-5 epidural steroid injection. After informed consent was obtained, she was placed in the sitting position. The L4-5 interspace was identified and a sterile Betadine prep was applied. 1% lidocaine was used for local anesthesia. An 18-gauge Tuohy needle was then introduced in the epidural space using the loss-of-resistance technique. Several re-directions of the needle were necessary due to probable osteophyte formation in the intraspinous and intralaminar spaces. Ultimately, the epidural space was found nicely at a depth of approximately 5 centimeters, and after negative aspiration times two,

GODFREY REGIONAL HOSPITAL
123 Main Street • Aldon, FL 77714 • (407) 555-1234

Continued

PAIN CONSULTATION PROCEDURE NOTE

Patient information:

Patient name:	Date:
DOB:	Surgeon:
MR#:	Anesthetist:

Preoperative diagnosis:

Postoperative diagnosis:

Procedure(s) performed:

Anesthesia:

Assistant surgeon:

Description of procedure:

the patient received a total of 80 mg of sterile methylprednisolone acetate in addition to 4 ccs of 0.5% lidocaine, which was used as a carrier. She tolerated the injection well without any systemic side effects. She was monitored in the preoperative holding area for a period of approximately 20 minutes, and then was discharged home in her stable pre-procedure condition.

From an empiric standpoint, it appears that the patient has some nerve root irritation and possible concomitant spinal stenosis at the lower lumbar sacral interface. We will see how she does with this empiric injection at L4-5. To be absolutely certain of the extent of the degenerative processes that are going on in her lower back, of course, we would have to get an MRI or a CAT scan of her back. Hopefully, with this empiric injection we will find significant improvement in her symptomatology and we can follow her on a PRN basis when she has exacerbations and flare-ups. She will follow up with her family doctors in the near future and she will continue on with all her previously prescribed therapies and medications as prescribed by his office. It should be noted that I also advised her to re-start her Plavix in the morning.

Rachel Perez MD

GODFREY REGIONAL HOSPITAL
123 Main Street • Aldon, FL 77714 • (407) 555-1234

EXERCISE 20

Level I

OPERATIVE REPORT

Patient information:

Patient name:
DOB:
MR#:

Date:
Surgeon:
Anesthetist:

Preoperative diagnosis:

Carpal tunnel syndromes, thenar paresis, right

Postoperative diagnosis:

Carpal tunnel syndromes, thenar paresis, right

Procedure(s) performed:

Carpal tunnel release, with median external neurolysis and release motor branch (right)

Anesthesia:

Assistant surgeon:

Description of procedure:

OPERATION:
After informed consent and complete discussion of the alternatives, potentials, and complications, and no guarantees implied or given, the patient was taken to the operating room. After an adequate level of regional and intravenous anesthesia had been obtained, the patient's upper extremity was surgically scrubbed with Betadine soap and prepped with Betadine solution. Draping occurred in the usual sterile fashion. Following Esmarch exsanguination, the forearm tourniquet was elevated to 150 mm Hg above systolic pressure.

A thenar incision was utilized. Dissection was carried down through the subcutaneous fat and fascia under 3 1/2 power loupe magnification. The superficial nerves were kept out of harm's way throughout the procedure.

The palmar fascia was divided longitudinally and the transverse carpal ligament was then carefully identified. A hemostat was placed under the ligament, and under direct visualization, the ulnar border of the transverse carpal ligament was released. Care was taken to release the most proximal border of the transverse carpal ligament by tunneling proximally with elevation of the proximal skin and speculum retractor until a complete release of the proximal carpal ligament and distal forearm fascia had been performed. Following this, a digit could be placed in the carpal tunnel, demonstrating complete release.

Next, the external neurolysis was performed with freeing of the scarred fascicles. Marked hourglass constriction and scarring were noted locally in the median nerve and motor branch. The sensory and motor branches were carefully dissected and released of the constricting

GODFREY REGIONAL HOSPITAL
123 Main Street • Aldon, FL 77714 • (407) 555-1234

Continued

OPERATIVE REPORT

Patient information:

Patient name:
DOB:
MR#:

Date:
Surgeon:
Anesthetist:

Preoperative diagnosis:

Postoperative diagnosis:

Procedure(s) performed:

Anesthesia:

Assistant surgeon:

Description of procedure:

tissue. The motor branch was identified and followed into the thickened abductor pollicis brevis fascia, and the constricting fascia was released.

Next, the thickened synovial layer between the medial nerve and tendons was released. The small finger could be placed in the carpal tunnel, demonstrating that the ligament was completely released over the median nerve, using the nasal speculum to directly view the ligament. Irrigation was carried out with triple antibiotic solution. Marcaine, 0.5%, and Decadron were instilled. The skin was re-approximated with subcuticular 3-0 Vicryl for the palmar fascia and interrupted 4-0 Prolene. Steri-Strips were applied. A bulky sterile hand dressing with volar and radial splint supports was applied with the thumb held in the protected position with adduction and opposition.

Following release of the tourniquet, good capillary fill was noted in the fingers. The patient tolerated the operative procedure and anesthesia satisfactorily. No breaks in sterile technique occurred. No complications occurred. The patient did receive cephalosporin antibiotics thirty minutes prior to the procedure prophylactically. The patient was taken to the recovery room with stable vital signs in satisfactory condition.

The patient was instructed preoperatively on the need for physiotherapy to maximize healing during the rehabilitation period.

Adm Westy MD

GODFREY REGIONAL HOSPITAL
123 Main Street • Aldon, FL 77714 • (407) 555-1234

EXERCISE 21

Level II

PAIN MANAGEMENT NOTE

Patient information:

Patient name: Date:
DOB: Surgeon:
MR#:   Anesthetist:

Preoperative diagnosis:

Postoperative diagnosis:

Procedure(s) performed:

Left stellate ganglion block

Anesthesia:

Assistant surgeon:

Description of procedure:

Mr. Donald Wilson is a 51-year-old man with possible sympathetic mediated pain in the left hand after a crush injury sustained at work, and then subsequent surgical repair and fusion of digits #2 and #5. He comes in for stellate ganglion block.

PROCEDURE:
Risks, benefits, options discussed; written consent obtained. Vital signs stable, afebrile. The patient placed supine on examination table under fluoroscopy. Sterile prep with Betadine, sterile drape and technique. Fluoroscopy was used to locate the C7 transverse process anteriorly. The patient received skin wheal local infiltration with a 26-gauge needle and lidocaine 1 cc 1%. An 18-gauge needle was used to perform a skin niche, then a 22-gauge blunt-tipped stellate ganglion block needle was placed through the skin niche and directed at the left transverse process. On aspiration, there was dark-colored blood (non-pulsatile) in the syringe. The needle was withdrawn. Pressure was applied to the neck. After approximately two minutes of mild pressure to the left side of the neck, the fluoroscope was used to visualize the transverse process of the C6 on the left. Then the skin was again anesthetized with lidocaine 1% 1 cc. Then the 18-gauge needle was used to perform a skin niche there. A 22-gauge stellate ganglion block blunt needle was then directed by fluoroscopy towards the transverse process. The needle came in contact with the transverse process, and aspiration during the insertion showed no EVL, and the patient experienced no paresthesias. Then 1 cc of Marcaine 0.25% with epinephrine 1/200,000 was injected after a negative aspiration. The patient did not show any signs of IT or IV injection. Then an additional 9 ccs was injected in increments of 2–3 ccs.

GODFREY REGIONAL HOSPITAL
123 Main Street • Aldon, FL 77714 • (407) 555-1234

Continued

PAIN MANAGEMENT NOTE

Patient information:	
Patient name: DOB: MR#:	Date: Surgeon: Anesthetist:

Preoperative diagnosis:

Postoperative diagnosis:

Procedure(s) performed:

Anesthesia:

Assistant surgeon:

Description of procedure:

The patient was then placed onto the recovery bed and placed sitting. He was monitored throughout the procedure and post-procedure, and he also had a peripheral IV in place prior to the procedure start. The patient tolerated the procedure well. The patient stated very good relief, but not complete relief in digits #5 and #2. The patient was told it was 5 p.m. when he received the injection and he is to let us know how long the injection lasts. He states that the previous injection only lasted three hours; it was given by a different doctor in a different clinic.

Fifty-one-year-old man with left-hand possible complex regional pain syndrome after crush injury and subsequent surgeries to repair it. The patient has undergone one stellate ganglion block at a different institution. Now, he has received a second stellate ganglion block at this pain clinic. He is to return to clinic for repeat stellate ganglion block next week under fluoroscopy.

He states he is having problems with the Neurontin. He is to go ahead and discontinue that medication. He is to continue the other medications as prescribed.

The patient was given an injection at 5 p.m. today and we will see how long this injection lasts.

Adm Westy MD

GODFREY REGIONAL HOSPITAL
123 Main Street • Aldon, FL 77714 • (407) 555-1234

EXERCISE 22

Level II

PAIN MANAGEMENT NOTE

Patient information:

Patient name: Date:
DOB: Surgeon:
MR#:   Anesthetist:

Preoperative diagnosis:

Postoperative diagnosis:

BRIEF INTERVAL HISTORY: This 35-year-old male has been complaining of low back pain without much radiation into the lower extremities. The patient has had about two diagnostic facet median nerve blocks so far, and following each of these procedures, the patient has reported excellent pain relief for a few weeks. Since the last procedure, the patient was apparently doing very well until about two days ago. The pain has gradually returned and has returned his back to the baseline. The patient does not report any weakness or numbness in his lower extremities and denies any bladder or bowel problems. The patient is here today for a possible facet denervation of the lumbar levels. Risks, benefits, and alternatives of the procedure were once again explained to the patient. The patient understands and agrees to the procedure as planned.

Procedure(s) performed:

Anesthesia:

Assistant surgeon:

Description of procedure:

After an IV was started, the patient was taken to the fluoroscopy suite and placed prone on the fluoroscopy table. The lumbar area was prepped and draped in the usual sterile fashion and L2-3, 3-4, 4-5, and L5-S1 levels were identified and marked. The patient was given 2 mg of Versed IV at the start of the procedure and during the procedure. The patient received intermittent doses of fentanyl, 25 micrograms at a time for a total of 75 micrograms.

The junctions between the transverse process and the body of the vertebrae were identified and marked under fluoroscopy at each level. The skin at this point was infiltrated with 1% lidocaine. A needle was inserted perpendicular to the skin and advanced gradually under fluoroscopy until contact was made at the bone at the junction between the transverse process and the body of the vertebrae at the superior medial aspect. The position of the needle was confirmed both in the AP and the oblique views. The radiofrequency catheter was then inserted through this needle and the facet median nerve was identified by stimulating at 50 hertz. The patient was also tested for any motor sensations by stimulating at 2 hertz. After the positioning of the needle was confirmed, the radiofrequency probe was applied to the lesion for 70 seconds at 90 degrees Fahrenheit. This procedure was repeated at each of these levels and the patient tolerated the procedure well. The patient was observed in the recovery area for a few minutes before being discharged home according to the usual discharge criteria.

FOLLOW-UP PLAN: The patient is to follow up in the pain clinic in 2-3 weeks, at which time we will consider further treatment options. The patient is to continue current medications and will take Percocet 1-2 tablets po q4-6h prn for any breakthrough pain. *Rachel Perez* MD

GODFREY REGIONAL HOSPITAL
123 Main Street • Aldon, FL 77714 • (407) 555-1234

Level II

PAIN MANAGEMENT NOTE

Patient information:	
Patient name: DOB: MR#:	Date: Surgeon: Anesthetist:

Preoperative diagnosis:

The patient is a 40-year-old lady from the military with low back pain with symptoms into the right hip and legs worsening over the past year. She has been treated with physical therapy in the past. Also, she had previous SI joint injections and epidural injections. She comes in for diagnostic facet block for possible facet pain syndrome.

Postoperative diagnosis:

Procedure(s) performed:

Anesthesia:

Assistant surgeon:

Description of procedure:

Risks, benefits, options discussed; written consent obtained. Vital signs stable, afebrile. The patient had peripheral IV in place. The patient was prone on the fluoroscopy table. Sterile prep with Betadine, sterile drape and technique. Fluoroscopy was used to locate the L3 transverse processes and the L4-L5 transverse processes also, and at the sacral ala area. The patient received skin wheal local infiltration leading to the medial superior aspect of the transverse processes bilaterally at L3, L4, and L5. She also received skin wheal local infiltration leading to the sacral ala bilaterally. A 22-gauge spinal needle was directed by fluoroscopy toward the medial superior aspect of the transverse process bilaterally. After a negative aspiration, 0.5 to 1 cc of Marcaine 0.5% with Depo-Medrol 4 mg per cc was given into each site. A total of eight injections. A total of approximately 4–8 ccs of the 0.5% Marcaine with Depo-Medrol was injected.

ASSESSMENT AND PLAN:
1. Possible facet pain syndrome. The patient presented today for diagnostic facet block. She is to return to clinic next week for repeat diagnostic facet block for possible future percutaneous radiofrequency denervation of the medial branch nerves.
2. Currently, unlikely diskogenic pain. The patient has had diskogram and CT of the diskogram, which were both negative.

GODFREY REGIONAL HOSPITAL
123 Main Street • Aldon, FL 77714 • (407) 555-1234

Continued

PAIN MANAGEMENT NOTE

Patient information:

Patient name: Date:
DOB: Surgeon:
MR#:   Anesthetist:

Preoperative diagnosis:

Postoperative diagnosis:

Procedure(s) performed:

Anesthesia:

Assistant surgeon:

Description of procedure:

3. Currently, unlikely sacroiliitis at this time. The patient states she had previous SI joint injections and they helped for approximately three days to one week.
4. Patient states that she has had previous epidural steroid injections and some injections had helped for approximately three weeks to one month.

The patient is to return to clinic for her second diagnostic facet block next week.

Adam Westy, MD

GODFREY REGIONAL HOSPITAL
123 Main Street • Aldon, FL 77714 • (407) 555-1234

EXERCISE 24

Level II

OPERATIVE REPORT

Patient information:

Patient name: ,   Date:
DOB: Surgeon:
MR#:   Anesthetist:

Preoperative diagnosis:

1. Malfunction of implanted Medtronic pump
2. Failed back surgery syndrome

Postoperative diagnosis:

1. Malfunction of implanted Medtronic pump
2. Failed back surgery syndrome

Procedure(s) performed:

1. Implantation of intrathecal Arrow catheter with tunneling and connection to the existing Medtronic pump
2. Pump refill with morphine sulfate, concentration 5 mg per cc, 18 cc volume
3. Pump review with reprogramming
4. Intraoperative fluoroscopy
5. Intrathecal myelography

Anesthesia:

Assistant surgeon:

Description of procedure:

COMPLICATIONS: None

Following informed consent after detailed description of the procedure and its rationale, complications, benefits, alternatives, and risks, the patient understands and accepts the risks and complications and wishes to proceed.

The patient was taken to the operating suite and positioned prone on the fluoro table. Monitored anesthesia care was established. The mid to lower back area was prepped with Betadine and draped in the usual sterile fashion. Under continuous fluoroscopy, the Medtronic catheter was identified and an incision was made along the previous scar. Tissues were dissected down to the fascial plane and the catheter was dissected out and identified. At this time a 17-gauge Arrow intrathecal needle was introduced under continuous fluoroscopy into the intrathecal space at the level of L3-L4. The intrathecal Arrow catheter was then advanced under continuous fluoroscopy to the lower border of T11. At this time the distal end of the catheter was accessed and approximately 3 cc of Isovue 200-M was injected with visualization of intrathecal myelogram, which was seen to extend from the upper thoracic regions down to the upper lumbar region, primarily to the left side of the midline. Following this, the needle was partially removed and a 3-0 Prolene purse-string suture was taken around the catheter and tied from lead to the underlying tissues after removal of the intrathecal needle. The catheter was then secured to the underlying fascia using the anchor provided in the Arrow kit. The Arrow catheter was tunneled underneath the skin and connected to the existing Medtronic catheter

GODFREY REGIONAL HOSPITAL
123 Main Street • Aldon, FL 77714 • (407) 555-1234

Continued

OPERATIVE REPORT

Patient information:	
Patient name: DOB: MR#:	Date: Surgeon: Anesthetist:

Preoperative diagnosis:

Postoperative diagnosis:

Procedure(s) performed:

Anesthesia:

Assistant surgeon:

Description of procedure:

using the special Arrow connector, and the wound was closed in two layers using 3-0 Vicryl sutures and two layers for subcutaneous closure and staples for the skin. Betadine ointment and a sterile dressing were applied.

The patient was transferred to the recovery room in stable condition. In the recovery room, with the patient supine, the area over the existing Medtronic pump was prepped with Betadine. The pump reservoir was accessed using a 22-gauge non-coring needle and the residual volume of approximately 1 cc was aspirated and removed. Subsequently, the pump was filled with a total of 18 cc of fresh preservative-free morphine sulfate at a concentration of 5 mg per cc. The pump was then programmed to begin at 0.25 mg per day, and a bridge bolus was calculated to accommodate the catheter space and was programmed as 2.5 mg to be delivered over 23 minutes.

The patient tolerated the procedure well without any complication. The patient will be discharged later today once she meets full ambulatory discharge criteria; will follow up and reassess her condition on an outpatient basis to check the wound and further adjust the intrathecal infusion therapy. She is continued on Percocet on an as-needed basis for incision pain control as well as Keflex orally.

Rachel Perez MD

GODFREY REGIONAL HOSPITAL
123 Main Street • Aldon, FL 77714 • (407) 555-1234

EYE EXERCISES

EXERCISE 1

Level II

OPERATIVE REPORT

Patient information:	
Patient name: DOB: MR#:	Date: Surgeon: Anesthetist:

Preoperative diagnosis:

Watery eyes since birth

Postoperative diagnosis:

Same

Procedure(s) performed:

Bilateral tear duct probing

HISTORY:
This young child has had watery eyes since birth. Massage and antibiotics controlled it somewhat, but eyes continued to be sticky, so it was elected to syringe and probe his ducts.

Anesthesia:

Assistant surgeon:

Description of procedure:

Under general anesthesia, the left eye was started and the lower canaliculus was dilated, but we were unable to pass along the duct into the lacrimal sac. So going through the upper canaliculus, which was narrow at the junction of the upper and lower canaliculi, I was able to enter the sac. Syringed and probed with a #2 probe. On the right, the inferior duct was opened into the lacrimal sac and syringed and probed with a #2. I discussed with the parents afterwards that the right eye looked like it was going to be okay, but the left one may well need tubes in the future. Patient is to be seen in a week in the office.

Linda Patrick MD

GODFREY REGIONAL HOSPITAL
123 Main Street • Aldon, FL 77714 • (407) 555-1234

EXERCISE 2

Level I

OPERATIVE REPORT

Patient information:	
Patient name:	Date:
DOB:	Surgeon:
MR#:	Anesthetist:

Preoperative diagnosis:

Cicatricial ectropion, left lower lid

Postoperative diagnosis:

Same

Procedure(s) performed:

Lidocaine injection of left lower lid
BRIEF HISTORY:
Please see preoperative note

Anesthesia:

Assistant surgeon:

Description of procedure:

The patient was taken to the operating room. She was prepped and draped in the usual manner. A pledget with 4% Xylocaine was placed on the lower lid. This was allowed to sit for 10 minutes. An anesthetic solution was prepared using 0.75% Marcaine mixed one to one with 2% Xylocaine added. This was labeled "strong solution." Then 1 cc of this solution was placed in an additional syringe with 9 cc of balanced salt solution; this was labeled "dilute solution."

The patient was given an inferior lower lid injection using 1 cc of the dilute solution. This was extended as an inferior orbital nerve block. This was allowed to sit for two minutes. The patient was then given an additional 1 cc of the anesthetic mixture in a similar fashion. The lower lid was seen to swell, become black and blue, and the patient developed an intralid hemorrhage—quite extensive.

Pressure was then placed on the area, and we observed for approximately 15 minutes. The globe appeared unaffected, but there is a marked ecchymosis of the lower lid, with marked distortion of landmarks. It was felt that the case should be canceled.

On extensive questioning of this patient, she states she took Goody's powder despite her instructions one week ago. We will place ice on the area, and she will be seen tomorrow morning at 9:00 a.m. for her first postoperative visit. We will reschedule her surgery when the hemorrhage has resolved.

Linda Patrick, MD

GODFREY REGIONAL HOSPITAL
123 Main Street • Aldon, FL 77714 • (407) 555-1234

EXERCISE 3

Level II

OPERATIVE REPORT

Patient information:	
Patient name: DOB: MR#:	Date: Surgeon: Anesthetist:

Preoperative diagnosis:

Primary open-angle glaucoma, left eye

Postoperative diagnosis:

Primary open-angle glaucoma, left eye

Procedure(s) performed:

Trabeculectomy, left eye

Anesthesia:

Assistant surgeon:

Description of procedure:

The eye was dilated with three drops of Cyclogyl along with drops of Ocufen and Ocuflox. In the surgery room, I added a drop of Neo-Synephrine 10%. Betadine was applied to the lid, lashes, and conjunctiva. She was sedated per Vanlint and peribulbar block of the usual anesthetic mixture minus Wydase, administered by me. This was followed with a full Betadine prep and the usual sterile drape. 50 mg of cefazolin was injected into the subconjunctiva and/or applied to the ocular surface. A traction suture was placed under the superior rectus tendon about 12 mm superior to the limbus. A limbus-based conjunctival incision was cut approximately 9–10 mm superior to the limbus, and the conjunctiva was turned back to the limbus. This proceeded very easily. A pledget soaked in 5-FU was applied to the planned trabeculectomy site. This was allowed to touch the tendinous layer over the trabeculectomy site, but not at the conjunctiva wound margin. This was held in place for three minutes and then the dissection bed was thoroughly irrigated. A 4-mm rectangular trabeculectomy flap was cut using a guarded diamond blade at a depth of 0.25 mm. The dissection was carried forward into the clear cornea. Paracentesis was cut at 1:30 and the chamber was filled with viscoelastic. The incision was cut with a 3.0-mm diamond keratome. The trabeculectomy was then fashioned using a series of 5 overlapping punches with a Kelly punch, 3 radial oriented and 2 circumferentially oriented. Corresponding peripheral iridectomy was cut. The trabeculectomy flap was

GODFREY REGIONAL HOSPITAL
123 Main Street • Aldon, FL 77714 • (407) 555-1234

Continued

OPERATIVE REPORT

Patient information:	
Patient name:	Date:
DOB:	Surgeon:
MR#:	Anesthetist:

Preoperative diagnosis:

Postoperative diagnosis:

Procedure(s) performed:

Anesthesia:

Assistant surgeon:

Description of procedure:

sutured down with 2 interrupted 10-0 nylons, which clearly allowed filtration. The conjunctiva and tendons were then closed with running sutures of 10-0 nylon. They were closed in two separate layers. 0.1 cc of 5-FU was injected subconjunctivally and internasally. The eye was dressed with a collagen shield soaked in Ocuflox, and Maxitrol was applied to the lid, which was closed with a Steri strip, followed by a sterile pad and metal shield.

She tolerated the procedure extremely well. At the close of the case, filtration was clearly established with irrigation in the paracentesis. The eye would hold soft to normal pressure as estimated digitally. Conjunctiva was intact and the suture line was secure. The cornea and chamber were clear. A modest amount of viscoelastic was left in the chamber.

Linda Patrick MD

GODFREY REGIONAL HOSPITAL
123 Main Street • Aldon, FL 77714 • (407) 555-1234

EXERCISE 4

Level I

OPERATIVE REPORT

Patient information:	
Patient name: DOB: MR#:	Date: Surgeon: Anesthetist:

Preoperative diagnosis:

Cataract, right eye

Postoperative diagnosis:

Cataract, right eye

Procedure(s) performed:

Phacoemulsification of the lens of the right eye, with posterior chamber intraocular lens implant

Anesthesia:

Topical

Assistant surgeon:

Description of procedure:

The patient was brought to the anesthesia waiting area and administered a drop of tetracaine in the eye. The patient was then taken into the operating room and placed in the supine position. Two drops of viscous lidocaine were placed in the conjunctival cul-de-sac of the eye. The patient was administered a mild sedative intravenously. The patient was then prepared and draped in the usual sterile fashion.

A 15-degree blade was used to make a stab incision at approximately two o'clock to the left of the temporal meridian. One-half cc of unpreserved 1% lidocaine was then irrigated into the anterior chamber. The anterior chamber was filled with Vitrax. A 2.65-mm keratome was advanced through the temporal limbus into the anterior chamber. A stab capsulotomy was then made with a 25-gauge bent-tip cystotome. Forceps were used to complete the circular capsulorrhexis.

The nucleus of the lens was hydrodissected with balanced salt solution. Phacoemulsification of the nucleus of the lens was carried out using a phaco chop method in 1 minute and 17 seconds with an EPT of 33 seconds. The residual cortex was aspirated from the cul-de-sac. The posterior capsule was polished. The capsular bag was filled with BioLon. An Allergen model AR 40, 20 diopter posterior chamber lens was then introduced into the capsular bag. The residual BioLon was removed from the eye.

GODFREY REGIONAL HOSPITAL
123 Main Street • Aldon, FL 77714 • (407) 555-1234

Continued

OPERATIVE REPORT

Patient information:

Patient name:	Date:
DOB:	Surgeon:
MR#:	Anesthetist:

Preoperative diagnosis:

Postoperative diagnosis:

Procedure(s) performed:

Anesthesia:

Assistant surgeon:

Description of procedure:

The wound was hydrated with balanced salt solution. The wound was stable without leakage. Drops of Ocuflox, Pred Forte, and Timoptic 0.5% were placed in the eye. The patient was taken to the recovery area in a stable condition.

ADDENDUM: Because of preexisting extreme density of the nucleus, BSS 1 was employed. Following the emulsification of half of the nucleus, additional Vitrax was placed into the anterior chamber. The cornea was clear at the end of the case.

Linda Patrick MD

GODFREY REGIONAL HOSPITAL
123 Main Street • Aldon, FL 77714 • (407) 555-1234

EXERCISE 5

Level II

OPERATIVE REPORT

Patient information:	
Patient name:	Date:
DOB:	Surgeon:
MR#:	Anesthetist:

Preoperative diagnosis:

Anisometropia, status post inaccurate intraocular lens implantation one month ago

Postoperative diagnosis:

Same

Procedure(s) performed:

Intraocular lens exchange, posterior chamber—left eye

ESTIMATED BLOOD LOSS: Less than 0.1 cc

COMPLICATIONS: None

INDICATIONS FOR SURGERY: This 76-year-old patient had an inaccurate intraocular lens calculation that resulted in four diopters of anisometropia. This is not tolerable to the patient as she likes to get up in the evening without needing her glasses. The risks and benefits of the exchange were discussed. A consent was signed. Her physical was updated.

Anesthesia:

Local retrobulbar with modified lid block

Assistant surgeon:

Description of procedure:

The patient was taken to the operating room and given IV sedation. She was given a four-cc volume of the standard mixture as a retrobulbar block with a modified lid block. The surgeon massaged the eye for four minutes. The patient was prepped and draped. The eyelashes were taped off the field. A speculum was placed. A peritomy was made superiorly. Cautery was used. A 5.2 millimeter incision was made 1.5 millimeters from the limbus. This was tunneled into clear cornea superiorly. The chamber was entered. Viscoat on a cannula was used to dissect the capsular bag away from the intraocular lens. The intraocular lens was then dialed out of the bag. The wound was expanded to 5.2 millimeters. The implant was removed with a forceps. Part of the wound was closed with a 10-0 nylon suture. A 17 diopter AMQSI40NB was inserted into the capsular bag and dialed into the 3 and 9 o'clock positions. The residual Viscoat was removed in its entirety using an automated irrigation aspiration set-up. Miochol was used to bring the pupil to a small round size. The wound was sutured with a second 10-0 nylon suture. The conjunctiva was sutured with 8-0 Vicryl. The patient received an inferior injection of Kenalog and gentamicin. TobraDex ointment was placed. The eye was patched.

The patient tolerated the procedure well. There were no complications. She will receive a Diamox sequel x one. She will leave her eye patched until the morning and then she will start her TobraDex four times a day. I will see her tomorrow.

Linda Patrick, MD

GODFREY REGIONAL HOSPITAL
123 Main Street • Aldon, FL 77714 • (407) 555-1234

EXERCISE 6

Level II

OPERATIVE REPORT

Patient information:	
Patient name:	Date:
DOB:	Surgeon:
MR#:	Anesthetist:

Preoperative diagnosis:

Lower lid ectropion and punctual stenosis, bilateral

Postoperative diagnosis:

Procedure(s) performed:

Bilateral punctoplasty also with a bilateral ectropion repair via a medial spindle procedure, also known as a lower lid shortening procedure

Anesthesia:

Assistant surgeon:

Description of procedure:

The family was informed of the risks and benefits of the procedure, and informed consent was placed in the chart. The patient was brought back to the operating room. Vital signs were noted to be stable. The patient is given local anesthesia using a 50/50 mixture of 0.75% Marcaine, 2% lidocaine with epinephrine, and Wydase. 0.5 cc of the solution was injected into the lower lids of both eyes. The patient was prepped and draped in a sterile fashion. Using a long Vannas scissors, a 1-snip punctoplasty was performed in both lower canaliculi. I then turned my attention to the lower lid. I removed a wedge of conjunctiva as well as underlying muscle and re-approximated the wedge using interrupted 8-0 Vicryl sutures. This turned the lower lid in nicely, medially. Both eyes were done in the exact same manner.

Patient tolerated the procedure well. Estimated blood loss was less than 5 ccs. Patient is to use TobraDex drops 4 times a day for approximately 1 week and follow up in 1 month or sooner if she is having problems. No complications.

Linda Patrick MD

GODFREY REGIONAL HOSPITAL
123 Main Street • Aldon, FL 77714 • (407) 555-1234

EXERCISE 7

Level II

OPERATIVE REPORT

Patient information:

Patient name:

DOB:

MR#:

Date:

Surgeon:

Anesthetist:

Preoperative diagnosis:

Keyhole iris due to previous cataract surgery

Postoperative diagnosis:

Same

Procedure(s) performed:

Suture of iris, left eye

Anesthesia:

Assistant surgeon:

Description of procedure:

Stab incision done at 2 o'clock and another one at 4:30 and at 3. 1 blade incision at 3 o'clock using a 16-mm straight needle. This was passed through the 2 o'clock incision into a hollow-bore needle through the 4:30 incision, having passed through 1 flap of the iris on the way through the anterior chamber. The needle was then turned, re-passed through this incision and through the other flap of the iris, and out through the 2 o'clock incision. The loose ends of the sutures were then drawn through the 3 o'clock incision. The needles were cut off. The suture was tied at the 3 o'clock position, opposing the two parts of the sphincter pupil, and these sutures were then cut flush with the iris. The chamber was reformed, and the patient was patched with Maxidex for a couple of hours. As he hadn't had a retrobulbar, he did not have to leave the patch on overnight. The patient was discharged from the theater in good condition.

Linda Patrick, MD

GODFREY REGIONAL HOSPITAL

123 Main Street • Aldon, FL 77714 • (407) 555-1234

EXERCISE 8

Level II

OPERATIVE REPORT

Patient information:	
Patient name: DOB: MR#:	Date: Surgeon: Anesthetist:

Preoperative diagnosis:

Ectropion, left lower lid

Postoperative diagnosis:

Same

Procedure(s) performed:

Wedge resection, left lower lid
COMPLICATIONS:
None

Anesthesia:

Local, with standby

Assistant surgeon:

Description of procedure:

NARRATIVE DESCRIPTION:
The patient was brought to the operating room directly from outpatient status. He was placed on the operating table and made secure and comfortable. Anesthesia administered medication that produced profound sedation. While sedated, he was given a local injection in the left lower lid of 2% Xylocaine with epinephrine. Prepping and draping were carried out in the usual manner. The globe was anesthetized with tetracaine so that the patient would not be uncomfortable when we touched the eye. Stevens scissors was used to resect a large-base triangular wedge between the medial and the lateral thirds of the lower lid close to the end of the tarsal plate. Hemostasis was obtained with cautery. The defect was then closed with interrupted 6-0 Vicryl. Two sutures were put through the tarsal plate and securely tied, giving good apposition. A third suture was placed through the grey line, reestablishing the lid margins, and three sutures were placed to close the skin. The wound was medicated with Maxitrol ointment. The eye was left open and without a patch. The patient was awake and alert and appeared to tolerate the procedure well.

There was no evidence of any surgical or anesthetic complications, and he left the operating room awake, alert, and in good condition.

Linda Patrick MD

GODFREY REGIONAL HOSPITAL
123 Main Street • Aldon, FL 77714 • (407) 555-1234

EAR EXERCISES

EXERCISE 1

Level I

OPERATIVE REPORT

Patient information:
Patient name: DOB: MR#:

Preoperative diagnosis:
29-year-old female with history of recurrent episodes of otitis media. She now has a chronic right otitis media with effusion and mild right conductive hearing loss. Patient presents now for right PE tube per discussion. 1) Recurrent right otitis media with effusion. 2) Right mild conductive hearing loss. 3) Sclerotic right tympanic membrane.

Postoperative diagnosis:
Same

Procedure(s) performed:
Right myringotomy with tympanostomy tube placement

Anesthesia:

Assistant surgeon:

Description of procedure:
After consent was obtained, the patient was taken to the operating room and placed on the operating table in the supine position. After an adequate level of IV sedation was obtained, the patient was draped in the appropriate manner for right PE tube. Utilizing the ear speculum and ear microscope, the external canal was cleared of cerumen. The tympanic membrane was very sclerotic in the posterior aspect. As such, a myringotomy incision was placed in the anterior quadrant. Serous effusion was suctioned. A Bobbin tympanostomy tube was then placed without difficulty. Cortisporin otic suspension and cotton ball were then placed. The patient tolerated the procedure well; there was no break in technique. The patient was awakened and taken to the recovery room in good condition. *James Elliott MD*

GODFREY REGIONAL HOSPITAL
123 Main Street • Aldon, FL 77714 • (407) 555-1234

EXERCISE 2

Level II

OPERATIVE REPORT

Patient information:

Patient name:
DOB:
MR#:

Preoperative diagnosis:

51-year-old female with severe mental retardation. She has bilateral ear disease with cerumen impactions unable to be cleaned at the clinic.
1) Mental retardation.
2) Bilateral cerumen impaction.

Postoperative diagnosis:

Same

Procedure(s) performed:

Bilateral microscopic ear examination and removal of bilateral cerumen impactions

Anesthesia:

Assistant surgeon:

Description of procedure:

After consent was obtained, the patient was taken to the operating room and placed on the operating room table in the supine position. After an adequate level of IV sedation was obtained, the patient was draped in the appropriate manner for ear cleaning. Attention was first focused on the right ear.

Utilizing the ear speculum and ear microscope, the external canal was cleared of firm cerumen. Subsequent examination showed narrow ear canals. There was no swelling or tenderness. The tympanic membrane was sclerotic and intact. There was no granulation tissue or discharge. There were similar findings in the left ear, and similar procedure was then performed on the left ear. There was a small patch of some granulation on the posterior aspect of the tympanic membrane. Cortisporin otic suspension and cotton ball were placed in the left ear. The patient tolerated the procedure well, there was no break in technique, and the patient was awakened and taken to the recovery room in good condition.

James Ellicott MD

GODFREY REGIONAL HOSPITAL
123 Main Street • Aldon, FL 77714 • (407) 555-1234

EXERCISE 3

Level II

OPERATIVE REPORT

Patient information:

Patient name:
DOB:
MR#:

Preoperative diagnosis:

1. Chronic otitis media left
2. Chronic mastoiditis on the left

Postoperative diagnosis:

Same

Procedure(s) performed:

Left simple mastoidectomy with ossiculoplasty

TISSUE TO PATHOLOGY: None

Anesthesia:

Assistant surgeon:

Description of procedure:

The patient was brought to the operating room and placed in the supine position. General endotracheal anesthesia was administered without difficulty. The table was turned 180 degrees and the head was turned to the right. Exam of the left ear was performed. We had to shave and prep the left ear and postauricular area in the standard fashion. A postauricular and endaural injection of 1% Xylocaine with 1:100,000 epinephrine was accomplished without difficulty. Approximately 3 cc–4 cc was utilized. Examination of the external canal revealed it was filled with pulsating pus emanating from a polyethylene tube placed in the anterior inferior quadrant by this surgeon months ago. The ear has continued to drain copiously for the last year despite myringotomy and tubes and a repeat adenoidectomy and myringotomy and tubes. CT scan was indicative of chronic bilateral mastoiditis with coalescence. The child most likely has a conductive hearing loss as well. We have been unable to get an exact hearing test on her due to her age and lack of ability to do an otoacoustic emission test. After waiting an appropriate period of time, a postauricular incision through the skin, dermis, subcutaneous tissue, and postauricular muscles and periosteum was accomplished with a #15 blade. Cauterization was used to cut through the periosteum in a T-shaped fashion so as to retract the ear pinna forward. We scraped the periosteum off the mastoid bone and retracted the posterior membranous canal skin forward. Using a #11 blade, we cut across the posterior external canal skin, passed a Penrose drain through this incision, and retracted the pinna and the lateral canal forward so as to gain a good posterior and anterior view of the external canal. We cleaned out and removed the tube, noting massive granulation tissue in the middle ear. A nose-and-toes incision was made in the external canal, creating a vascular flap. Elevating the skin forward and the annulus out of the annular groove, we retracted the eardrum forward. The entire middle ear space was completely filled up with granulation tissue. I could see it emanating from the eustachian tube orifice back posterior and superiorly into the epitympanum. The ossicles were completely enveloped in this granulation tissue, as was the corde tympanic nerve. No middle ear

GODFREY REGIONAL HOSPITAL
123 Main Street • Aldon, FL 77714 • (407) 555-1234

Continued

OPERATIVE REPORT

Patient information:

Patient name:
DOB:
MR#:

Preoperative diagnosis:

Postoperative diagnosis:

Procedure(s) performed:

Anesthesia:

Assistant surgeon:

Description of procedure:

structures could be identified. We started removing granulation tissue just as gently as possible and removed tissue out of the hypotympanum around the ossicles, anterior to the malleus, around the eustachian tube orifice, and in the retrofacial area. We then started to perform the mastoidectomy. We took large to small cutting burs and following the usual landmarks—the spine of Henle, the superior temporal line, the posterior bony canal wall—we removed the cortex of bone off the mastoid. We immediately encountered granulation tissue inside of a fairly well aerated mastoid. We took the bone down from the tegmen down to the digastric ridge, took down the sinodural angle, and identified the transverse sinus. I removed as many air cells as I felt necessary. All were obviously inflamed and were filled with granulation tissue. I took down the area of bone overlying the head of the incus and identified the horizontal semicircular canal. As I was cleaning granulation tissue, it was just impossible to clean all this and aerate the epitympanum without involvement of the corde tympanic nerve. Once this was removed along with all the inflammatory tissue, it was noted that the incudostapedial joint appeared to be disrupted. While it lay adjacent when the chain was tested, the incus and long process of the incus could be moved, but the head of the stapes did not appear to be mobile. There appeared to be no direct connection between the two. I therefore decided to use some Dermabond tissue adhesive, and on a 1-mm angled pick, I placed the most minuscule amount I could around the connection between incus tip and the head of the stapes. This appeared to have a little bit better bonding and movement than before. I was very careful to only place the tissue adhesive on the joint itself. None of it was on the crest of the stapes or on the promontory or near the oval window. The material dried instantly and was only on the joint itself. The majority of time was spent removing granulation tissue, especially around the head of the incus, so that there would be good aeration and flow of fluid as well as air from the epitympanum and mastoid air cells into the middle ear space. The footplate of the stapes appeared to be intact. The facial nerve appeared to run in its bony canal. I had to harvest the temporalis fascia graft and support it in

GODFREY REGIONAL HOSPITAL
123 Main Street • Aldon, FL 77714 • (407) 555-1234

Continued

OPERATIVE REPORT

Patient information:

Patient name:
DOB:
MR#:

Preoperative diagnosis:

Postoperative diagnosis:

Procedure(s) performed:

Anesthesia:

Assistant surgeon:

Description of procedure:

the middle ear with Gelfoam and repair the eardrum from the posterior inferior quadrant. I had to remove a lot of bone over the posterior superior bony canal wall so as to open up the area lateral to the head of the incus. This created a cavitation in the posterior bony superior canal wall, which caused me to place my temporalis fascia graft not only in the posterior inferior quadrant but in the posterior superior quadrant and cover this area completely. When I had finished the case, I was able to drain the mastoid by sucking fluid out of the hypotympanum so that I knew that there was a good flow of air and water from this area. I put the ear back in its original position and sutured it in place with interrupted 3-0 undyed Vicryl and 4-0 running locking Prolene. The external canal was filled with Gelfoam laterally to support the graft. A mastoid pressure dressing was placed. I then turned my attention to the right ear. Using an otic speculum and operative microscope, an anterior inferior quadrant incision was made through a thickened eardrum, which rendered secretory middle ear fluid. We placed a cotton ball in the ear. I let the wide myringotomy incision suffice.

The patient was awakened, extubated, and brought to the recovery room in stable condition with an intact facial nerve. She was given steroids and antibiotics during the surgical procedure.

James Elliott MD

GODFREY REGIONAL HOSPITAL
123 Main Street • Aldon, FL 77714 • (407) 555-1234

EXERCISE 4

Level II

OPERATIVE REPORT

Patient information:

Patient name:
DOB:
MR#:

Preoperative diagnosis:

Conductive hearing loss and external auditory canal stenosis

CLINICAL NOTE: The patient is a 27-year-old white male who has soft tissue stenosis involving approximately 95% of his external auditory canal. He also has a significant conductive hearing loss. He has had surgery in the past by my associate, Dr. Hirsch. Dr. Hirsch recently took ill with an extended absence just prior to the patient's surgery. I was asked to perform the surgery on this patient.

Postoperative diagnosis:

External auditory canal stenosis of the left ear with conductive hearing loss/tympanic membrane perforation, middle ear and ossicular chain adhesions. Foreign body (old PE tube) within fibrotic tissue capsule between manubrium of malleolus and medial wall of the middle ear also interfering with the patient's hearing.

Procedure(s) performed:

Left canal plasty, left tympanoplasty. Middle ear exploration with lysis of adhesions, foreign body removal from middle ear, temporalis fascia graft and split-thickness skin graft reconstructions of the tympanic membrane perforation.

Anesthesia:

General

Assistant surgeon:

Description of procedure:

The patient was brought in the operating room and placed on the operating room table in a supine position. General endotracheal anesthesia was performed. Postauricular endaural injections were made with 1% lidocaine with 1:100,000 parts epinephrine. The left ear was prepped and draped in sterile fashion, and the patient received prophylactic dose of IV antibiotics perioperatively.

Using microscope and speculum, the left external auditory canal was examined. Using a cycle knife, incisions were made at 11 o'clock and 5 o'clock within the soft tissue stenosis. Using a #2 round knife, an incision was made lateral to the stenosis between these two incisions along the posterior ear canal wall. This was undermined proximally and the ear stenosis was removed. Similar incisions at 11 o'clock and 7 o'clock anteriorly were also made and stenosis was removed in similar fashion. Using the #2 round knife, the canal skin was then elevated down to the region of the annulus, but there was a lot of reactive and fibrotic tissue present and it was difficult to ascertain even location of the ossicles. Postauricular incision was made with a 15-blade scalpel and carried down to the mastoid bone with Bovie cautery. The temporalis fascia was exposed superiorly and harvested in standard fashion. The fascia was cleaned of soft tissue and subcutaneous fat and placed in the fascial press and allowed to air dry. The postauricular incision was connected to the endaural incision and the ear was retracted anteriorly with Weitlaner retractors. This allowed true visualization.

Next, dissection was carried down into the middle ear space through the granulation tissue using a Rosen pick and Bellucci scissors cut areas of fibrosis. The manubrium of the malleolus was identified and there were several adhesions between this and the middle ear, which were removed with microcup forceps and Bellucci scissors. Further adhesions between the incus and medial wall of the middle ear were also encountered and removed in similar fashion. There was a bulging present between the incus and medial wall of the middle ear that was restricting ossicular mobility, and using the

GODFREY REGIONAL HOSPITAL
123 Main Street • Aldon, FL 77714 • (407) 555-1234

Continued

OPERATIVE REPORT

Patient information:

Patient name:
DOB:
MR#:

Preoperative diagnosis:

Postoperative diagnosis:

OPERATIVE FINDINGS: The canal stenosis with area deep to this involving 80% perforation of the tympanic membrane with only the annulus and anterior remnant of the original tympanic membrane present. The patient had significant adhesions of the middle ear adjacent to the ossicles. The ossicles were mobile once the adhesions were removed. There was a fibrotic capsule that was present as described above that encased the previously placed collar button PE tube that had migrated into the middle ear.

Procedure(s) performed:

Anesthesia:

Assistant surgeon:

Description of procedure:

Rosen pick, this was palpated and dissected open and was found to contain within it a previously placed PE tube from a prior operative procedure. The PE tube was teased out and removed. Palpation of the manubrium of the malleolus showed normal mobility of the incus and stapes with round window reflex. Further granulation tissue present in the middle and towards the eustachian tube orifice was removed with microcup forceps. Hemostasis was obtained with Merocel impregnated with 1:100,000 epinephrine. The remnant of the tympanic membrane was de-epithelialized with Rosen pick and microcup forceps, and although exhibiting some mild sclerosis, it appeared to be well vascularized. The medial wall of the middle ear towards the eustachian tube was packed with trimmed Gelfilm. This was followed by Gelfoam impregnated with pressed dry 1:100,000 parts epinephrine. A split-thickness skin graft was shaved with 15-blade scalpel from behind the left ear and placed aside. Gelfilm was cut to size and placed medial to the remnant of the tympanic membrane, and underneath the manubrium of the malleolus, tympanic membrane was still present. The fascial graft was cut to size, placed as an underlay graft, and draped onto the region of the annulus and posterior ear canal bony wall. This was followed by split-thickness skin graft laterally and then an overlay graft of fascia. Gelfilm was cut to size and placed lateral to the overlay temporalis graft. The remainder of the ear was packed with Gelfoam impregnated with Cortisporin otic suspension. The left postauricular incision was closed with inverted interrupted 3-0 chromic sutures for periosteum and soft tissue, followed by inverted interrupted 4-0 chromic sutures subcuticularly. Running interlocking 5-0 nylon sutures were used to close the skin postauricularly. The ear was packed with cotton impregnated with Bacitracin ointment at the external auditory canal meatus, and Bacitracin ointment was placed over the postauricular incision in the region of the split-thickness skin graft donor site. This was dressed with Telfa, and a Glasscock mastoid pressure dressing was placed.

The patient was awakened from general anesthesia, extubated, and brought to the recovery room in stable condition, having tolerated the procedure well.

James Ellicott MD

GODFREY REGIONAL HOSPITAL
123 Main Street • Aldon, FL 77714 • (407) 555-1234

EXERCISE 5

Level II

OPERATIVE REPORT

Patient information:

Patient name:
DOB:
MR#:

Preoperative diagnosis:

Left tympanic membrane perforation

CLINICAL NOTE:
The patient is a 79-year-old white male with left tympanic membrane perforation involving the inferior half of the tympanic membrane, central in location. He is being brought to the operating room for repair of the tympanic membrane perforation.

Postoperative diagnosis:

Left tympanic membrane perforation

Procedure(s) performed:

Left tympanoplasty. Temporalis fascia graft. Split-thickness skin graft taken from left postauricular ear to reconstruct tympanic membrane perforation.

ESTIMATED BLOOD LOSS: Negligible

Anesthesia:

General

Assistant surgeon:

SURGEON: Faisal Mahmood, MD

Description of procedure:

The patient was brought to the operating room and placed on the operating table in a supine position. General endotracheal anesthesia was performed. The left ear was injected with 1% lidocaine with 1:100,000 parts epinephrine in the bony cartilaginous junction endaurally and postauricularly. The left ear was prepped and draped in a sterile fashion.

Using a microscope for visualization, the left middle ear was examined. There was some erosion of the manubrium of the malleus, but ossicles appeared to be intact on visualization of the stapes superstructure. Using an otic pick and microcup forceps, the tympanic membrane perforation was de-epithelialized around its circumference. There were no middle ear adhesions seen.

Left superior postauricular incision was made with a 15-blade scalpel and dissection was carried down to the temporalis fascia using Bovie cautery. Temporalis fascia was harvested in a standard fashion and placed in a fascia press and allowed to dry. Using a 15-blade scalpel, a split-thickness skin graft was taken from behind the left ear. The donor site was cauterized for hemostasis. A skin graft was also placed in a fascia press and allowed to air dry.

GODFREY REGIONAL HOSPITAL
123 Main Street • Aldon, FL 77714 • (407) 555-1234

Continued

OPERATIVE REPORT

Patient information:

Patient name:
DOB:
MR#:

Preoperative diagnosis:

Postoperative diagnosis:

Procedure(s) performed:

Anesthesia:

Assistant surgeon:

Description of procedure:

The left middle ear was then packed with a layer of Gelfilm along the medial wall of the middle ear, followed by Gelfoam, impregnated with 1:100,000 parts epinephrine squeeze-dried, up to the level of the tympanic membrane perforation. Temporalis fascia graft was cut to size and placed as an underlay graft. Split-thickness skin graft was placed lateral to the tympanic membrane perforation and directly over the underlay graft, followed by an overlay graft of larger temporalis fascia. A second layer of Gelfilm was placed lateral to the overlay graft, followed by Gelfoam impregnated with Cortisporin otic suspension to completely fill the ear canal. A cotton ball dressing with Bacitracin ointment was placed in the left ear. A postauricular incision was closed with inverted interrupted 4-0 chromic sutures for the subcutaneous layer, followed by interrupted 5-0 nylon sutures for the skin. A mastoid pressure dressing was placed.

The patient was awakened from general anesthesia, extubated, and brought to the recovery room in stable condition, having tolerated the procedure well.

James Elliott MD

GODFREY REGIONAL HOSPITAL
123 Main Street • Aldon, FL 77714 • (407) 555-1234

EXERCISE 6

Level I

OPERATIVE REPORT

Patient information:

Patient name:
DOB:
MR#:

Preoperative diagnosis:

CC: Here to have wax cleaned from left ear
ROS: Negative ear pains, positive decreased authority acuity, Negative chills, fever
PMH/SH: Unremarkable

Postoperative diagnosis:

Cerumen Impaction, Ear

Procedure(s) performed:

Cerumen was removed from both ears. Patient tolerated the procedure well.

Anesthesia:

Assistant surgeon:

Description of procedure:

EXAM:
HEENT: Left Ear, Canal with large amount of dry cerumen. Right ear, normal. Nose, normal external appearance.
Septum midline and intact. Pharynx normal in appearance.
Respiratory: No respiratory distress. Lungs clear.
CV: Unremarkable
Skin: Warm, dry, with normal turgor
Neuro: Oriented to person, time, and place

James Ellicott MD

GODFREY REGIONAL HOSPITAL
123 Main Street • Aldon, FL 77714 • (407) 555-1234

EXERCISE 7

Level I

OPERATIVE REPORT

Patient information:

Patient name:
DOB:
MR#:

Preoperative diagnosis:

8-year-old brought in to the emergency room by father after child accidentally put foreign body in left ear. Denies any hearing problem. No drainage apparent from the ear.

ALLERGIES: none

Postoperative diagnosis:

Procedure(s) performed:

Anesthesia:

Assistant surgeon:

Description of procedure:

Alert, oriented $\times$ 3. Temp 98.1, pulse 100, respiratory rate 20. Does not appear to be in any distress.

Ear exam revealed left ear canal with a small plastic object. Right ear within normal limited.

FB in left ear with auditory canal which was removed after washing and using Alligator forceps. Under direct visual guidance, object was grasped and taken out in one piece. Reexam reveals no ulcers, slight erythema around the area where the item was sitting. Rest of the exam is unremarkable.

Patient was discharged in the care of the father in stable condition.

Nancy Cauly MD

GODFREY REGIONAL HOSPITAL
123 Main Street • Aldon, FL 77714 • (407) 555-1234

EXERCISE 8

Level II

OPERATIVE REPORT

Patient information:
Patient name: DOB: MR#:

Preoperative diagnosis:
6-year-old male with prior history of PE tube placement. Since extrusion of his PE tubes, he has had recurrent episodes of otitis media and otitis media with effusion. Patient has retention of the right PE tube in the posterior tympanic membrane. 1) Recurrent otitis media and otitis media with effusion after extrusion of PE tubes. 2) Retained right PE tube.

Postoperative diagnosis:
Same

Procedure(s) performed:
1) Removal of right retained PE tube. 2) Bilateral myringotomy with tympanostomy tube placement.

Anesthesia:

Assistant surgeon:

Description of procedure:
After consent was obtained, the patient was taken to the operating room and placed on the operating room table in the supine position. After an adequate level of general inhalational anesthesia was obtained, patient was prepped and draped in the appropriate manner for PE tubes. Attention was first focused on the right ear. Utilizing the ear speculum and ear microscope, the external canal was cleared of cerumen. The retained PE tube was freed from the surrounding tympanic membrane at the posterior aspect. This was then removed. There was no perforation. A small amount of granulation tissue was also removed. A myringotomy incision was then placed in the anterior inferior quadrant. Serous effusion was suctioned. A Bobbin tympanostomy tube was then placed without difficulty. Cortisporin otic suspension and cotton ball was then placed. Attention was then focused on the left ear. The ear canal was cleared of cerumen. A myringotomy incision was placed in the anterior-inferior quadrant. Serous effusion was suctioned. A Bobbin tympanostomy tube was then placed without difficulty. Cortisporin otic suspension on a cotton ball was then placed in the left ear. The patient tolerated the procedure well; there was no break in technique. The patient was awakened and taken to the postanesthesia care unit in good condition.

Maurice Doater, MD

GODFREY REGIONAL HOSPITAL
123 Main Street • Aldon, FL 77714 • (407) 555-1234

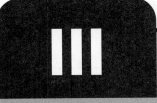

RADIOLOGY

All exercises in the Radiology Section serve as exercises for the student or for certification review.

EXERCISE 1

RADIOLOGY REPORT

MR#:
DOB:
Dr.

Clinical summary:

CLINICAL DIAGNOSIS:
Atypical headaches

PART TO BE EXAMINED:
CT head with and without contrast

Abdomen:

Conclusion:

HEAD CT:

INDICATIONS:
Atypical headaches

REPORT:
CT of the head performed without and with IV contrast. Demonstrates no evidence of intracranial hemorrhage, mass effect, or midline shift. There are no enhancing cerebral masses.

IMPRESSION:
Negative head CT

Ddt/mm

D:
T:

_____
Lisa Valhas, M.D.   Date

GODFREY REGIONAL HOSPITAL
123 Main Street • Aldon, FL 77714 • (407) 555-1234

EXERCISE 2

RADIOLOGY REPORT

MR#:
DOB:
Dr.

Clinical summary:

DIAGNOSIS:
Constipation

PART TO BE EXAMINED:
Barium enema

Abdomen:

Conclusion:

BARIUM ENEMA:
Negative colon and terminal ileum

Ddt/mm

D:
T:

_____
Lisa Valhas, M.D.   Date

GODFREY REGIONAL HOSPITAL
123 Main Street • Aldon, FL 77714 • (407) 555-1234

EXERCISE 3

RADIOLOGY REPORT

MR#:
DOB:
Dr.

Clinical summary:

DIAGNOSIS:
Abdominal/pelvic pain

PART TO BE EXAMINED:
Abdomen/pelvis

Abdomen:

Conclusion:

TRANSABDOMINAL PELVIC ULTRASOUND:
Transabdominal pelvic ultrasound was performed by the ultrasound technologist. Thirty static images are submitted for review. Without the benefit of endovaginal scanning of the pelvis, this exam is incomplete. The uterus was of normal size. Uterus is grossly negative for mass. The endometrium is not well visualized on any of the images. On one static image, the endometrial thickness is measured at approximately 5 mm. In the postmenopausal patient, this is at the upper limits of normal. If the patient is having vaginal bleeding, this finding should be further evaluated with follow-up ultrasound. Neither ovary is definitively identified. The visualized portions of both adnexa are very grossly negative for mass or fluid collections. If pelvis mass is a consideration, I would recommend an endovaginal ultrasound examination of the pelvis or a CT scan.

Ddt/mm

D:
T:

_____
Lisa Valhas, M.D.   Date

GODFREY REGIONAL HOSPITAL
123 Main Street • Aldon, FL 77714 • (407) 555-1234

EXERCISE 4

RADIOLOGY REPORT

MR#:
DOB:
Dr.

Clinical summary:

ABDOMINAL ULTRASOUND

INDICATION:
Nausea and abdominal pain

Abdomen:

Conclusion:

REPORT:
Abdominal ultrasound demonstrates normal echogenicity of the liver with no focal masses. No evidence of intra- or extrahepatic bile duct dilation. The gallbladder is normal. The pancreatic head appears normal. The body and tail of the pancreas are not well seen due to overlying bowel gas. Proximal aorta appears normal. The distal aorta is poorly visualized due to bowel gas. Both kidneys are negative for hydronephrosis. The right kidney measures 10.5 cm and the left 9.4 cm pole to pole. Normal spleen.

Ddt/mm

D:
T:

_____
Lisa Valhas, M.D.   Date

GODFREY REGIONAL HOSPITAL
123 Main Street • Aldon, FL 77714 • (407) 555-1234

EXERCISE 5

RADIOLOGY REPORT

MR#:
DOB:
Dr.

Clinical summary:

DIAGNOSIS:
Abdominal pain, nausea

PART TO BE EXAMINED:
UGI

Abdomen:

Conclusion:

UPPER GI:
There is mild esophageal dismotility, with loss of the primary peristalsis, followed by multiple non-propulsive tertiary contractions in the distal esophagus. The esophageal mucosa appears normal. Small sliding-type esophageal hiatal hernia. No evidence of esophagitis at this time. The stomach is negative. There are mild to moderately thickened folds in the duodenal bulb, consistent with duodenitis. No ulcer demonstrated.

Ddt/mm

D:
T:

_____
Lisa Valhas, M.D.   Date

GODFREY REGIONAL HOSPITAL
123 Main Street • Aldon, FL 77714 • (407) 555-1234

RADIOLOGY REPORT

MR#:
DOB:
Dr.

Clinical summary:

DIAGNOSIS:
Weight loss

PART TO BE EXAMINED:
CXR

Abdomen:

Conclusion:

PA AND LATERAL CHEST:
Normal heart size and pulmonary vascularity. A small amount of pleural fluid or pleural thickening has developed bilaterally since the previous exam of three years ago. There is also mild bibasilar atelectasis. The remainder of the exam is unchanged. There are old bilateral rib fractures. Mildly tortuous thoracic aorta.

Ddt/mm

D:
T:

_____
Lisa Valhas, M.D.   Date

GODFREY MEDICAL ASSOCIATES
1532 Third Avenue, Suite 120 • Aldon, FL 77713 • (407) 555-4000

EXERCISE 7

RADIOLOGY REPORT

MR#:
DOB:
Dr.

Clinical summary:

OB ULTRASOUND

INDICATION:
Size and dates, history of hypertension

Abdomen:

Conclusion:

REPORT:
Single intrauterine viable pregnancy with the fetus in the cephalic position. The placenta is located anteriorly in the upper uterine segment. Normal amount of amniotic fluid. Fetal cardiac motion observed by the technologist with rate of approximately 137 beats per minute. Fetal anatomy appears normal on the images provided. The estimated ultrasound due date is 4/15/xx. Please see obstetrical worksheet for measurements.

Ddt/mm

D:
T:

_____
Lisa Valhas, M.D.   Date

GODFREY REGIONAL HOSPITAL
123 Main Street • Aldon, FL 77714 • (407) 555-1234

RADIOLOGY REPORT

MR#:
DOB:
Dr.

Clinical summary:

DIAGNOSIS:
Follow-up, both-bone forearm fracture

PART TO BE EXAMINED:
Right forearm

Abdomen:

Conclusion:

TWO VIEWS OF THE RIGHT FOREARM:
Comparison is made with previous views of the right forearm dated 7-3-xx. On today's exam an overlying cast obscures bony detail. The previously described fractures of the distal right radial and ulnar shafts are again demonstrated. The fracture involving the distal right radial shaft has been reduced, and the previously described significant palmar angulation is no longer present. Alignment of the radial fracture fragment is satisfactory. As previously described, the distal right ulnar shaft fracture is an incomplete fracture. Once again, I can only confirm normal alignment of the radial head with the capitellum on one view, and thus if radial head dislocation is a clinical consideration, I would recommend AP and lateral views of the right elbow in further evaluation.

Ddt/mm

D:
T:

_____
Lisa Valhas, M.D.   Date

GODFREY REGIONAL HOSPITAL
123 Main Street • Aldon, FL 77714 • (407) 555-1234

E X E R C I S E 9

RADIOLOGY REPORT

MR#:
DOB:
Dr.

Clinical summary:

DIAGNOSIS:
Fell; pain, left knee

PART TO BE EXAMINED:
Left knee

Abdomen:

Conclusion:

EMERGENCY ROOM

LEFT KNEE:
AP and lateral views of the left knee obtained. Total knee replacement, left, in satisfactory position. No fracture or subluxation. No change from the previous exam.

Ddt/mm

D:
T:

_____
Lisa Valhas, M.D.   Date

GODFREY MEDICAL ASSOCIATES
1532 Third Avenue, Suite 120 • Aldon, FL 77713 • (407) 555-4000

EXERCISE 10

RADIOLOGY REPORT

MR#:
DOB:
Dr.

Clinical summary:

Abdomen:

Conclusion:

OB ULTRASOUND EXAMINATION:
The technologist performed the exam and hard-copy images were reviewed.

Single intrauterine pregnancy with fetus in the breech position. The placenta is located anteriorly and to the right. The lower margin of the placenta covers or partially covers the internal cervical os and this is considered to represent a "partial placenta previa."

Fetal cardiac motion observed by the technologist. Fetal anatomy is within normal limits on the images provided. Average ultrasound age estimated to be 21 weeks and 9 days.

The technologist estimates amniotic fluid index at 17.2 cm, which is in the 90th percentile for known gestational age.

Refer to the obstetrical worksheet for other measurements.

Ddt/mm

D:
T:

_____
Lisa Valhas, M.D.   Date

GODFREY REGIONAL HOSPITAL
123 Main Street • Aldon, FL 77714 • (407) 555-1234

EXERCISE 11

RADIOLOGY REPORT

MR#:
DOB:
Dr.

Clinical summary:

PROCEDURE:
Abdominal and pelvic CT

Abdomen:

Oral and IV contrast material used. Nonenhanced sections made of the liver.

Since 7/21/xx, the ion density mass described in the upper left abdomen has been resected. The patient has a history of gastric sarcoma. There are surgical staples at the greater curvature of the stomach. The bowel is not dilated. The bolus of contrast material is relatively weak, but the liver appears uniform in density. 2-cm low-density mass in posterior left kidney, probably a cyst. Small cortical cyst, right kidney. Atheromatous changes, abdominal aorta. No evidence of retroperitoneal adenopathy.

PELVIC CT:
Oral and IV contrast material used. Moderate enlargement of the prostate gland. No other evidence of a pathologic pelvic mass.

Conclusion:

Ddt/mm

D:
T:

_____
Lisa Valhas, M.D.   Date

GODFREY REGIONAL HOSPITAL
123 Main Street • Aldon, FL 77714 • (407) 555-1234

EXERCISE 12

RADIOLOGY REPORT

MR#:
DOB:
Dr.

Clinical summary:

Abdomen:

Conclusion:

LUMBAR SPINE MRI:
T1 and T2 sagittal and selected axial images
The sagittal images demonstrate anterior spondylolisthesis of L5, displaced forward by approximately 9 mm relative to the sacrum and 4–5 mm relative to L4. There is evidence of bilateral spondylolysis at L5. The findings cause deformity of the spinal canal at LS-S1 with increase in AP diameter. Degenerative disk disease with narrowing at L5-S1 interspace. Moderate posterior bulging of the disks at L1, L2, and L3 interspaces associated with degenerative changes in the facet joints. This results in spinal stenosis, moderately severe at L2-L3 and moderate at L1-L2 and L3-L4. Moderate degenerative changes in the interspaces anteriorly. Anterior wedging of the body of T12 with mild to moderate bulging of the disk at this level.

SUMMARY:
Significant spondylolisthesis of L5 with forward subluxation. Moderately severe spinal stenosis at L1-L2 and L3-L4. There is high-signal material associated with the right kidney on the T2 images. Suggest obtaining an ultrasound exam to evaluate further.

Ddt/mm

D:
T:

_____
Lisa Valhas, M.D.   Date

GODFREY REGIONAL HOSPITAL
123 Main Street • Aldon, FL 77714 • (407) 555-1234

EXERCISE 13

RADIOLOGY REPORT

MR#:
DOB:
Dr.

Clinical summary:

Abdomen:

Conclusion:

RIGHT KNEE MRI:
Selected sagittal, axial, and coronal images obtained without additional contrast. Most of the medial meniscus is absent. Lateral meniscus intact. The anterior cruciate ligament is not visualized clearly but it is most likely intact. Posterior cruciate ligament intact. Collateral ligaments intact. Moderately degenerative changes, medial compartment of the knee with moderate narrowing of the joint space and with at least a moderate amount of loss of articulating cartilage. A small to moderate sized nonspecific joint effusion.

IMPRESSION:
Extensive degenerative tear involving the medial meniscus. Moderate degenerative changes, medial compartment of the right knee.

Ddt/mm

D:
T:

_____
Lisa Valhas, M.D.   Date

GODFREY REGIONAL HOSPITAL
123 Main Street • Aldon, FL 77714 • (407) 555-1234

EXERCISE 14

RADIOLOGY REPORT

MR#:
DOB:
Dr.

Clinical summary:

Abdomen:

Conclusion:

PELVIC ULTRASOUND:
Retroverted uterus is slightly enlarged in a generalized manner, measuring 9.0 cm in length and 7 cm in its AP and width. Thickness of the endometrium 1.0 cm. There is a light nonhomogenicity to the parenchymal pattern within the uterus, but subtle 4.7-cm × 3.6-cm area of slightly increased echogenicity anteriorly in the lower body area of the uterus, which could represent a uterine fibroid. Both ovaries are top normal in size, with the right ovary measuring 4.3 cm in its greatest dimension, and it contains a 1.8-cm cyst. Left ovary measures 4.1 cm and contains two cysts, measuring 1.6 cm and 1.7 cm in their greatest dimensions. No free fluid in the pelvis.

Ddt/mm

D:
T:

_____
Lisa Valhas, M.D.   Date

GODFREY REGIONAL HOSPITAL
123 Main Street • Aldon, FL 77714 • (407) 555-1234

EXERCISE 15

RADIOLOGY REPORT

MR#:
DOB:
Dr.

Clinical summary:

Abdomen:

Conclusion:

MRA EXAMINATION OF THE CAROTID ARTERIES:
Time-of-flight and phase-contrast technique used. There is mild to moderate motion artifact, which compromises the images. The common external and internal carotid arteries bilaterally do contain signal and no gross abnormality is noted. The vertebral arteries bilaterally also contain flow.

MRI EXAMINATION OF THE CIRCLE OF WILLIS:
Right and left carotid arteries, proximal anterior, middle, and posterior cerebral arteries, and distal basilar artery are imaged and these vessels contain flow. No definite evidence of a focal aneurysm by this method of imaging.

The internal carotid arteries near the base of the skull on either side not well imaged on the MRA examination.

Ddt/mm

D:
T:

_____
Lisa Valhas, M.D.   Date

GODFREY REGIONAL HOSPITAL
123 Main Street • Aldon, FL 77714 • (407) 555-1234

EXERCISE 16

RADIOLOGY REPORT

MR#:
DOB:
Dr.

Clinical summary:

US BILAT LOWER EXT ARTERIAL

REASON FOR EXAM:
Claudication, calf pain

Abdomen:

Conclusion:

FINDINGS:
Right common femoral artery, proximal, mid, and distal superficial femoral arteries, popliteal artery, and posterior tibial artery show triphasic wave signals. Dorsalis pedis shows the same. Left common femoral artery, proximal, mid, and distal superficial femoral arteries, popliteal artery, posterior tib, and dorsalis pedis show triphasic signal also. ABI at the right ankle is 1.19; at the right dorsalis pedis, 1.04. On the left, 1.17 and 1.19 respectively. These are normal ratios. Velocities on the right show a mild gradient in proximal superficial femoral artery to the mid superficial femoral artery on the right only. The mid superficial femoral artery to the distal superficial femoral artery shows a small gradient.

The color Doppler images are not showing any high-grade stenosis.

IMPRESSION:
No evidence of any arterial stenosis. Normal triphasic signals and ABIs throughout both lower extremities.

Ddt/mm

D:
T:

_____

Lisa Valhas, M.D.   Date

GODFREY REGIONAL HOSPITAL
123 Main Street • Aldon, FL 77714 • (407) 555-1234

EXERCISE 17

RADIOLOGY REPORT

MR#:
DOB:
Dr.

Clinical summary:

UPPER GI WITH AIR CONTRAST

REASON FOR EXAM:
Abdominal pain, nausea daily off and on

Abdomen:

Conclusion:

Patient ingested gas crystals, then barium. Multiple spot and overhead images were obtained of the upper GI tract.

Stomach is normal in shape, size, and contour. There is mild irregularity of the duodenal wall folds, small lucent filling defects in the base of the duodenum. Duodenal sweep is remarkable for the second part showing a little spiculation of the folds; the third part of the sweep, the fourth, and the jejunum appear normal. GE reflux is demonstrated into the lower esophagus. Neither hernia nor stricture.

IMPRESSION:
Films suggest mild duodenitis affecting the bulb and the second part of the sweep, GE reflux into the lower esophagus.

Ddt/mm

D:
T:

_____
Lisa Valhas, M.D.   Date

GODFREY REGIONAL HOSPITAL
123 Main Street • Aldon, FL 77714 • (407) 555-1234

EXERCISE 18

RADIOLOGY REPORT

MR#:
DOB:
Dr.

Clinical summary:

CT ABDOMEN WITH CONTRAST

CT PELVIS WITH CONTRAST

REASON FOR EXAM:
LLQ pain

Abdomen:

Conclusion:

CT (spiral, 8-mm collimation) through the abdomen and pelvis with oral and IV contrast, 150 ml of Omnipaque 300.

The study is abnormal because there is a thickened abnormal loop of bowel in the left lower quadrant of the abdomen. The bowel wall is clearly thickened, with small air lucencies around it, and there is blurred definition with pericolonic hazy soft tissue attenuating inflammatory changes. There is about a 4-cm fluid attenuating density in the left parametrial level near the fundus; this could represent fluid-filled focus of colon, early formation of abscess (no air in it), ovarian cyst; it's probably part of the inflammatory colonic process. There is no free fluid.

Punctate 5–7 mm nodule in the right lung base, probably a granuloma but it should be followed up with CAT scan.

The liver has a uniform attenuation; small contracted gallbladder; the spleen is normal. Pancreas, kidneys, stomach are normal. Small and large bowel are as described. There are tiny studs of lymph nodes in the periaortic retroperitoneum, but they are not pathologically enlarged; they may be a response to this inflammatory process in the abdomen. There is no clear approachable area of abscess formation. The uterus is unremarkable, as are the urinary bladder and the inguinal region.

IMPRESSION:
Abnormal left lower quadrant inflammatory process, at least a 10-cm segment of inflamed thickened colon; differential includes diverticulitis, colitis, possible early abscess formation (not approachable by CT). GYN etiology for inflammation can also cause a similar presentation.

Ddt/mm

D:
T:

_____
Lisa Valhas, M.D.   Date

GODFREY REGIONAL HOSPITAL
123 Main Street • Aldon, FL 77714 • (407) 555-1234

EXERCISE 19

RADIOLOGY REPORT

MR#:
DOB:
Dr.

Clinical summary:

UGI/AIR CONTRAST WITH SBFT

REASON FOR EXAM:
Abdominal pain

Abdomen:

Conclusion:

Patient ingested gas crystals, then barium. Multiple spot and overhead images were obtained of the upper GI tract. Patient ingested two more cups of barium, and the small bowel was followed through to the terminal ileum.

The stomach is normal in shape, size, and contour. Gastric rugae are moderately thickened throughout in a diffuse pattern. On one view, there is slight narrowing of the distal body where it becomes confluent with the antrum, but it completely remits on another overhead image. The duodenal bulb maintains a normal arrowhead configuration. The most proximal second part of the sweep has mild thickening of the duodenal folds, and they are spiculated and irregular, involving several centimeters of the second part of the sweep. Multiple images were obtained of the duodenum, and the second part maintains its irregular narrowing. This is suggestive of duodenitis; other entities can cause this appearance, including pancreatic head changes.

Looking back on a prior CAT scan, there was some fluid in the duodenum as it coursed around the pancreatic head. The uncinate process was sharp; however, given this focus of fluid in the second part of the duodenum and the upper GI and small bowel follow-through today, would recommend the patient return for CAT scan of the abdomen with thin cuts through the pancreas with optimal duodenal opacification. An ERCP may be indicated. The body of the pancreas appears normal, but a thin-sliced CT will better delineate the head from the duodenal sweep. There was not a clear delineation of a pancreatic head mass but further studies are warranted.

Back to the barium study, the jejunal loops are normal. The ileal loops are normal.

Ddt/mm

D:
T:

_____
Lisa Valhas, M.D.   Date

GODFREY REGIONAL HOSPITAL
123 Main Street • Aldon, FL 77714 • (407) 555-1234

EXERCISE 20

RADIOLOGY REPORT

MR#:
DOB:
Dr.

Clinical summary:

US CYST ASPIRATION

REASON FOR EXAM:
Adnexal cyst

AREA/JOINT:
Ovarian cyst

CLINICAL HISTORY:
Adnexal cyst drainage

Abdomen:

Conclusion:

FINDINGS:
Pre-drainage sonographic evaluation demonstrates a large pelvic sonolucent fluid collection with an estimated volume of 44/46 cc.

Using sterile technique and an 18-gauge spinal needle under sonographic guidance, approximately 6500 cc of slightly yellow tinged fluid was aspirated without complication.

Ddt/mm

D:
T:

_____

Lisa Valhas, M.D.   Date

GODFREY REGIONAL HOSPITAL
123 Main Street • Aldon, FL 77714 • (407) 555-1234

EXERCISE 21

RADIOLOGY REPORT

MR#:
DOB:
Dr.

Clinical summary:

ABD FLAT/UPRIGHT

REASON FOR EXAM:
Abdominal pain

CLINICAL HISTORY:
Abdominal pain

Abdomen:

Conclusion:

FINDINGS:
There is a 4-cm round bony deformity in left lateral iliac crest; correlate for intervention here versus exostoses or primary bone process. Bowel pattern is negative; lung bases are clear. No pathologic calcifications; punctate pelvic phleboliths on the left.

IMPRESSION:
Punctate pelvic phleboliths on the left just below the level of the ischial spine. Deformity in left lateral iliac crest; exostoses/bone process versus postbiopsy site.

Ddt/mm

D:
T:

_____
Lisa Valhas, M.D.   Date

GODFREY MEDICAL ASSOCIATES
1532 Third Avenue, Suite 120 • Aldon, FL 77713 • (407) 555-4000

EXERCISE 22

RADIOLOGY REPORT

MR#:
DOB:
Dr.

Clinical summary:

CT BRAIN WITHOUT CONTRAST

CLINICAL HISTORY:
Found on floor, passed out, left-side weakness, down unknown length of time, evaluate for bleed.

Abdomen:

Conclusion:

FINDINGS:
CT in sequential 4 and 8 mm axial images without IV contrast.

The study is remarkable for a large right temporoparietal lobe low-attenuating area somewhat geographically shaped extending to the calvaria; it completely effaces the right lateral ventricle in the mid and anterior region of the horn. The fourth ventricle is patent. There is no subfalcine herniation, no hemorrhage. Left side shows sharply demarcated, about 1-cm, low-attenuating change in the deep white matter of the left posterior parietal lobe; that's probably an old lacunar infarction. Suprasellar area shows the pituitary gland a little prominent.

There is a very large soft tissue scalp hematoma over the left parietal skull but there is no finding of fracture.

IMPRESSION:
Massive low-attenuating area in the right temporoparietal lobe. Differential includes a bland infarction; a malignancy can also have this appearance but the study was not done with contrast. Minimal subfalcine herniation. No downward transtentorial herniation. Effacement of the right lateral ventricle.

Ddt/mm

D:
T:

_____
Lisa Valhas, M.D.   Date

GODFREY REGIONAL HOSPITAL
123 Main Street • Aldon, FL 77714 • (407) 555-1234

E X E R C I S E   23

RADIOLOGY REPORT

MR#:
DOB:
Dr.

Clinical summary:

Abdomen:

EXCRETORY UROGRAPHY:
The plain film of the abdomen demonstrates a considerable amount of stool throughout the colon, although the patient reports having received a colon prep last night.

Intravenous injection of 100 ccs of Isovue produced no adverse reaction. There is a prominent symmetrical nephrogram demonstrating normal, smoothly marginated kidneys. This is best seen on the nephrotomography.

Contrast appears in the collecting structures at two minutes bilaterally.

Conclusion:

1. Normal excretory urography
2. Minimal bladder trabeculation

Ddt/mm

D:
T:

_____
Lisa Valhas, M.D.   Date

GODFREY REGIONAL HOSPITAL
123 Main Street • Aldon, FL 77714 • (407) 555-1234

RADIOLOGY REPORT

MR#:
DOB:
Dr.

Clinical summary:

CLINICAL INFORMATION:
Chest nodule

Abdomen:

Conclusion:

CT OF THE CHEST:
There is a prior chest radiograph obtained four years ago. The patient's recent chest radiograph, obtained at a Godfrey Regional Hospital, has not been delivered for review.

Axial scans were obtained through the chest at 10-mm intervals. Subsequently, 2-mm scans were obtained though a 10-mm nodule in the left upper lobe. Subsequently, the patient was given 150 ccs of Isovue intravenously, and axial scans were obtained through the chest at 7-mm intervals. Following this, 2-mm scans were obtained through the nodular density in the left upper lobe.

The slightly ovoid lobule in the left upper lobe measures 10 mm in diameter. It has a Hounsfield density of 27 on the pre-enhanced images and approximately 28 on the post-enhanced images. This indicates that it is not enhancing.

Since the nodule was apparently identifiable on a chest radiograph, it must contain sufficient calcification to be identifiable at this small size. Hounsfield measurements are probably artifactually low due to partial volume affect. For this reason, the finding is most consistent with small granuloma. Review of an old chest radiograph obtained here two years ago shows a marginal density overlying the left 7th rib in about this location, so it has probably been present since that time.

When the old chest radiograph arrives, we will compare it with the current study.

No additional pulmonary abnormality is identified. The major bronchi are normal. The hilar mediastinal structures are normal.

Scans into the upper abdomen show numerous calculi in the gallbladder. The adrenals are normal.

1. Small non-enhancing nodule left upper lobe (see discussion above)
2. The old radiographs will be reviewed when they arrive.
3. Cholelithiasis

Ddt/mm

D:
T:

_____
Lisa Valhas, M.D.   Date

GODFREY REGIONAL HOSPITAL
123 Main Street • Aldon, FL 77714 • (407) 555-1234

EXERCISE 25

RADIOLOGY REPORT

MR#:
DOB:
Dr.

Clinical summary:

CLINICAL INFORMATION:
Follow-up to a mammogram

Abdomen:

Conclusion:

Magnification views were obtained to evaluate a questioned area of spiculation on the upper, inner quadrant of the left breast described on the prior exam. On magnification views, this resolves into overlapping parenchyma. There are no radiographic signs of breast carcinoma.

CONCLUSION:
No radiographic signs of breast carcinoma

Ddt/mm

D:
T:

_____
Lisa Valhas, M.D.   Date

GODFREY REGIONAL HOSPITAL
123 Main Street • Aldon, FL 77714 • (407) 555-1234

EXERCISE 26

RADIOLOGY REPORT

MR#:
DOB:
Dr.

Clinical summary:

CLINICAL INFORMATION:
History of CVA

Abdomen:

Conclusion:

DUPLEX CAROTID ULTRASOUND:
Examination of the left carotid demonstrated extensive plaque formation in the bulb extending into the origin of the left internal carotid. Doppler frequency spectrum analysis demonstrated velocities of up to 344 cm per second within the left internal carotid. Systolic ratio is 6.7, indicating greater than 60% diameter stenosis. There is normal flow in the left vertebral artery.

Examination of the right carotid demonstrated moderate amount of plaque in the bulb extending into the origins of the internal and external carotids. Doppler frequency spectrum analysis, however, demonstrated no hemodynamically significant stenosis. There is normal flow in the right vertebral artery.

CONCLUSION:
Greater than 60% diameter stenosis of the left internal carotid

Ddt/mm

D:
T:

_____
Lisa Valhas, M.D.   Date

GODFREY REGIONAL HOSPITAL
123 Main Street • Aldon, FL 77714 • (407) 555-1234

EXERCISE 27

RADIOLOGY REPORT

MR#:
DOB:
Dr.

Clinical summary:

CLINICAL INFORMATION:
Right lobectomy 2 years ago, lung CA

Abdomen:

Conclusion:

CT OF THE CHEST:
Axial scans were obtained at 7-mm intervals through the lung fields. The patient was then given 150 ccs Isovue intravenously and axial scans were obtained at 7-mm intervals through the entire chest. Comparison is made with the prior exam.

There are changes from previous pulmonary resection on the right. The upper lobe bronchus is not present, so presumably the entire upper lobe was resected.

There is no pulmonary nodule. The major bronchi are otherwise normal. There is no adenopathy. There is no enhancing lesion.

Scans into the upper abdomen show no focal abnormality in the liver. The right adrenal is enlarged, as on the previous study. It measures about 3 cm in greatest dimension, unchanged.

CONCLUSION:
1. Stable appearance of CT of the chest when compared with the previous study
2. The enlarged right adrenal is stable as well

Ddt/mm

D:
T:

_____
Lisa Valhas, M.D.   Date

GODFREY REGIONAL HOSPITAL
123 Main Street • Aldon, FL 77714 • (407) 555-1234

EXERCISE 28

RADIOLOGY REPORT

MR#:
DOB:
Dr.

Clinical summary:

CLINICAL INFORMATION:
Bruise over third finger

Abdomen:

Conclusion:

RIGHT HAND, THREE VIEWS:
There is no fracture or dislocation. Degenerative changes are seen at the first metacarpal phalangeal joint with joint space narrowing and marginal osteophyte formation and subchondral sclerosis. Mild degenerative change is seen at the interphalangeal joints throughout.

CONCLUSION:
Degenerative changes; no fracture is identified

Ddt/mm

D:
T:

_____
Lisa Valhas, M.D.   Date

GODFREY MEDICAL ASSOCIATES
1532 Third Avenue, Suite 120 • Aldon, FL 77713 • (407) 555-4000

E X E R C I S E   29

RADIOLOGY REPORT

MR#:
DOB:
Dr.

Clinical summary:

CLINICAL INFORMATION:
Fell and injured right hand and rib area

Abdomen:

Conclusion:

THREE VIEWS OF THE RIGHT HAND:
There is a faint transverse lucency through the base of the 5th metacarpal. This may represent a small undisplaced and incomplete fracture, but could also simply be artifact. If the patient has symptoms in this area, one could obtain follow-up radiographs to further assess in several weeks' time. Elsewhere there is no focal bony abnormality. Degenerative changes are seen at the radiocarpal joint as well as the interphalangeal joints.

CONCLUSION:
Possible incomplete, undisplaced fracture base of the 54th metacarpal (see discussion above)

CHEST PA AND LATERAL:
The heart size and the vasculature are normal. There is neither infiltrate nor effusion. Degenerative changes are seen.

CONCLUSION:
No active disease in the chest

Ddt/mm

D:
T:

_____
Lisa Valhas, M.D.   Date

GODFREY MEDICAL ASSOCIATES
1532 Third Avenue, Suite 120 • Aldon, FL 77713 • (407) 555-4000

EXERCISE 30

RADIOLOGY REPORT

MR#:
DOB:
Dr.

Clinical summary:

CLINICAL INFORMATION:
Wrist pain

Abdomen:

Conclusion:

LEFT WRIST:
Three views of the left wrist were obtained. No acute fracture is identified. There is considerable degenerative change of the right carpal joint with joint space narrowing and subchondral sclerosis. Degenerative changes are seen at the articulation between the greater multiangular and the navicular bones. On the lateral view a dorsal osteophyte rises from the mid carpus, probably arising from the lunate. Moderate soft tissue swelling is seen dorsally and ventrally. There are a few small calcific densities in the soft tissue ventrally. I cannot determine whether these are vascular or soft tissue, or even small avulsions. At this age I would suspect they are vascular.

CONCLUSION:
Degenerative changes, no definite fractures

Ddt/mm

D:
T:

_____
Lisa Valhas, M.D.   Date

GODFREY MEDICAL ASSOCIATES
1532 Third Avenue, Suite 120 • Aldon, FL 77713 • (407) 555-4000

E X E R C I S E   31

RADIOLOGY REPORT

MR#:
DOB:
Dr.

Clinical summary:

CLINICAL INFORMATION:
SOB

Abdomen:

Conclusion:

CHEST PA AND LATERAL:
Comparison is made with the study of six years ago.

The heart size and the vasculature are normal. There is no infiltrate or effusion. Senescent changes are seen throughout the chest.

CONCLUSION:
No active disease in the chest

Ddt/mm

D:
T:

_____

Lisa Valhas, M.D.   Date

GODFREY MEDICAL ASSOCIATES
1532 Third Avenue, Suite 120 • Aldon, FL 77713 • (407) 555-4000

EXERCISE 32

RADIOLOGY REPORT

MR#:
DOB:
Dr.

Clinical summary:

CLINICAL INFORMATION:
Chest pain

Abdomen:

Conclusion:

MYOVIEW STRESS TEST:
The patient achieved maximum heart rate of 147 per minute.
Rest imaging was performed utilizing 9.8 mCi of stress-imaging 32.9 mCi Tc 99m tetrofosmin. Gated imaging demonstrates a left ventricular ejection fraction of 36%. End-systolic and end-diastolic images show decreased contractility.

On stress imaging there is symmetric perfusion of the left ventricle. There is no evidence of infarct or ischemia.

CONCLUSION:
Decreased ejection fraction at 36%. No evidence of infarct or ischemia.

Ddt/mm

D:
T:

_____
Lisa Valhas, M.D.   Date

GODFREY MEDICAL ASSOCIATES
1532 Third Avenue, Suite 120 • Aldon, FL 77713 • (407) 555-4000

EXERCISE 33

RADIOLOGY REPORT

MR#:
DOB:
Dr.

Clinical summary:

Abdomen:

Conclusion:

RADIONUCLIDE RENOGRAM:
10.2 millicuries of technetium 99m DTPA used.

On the perfusion scan over 60 seconds, the perfusion curve for each kidney is relatively flattened, with the curve for the right kidney reduced in amplitude compared with the left. The aortic bolus curve is normal in configuration; these findings are not specific, but could be seen with bilateral renal artery stenosis or nephrosclerosis. Suggest further evaluation with duplex ultrasound if not already done.

Considering the function study performed over 45 minutes, the renogram curve on the left is relatively flattened. The curves do decrease in amplitude over time, and percent contribution on the right is 44, and percent contribution on the left is 56. It may be helpful to repeat the study using Lasix if indicated clinically.

Ddt/mm

D:
T:

Lisa Valhas, M.D.   Date

GODFREY REGIONAL HOSPITAL
123 Main Street • Aldon, FL 77714 • (407) 555-1234

EXERCISE 34

RADIOLOGY REPORT

MR#:
DOB:
Dr.

Clinical summary:

Abdomen:

RETROGRADE PYELOGRAPHY RIGHT:
Preliminary film of the abdomen revealed a catheter in place in the right renal pelvis. Following injection of contrast into the renal pelvis, the pyelocaliceal system and ureter were visualized, revealing no evidence of obstructive uropathy or filling defects. Upright view showed contrast urine level in the urinary bladder, with emptying of the pyelocaliceal system and ureter to a high degree.

Conclusion:

IMPRESSION:
Normal retrograde pyelography on the right. Findings are compared with previous IVP. A total of 5 films were obtained for this examination.

Ddt/mm

D:
T:

_____
Lisa Valhas, M.D.   Date

GODFREY REGIONAL HOSPITAL
123 Main Street • Aldon, FL 77714 • (407) 555-1234

RADIOLOGY REPORT

MR#:
DOB:
Dr.

Clinical summary:

CLINICAL INFORMATION:
Fell; right wrist pain

Abdomen:

Conclusion:

THREE VIEWS OF THE RIGHT WRIST:
There is a slightly comminuted distal radial articular surface fracture. This primarily involves the metaphysis with the accessory fracture line extending into the articular surface. There is no displacement or angulation. The ulna appears normal. There are degenerative changes at the first metacarpal carpal joint.

CONCLUSION:
Distal radial articular surface fracture

Ddt/mm

D:
T:

_____
Lisa Valhas, M.D.   Date

GODFREY REGIONAL HOSPITAL
123 Main Street • Aldon, FL 77714 • (407) 555-1234

EXERCISE 36

RADIOLOGY REPORT

MR#:
DOB:
Dr.

Clinical summary:

DIAGNOSIS:
Follow-up abnormal chest

PART TO BE EXAMINED:
Chest

Abdomen:

Conclusion:

SINGLE PA VIEW OF THE CHEST:
The nodular opacity seen in the left lung base previously is not as well demonstrated on this exam. Although it may lie just beneath the nipple marker, I believe that this finding is still indeterminate. Would recommend CT of the chest to exclude a pulmonary nodule. Scattered interstitial infiltrate in the right mid lung and both costophrenic angles has not changed significantly. Tortuous aorta. Prominent fat pad at the cardiac apex. Focal eventration, right hemidiaphragm. Chest otherwise negative.

LIMITED CHEST FLUOROSCOPY:
This was performed to evaluate the indeterminate nodular opacity in left lung base seen on prior chest x-ray. Under fluoroscopy, I was unable to identify the vague nodular opacity seen on the previously described chest x-ray. Although this could represent a nipple shadow or a density in the chest wall soft tissues or bones, I still believe a pulmonary nodule cannot be excluded, and would recommend CT of the chest in further evaluation.

Ddt/mm

D:
T:

_____

Lisa Valhas, M.D.   Date

GODFREY REGIONAL HOSPITAL
123 Main Street • Aldon, FL 77714 • (407) 555-1234

EXERCISE 37

RADIOLOGY REPORT

MR#:
DOB:
Dr.

Clinical summary:

CLINICAL INFORMATION:
Right breast density

Abdomen:

Conclusion:

ADD VIEWS OF A RIGHT MAMMOGRAM:
CC and MLO magnification spot films of a nodular density in the lower outer quadrant of the right breast were obtained.

The density has somewhat lobular margins with some minimal breaking at one point. No unusual calcification is seen.

CONCLUSION:
Stable nodule in the right breast

ULTRASONOGRAPHY OF THE RIGHT BREAST: Right breast ultrasonography shows a 6-mm diameter hypodense nodule in the right breast at the 8 o'clock position. It does not contain any internal echoes. It does not, however, show significant enhancement through transmission. It probably corresponds to the nodule seen on mammography. One could attempt to aspirate this with ultrasound guidance to see if it is a cyst, but if it is not cystic or cannot be accurately aspirated, then excision would be recommended, as it has increased in size since the previous mammogram.

CONCLUSION: Ultrasonography shows a hypodense lesion in the right breast at the 8 o'clock position (see discussion above)

FDA CATEGORY:
4—Suspicious abnormality
Ddt/mm

D:
T:

_____
Lisa Valhas, M.D.   Date

GODFREY REGIONAL HOSPITAL
123 Main Street • Aldon, FL 77714 • (407) 555-1234

EXERCISE 38

RADIOLOGY REPORT

MR#:
DOB:
Dr.

Clinical summary:

CLINICAL INFORMATION:
Follow-up chest lesion

Abdomen:

Conclusion:

CT OF THE CHEST:
Axial scans were obtained at 7-mm intervals through the lung fields. The patient was then given 150 ccs Isovue intravenously and axial scans were obtained at 7-mm intervals through the entire chest. Additional 5-mm scans were obtained through the superior segment of the left lower lobe.

As on the previous exam, there is a small mass density in the superior segment of the left lower lobe adjacent to some pleural thickening laterally. This measures about 3 cm in greatest dimension, unchanged from the earlier study. A few small air collections are seen within it. Whether these are within a nodule or represent emphysematous bullae in the area of infiltrate, etc., is not determined.

Small, but slightly enlarged, lymph node, measuring about 1.6 cm in greatest dimension is again seen anterior to the carina. No new abnormality is identified. There is pleural and parenchymal scarring in the apices that is stable. No hilar adenopathy is seen.

CONCLUSION:
1. Stable lesions, superior segment of the left lower lobe
2. No definite free pleural fluid; pleural thickening is seen on the left
3. A single carinal lymph node is stable

Ddt/mm

D:
T:

_____
Lisa Valhas, M.D.   Date

GODFREY REGIONAL HOSPITAL
123 Main Street • Aldon, FL 77714 • (407) 555-1234

EXERCISE 39

RADIOLOGY REPORT

MR#:
DOB:
Dr.

Clinical summary:

CLINICAL INFORMATION:
Fell down stairs

Abdomen:

Conclusion:

AP UPRIGHT STANDING BOTH KNEES AND A LATERAL VIEW OF EACH KNEE:
The radiographs demonstrate no evidence of joint effusion on the right or on the left. There are early degenerative changes for a patient of this age group. Subchondral sclerosis is seen in the tibial plateaus and there are osteophytes arising from the tibial spines, the posterior aspect of each patella, and at the insertion of each quadriceps tendon.

CONCLUSION:
1. No acute fracture is identified
2. There is minimal degenerative change for a patient of this age group

Ddt/mm

D:
T:

_____
Lisa Valhas, M.D.   Date

GODFREY REGIONAL HOSPITAL
123 Main Street • Aldon, FL 77714 • (407) 555-1234

EXERCISE 40

RADIOLOGY REPORT

MR#:
DOB:
Dr.

Clinical summary:

DIAGNOSIS:
Injury

PART TO BE EXAMINED:
Left foot

Abdomen:

Conclusion:

TWO VIEWS OF THE LEFT FOOT:
Mildly displaced fracture at the base of the first metatarsal involving the metaphysis. Otherwise negative.

Ddt/mm

D:
T:

_____
Lisa Valhas, M.D.   Date

GODFREY MEDICAL ASSOCIATES
1532 Third Avenue, Suite 120 • Aldon, FL 77713 • (407) 555-4000

E X E R C I S E 41

RADIOLOGY REPORT

MR#:
DOB:
Dr.

Clinical summary:

DIAGNOSIS:
Menopausal, hypothyroid, breast CA

PART TO BE EXAMINED:
Bone density

Abdomen:

Conclusion:

DEXA BONE DENSITY:
T values obtained for the lumbar spine range from 11.1 to 20.0. At the hip, the values range from 20.2 to 20.6. No evidence of osteoporosis.

The standards for the T-scores are as follows:
    Osteopenia: 21 to 22.5 S.D.
    Osteoporosis: below 22.5 S.D.
    Established osteoporosis: below 22.5 S.D. plus fracture

Ddt/mm

D:
T:

_____
                  Lisa Valhas, M.D.   Date

GODFREY REGIONAL HOSPITAL
123 Main Street • Aldon, FL 77714 • (407) 555-1234

EXERCISE 42

RADIOLOGY REPORT

MR#:
DOB:
Dr.

Clinical summary:

DIAGNOSIS:
Injury

PART TO BE EXAMINED:
Right shoulder

Abdomen:

Conclusion:

RIGHT SHOULDER, TWO VIEWS:
0.4-cm area of calcification projected adjacent to the lateral aspect of the humeral head on the AP view. This is likely due to tendinous disease, or less likely, small avulsion fracture. Also, there is prominence of the inferior surface of the acromion that could be due to injury or anatomic variation. This projects into the upper aspect of the space between the acromion and humeral head. Evaluate further with MRI if indicated.

Ddt/mm

D:
T:

_____

Lisa Valhas, M.D.   Date

GODFREY MEDICAL ASSOCIATES
1532 Third Avenue, Suite 120 • Aldon, FL 77713 • (407) 555-4000

EXERCISE 43

RADIOLOGY REPORT

MR#:
DOB:
Dr.

Clinical summary:

DIAGNOSIS:
Increased kyphosis (thoracic)

PART TO BE EXAMINED:
Bone density

Abdomen:

Conclusion:

DEXA BONE DENSITY:
T values obtained for the lumbar spine range from 24.2 to 25.5, consistent with osteoporosis. At the hip, the values are from 22.0 to 22.8.

The standards for the T-scores are as follows:
    Osteopenia: 21 to 22.5 S.D.
    Osteoporosis: below 22.5 S.D.
    Established osteoporosis: below 22.5 S.D. plus fracture

Ddt/mm

D:
T:

_____
    Lisa Valhas, M.D.   Date

GODFREY REGIONAL HOSPITAL
123 Main Street • Aldon, FL 77714 • (407) 555-1234

EXERCISE 44

RADIOLOGY REPORT

MR#:
DOB:
Dr.

Clinical summary:

DIAGNOSIS:
Pain, heel

PART TO BE EXAMINED:
Rt. heel

Abdomen:

Conclusion:

TWO VIEWS RIGHT HEEL:
Moderate size spur planter aspect os calcis.

Ddt/mm

D:
T:

_____
Lisa Valhas, M.D.   Date

GODFREY MEDICAL ASSOCIATES
1532 Third Avenue, Suite 120 • Aldon, FL 77713 • (407) 555-4000

EXERCISE 45

RADIOLOGY REPORT

MR#:
DOB:
Dr.

Clinical summary:

DIAGNOSIS:
GB disease

PART TO BE EXAMINED:
Abdominal ultrasound

Abdomen:

Conclusion:

ABDOMINAL ULTRASOUND:
Gallbladder normal with no biliary ductal dilatation. Liver, spleen, and kidneys are normal. The pancreas was not optimally visualized, but no definite pancreatic abnormality. Abdominal aorta normal size. No ascites.

Ddt/mm

D:
T:

_____
Lisa Valhas, M.D.   Date

GODFREY REGIONAL HOSPITAL
123 Main Street • Aldon, FL 77714 • (407) 555-1234

EXERCISE 46

RADIOLOGY REPORT

MR#:
DOB:
Dr.

Clinical summary:

DIAGNOSIS:
Chronic parotitis

PART TO BE EXAMINED:
R sialogram

Abdomen:

Conclusion:

PAROTID SIALOGRAM:
After the exam was explained to the patient, it was carried out under sterile conditions. The tip of the sialogram catheter was positioned within the opening to the right parotid duct, and 2 ccs of Renografin 60 was gently injected under fluoroscopic visualization. The main right parotid duct is of normal size and without filling defect. The intraglandular branches are normal to slightly decreased in size. Would question possible displacement of the intraglandular branching ducts and might further evaluate with CT or MRI scan of the right parotid gland.

Ddt/mm

D:
T:

_____
Lisa Valhas, M.D.   Date

GODFREY REGIONAL HOSPITAL
123 Main Street • Aldon, FL 77714 • (407) 555-1234

E X E R C I S E   4 7

RADIOLOGY REPORT

MR#:
DOB:
Dr.

Clinical summary:

DIAGNOSIS:
UTI

PART TO BE EXAMINED:
VCUG

Abdomen:

Conclusion:

VOIDING CYSTOURETHROGRAM:
Scout film unremarkable. Following injection of contrast into the urinary bladder, urinary bladder is well distended, smooth in outline without filling defect. There is reflux up to the pelvic portion of the left ureter. There is complete emptying of the urinary bladder after voiding with no contrast remaining in the left ureter.

Ddt/mm

D:
T:

_____
Lisa Valhas, M.D.   Date

GODFREY REGIONAL HOSPITAL
123 Main Street • Aldon, FL 77714 • (407) 555-1234

EXERCISE 48

RADIOLOGY REPORT

MR#:
DOB:
Dr.

Clinical summary:

DIAGNOSIS:
Injured ribs

PART TO BE EXAMINED:
CXR and rt ribs

Abdomen:

Conclusion:

THREE VIEWS FOR RIGHT RIB DETAIL:
Recent fracture, anterior aspect of the right seventh rib and only slight displacement.

PA AND LATERAL CHEST:
Heart size and pulmonary vascularity normal. Lung fields are clear. No pleural fluid or pneumothorax. Harrington rods transfix the thoracolumbar spine. Previous coronary bypass procedure. No significant change since last CXR.

The recent fracture involving the anterior aspect of the right seventh rib, as noted on the right rib detail today, is not visualized clearly on the chest radiograph.

Ddt/mm

D:
T:

Lisa Valhas, M.D.   Date

GODFREY REGIONAL HOSPITAL
123 Main Street • Aldon, FL 77714 • (407) 555-1234

RADIOLOGY REPORT

MR#:
DOB:
Dr.

Clinical summary:

DIAGNOSIS:
Cyst on liver

PART TO BE EXAMINED:
CT abdomen

Abdomen:

Conclusion:

CT ABDOMEN:
Exam performed both with and without IV contrast. Oral contrast also given. Lung bases are clear. There is no pleural fluid.
Liver of normal size. There is a 3 1/2 × 3 centimeter benign cyst inferior on medial aspect of the right lobe of liver. Several
other additional small benign cysts measuring up to 0.9 centimeters are elsewhere on the right and left lobes of liver.
Recent ultrasound exam of the liver demonstrates a 1.3-centimeter focal area of increased echogenicity in left lobe of liver,
but this is not visualized with certainty on the CT exam. Might obtain follow-up ultrasound exam in three months or so to
make sure there is no interval change. Gallbladder is normal with no biliary ductal dilatation. Spleen and pancreas are
normal. Kidneys are normal except for several small benign cysts in the left kidney. Abdominal aorta normal size. No
ascites or adenopathy. No abnormality involved in the bowel.

Ddt/mm

D:
T:

_____
Lisa Valhas, M.D.   Date

GODFREY REGIONAL HOSPITAL
123 Main Street • Aldon, FL 77714 • (407) 555-1234

EXERCISE 50

RADIOLOGY REPORT

MR#:
DOB:
Dr.

Clinical summary:

DIAGNOSIS:
Chronic sinusitis

PART TO BE EXAMINED:
Sinus CT

Abdomen:

Conclusion:

CT PARANASAL SINUSES:
Coronal images without contrast obtained. The lower half or so of the right maxillary sinus is opacified and this is apparently secondary to mucous membrane thickening. Small amount of mucous membrane in the right ethmoidal sinus. Paranasal sinuses otherwise clear. No abnormality in the posterior nasopharyngeal area. A slight deviation of the nasal septum with slight prominence of the inferonasal turbinates bilaterally.

Ddt/mm

D:
T:

_____
Lisa Valhas, M.D.   Date

GODFREY REGIONAL HOSPITAL
123 Main Street • Aldon, FL 77714 • (407) 555-1234

EXERCISE 51

RADIOLOGY REPORT

MR#:
DOB:
Dr.

Clinical summary:

DIAGNOSIS:
Cough

PART TO BE EXAMINED:
Sinus series, chest

Abdomen:

Conclusion:

THREE VIEWS PARANASAL SINUSES:
Complete opacification of the right maxillary sinus and a moderate amount of mucous membrane thickening in the left maxillary sinus noted. No air fluid level.

PA AND LATERAL CHEST:
Heart size top normal. Pulmonary vascularity normal. Lung fields are clear and there is no pleural fluid.

Ddt/mm

D:
T:

_____

Lisa Valhas, M.D.   Date

GODFREY REGIONAL HOSPITAL
123 Main Street • Aldon, FL 77714 • (407) 555-1234

EXERCISE 52

RADIOLOGY REPORT

MR#:
DOB:
Dr.

Clinical summary:

DIAGNOSIS:
Size and dates

PART TO BE EXAMINED:
OB US

Abdomen:

Conclusion:

OB ULTRASOUND:
There is a single viable intrauterine pregnancy in a breech presentation. Average ultrasound age is 18 weeks 0 days. Normal amount of amniotic fluid. Placenta is posterior and to the right with no placenta previa abruptio. No fetal abnormality evident.

Ddt/mm

D:
T:

_____
Lisa Valhas, M.D.   Date

GODFREY REGIONAL HOSPITAL
123 Main Street • Aldon, FL 77714 • (407) 555-1234

EXERCISE 53

RADIOLOGY REPORT

MR#:
DOB:
Dr.

Clinical summary:

DIAGNOSIS:
Epigastric and RUQ pain

PART TO BE EXAMINED:
GUI, gallbladder US

Abdomen:

Conclusion:

UPPER GI SERIES:
Moderate amount of gastroesophageal reflux without associated hiatal hernia. Stomach normal. Mild duodenitis in first and second portions of the duodenum with no ulceration or mass. Proximal jejunum normal.

ABDOMINAL ULTRASOUND:
Gallbladder of normal size and with no evidence of calculus. There is a very small polyp along the inner wall of the gallbladder, which is most likely of no clinical significance. No biliary ductal dilatation. Liver, pancreas, and spleen normal. Kidneys are normal except for a 5-cm benign cyst, upper aspect of the left kidney. Abdominal aorta normal size. No ascites.

Ddt/mm

D:
T:

_____
Lisa Valhas, M.D.   Date

GODFREY REGIONAL HOSPITAL
123 Main Street • Aldon, FL 77714 • (407) 555-1234

RADIOLOGY REPORT

MR#:
DOB:
Dr.

Clinical summary:

DIAGNOSIS:
Pain—no injury, chronic sinusitis

PART TO BE EXAMINED:
Right shoulder, sinus CT

Abdomen:

Conclusion:

CT PARANASAL SINUSES:
Coronal images without contrast obtained. Paranasal sinuses well pneumatized and clear. No abnormality in the posterior nasopharyngeal area. No abnormality in the area of the nares other than very slight deviation of the nasal septum.

TWO VIEWS RIGHT SHOULDER:
There is a 1 1/2 centimeter by 1 centimeter separate calcification projecting along the superior lateral aspect of the head of the right humerus, which may be secondary to previous tendinitis. Correlate clinically.

Ddt/mm

D:
T:

_____
Lisa Valhas, M.D.   Date

GODFREY REGIONAL HOSPITAL
123 Main Street • Aldon, FL 77714 • (407) 555-1234

EXERCISE 55

(use Format 13)

RADIOLOGY REPORT

MR#:
DOB:
Dr.

Clinical summary:

DIAGNOSIS:
Chest pain, history of reflux

PART TO BE EXAMINED:
UGI

Abdomen:

Conclusion:

UPPER GI SERIES:
Moderate amount of gastroesophageal reflux associated with a very small sliding esophageal hiatus hernia. Stomach and esophagus otherwise normal. Duodenum and proximal jejunum normal. Surgical clips in right upper abdomen and presumably from previous cholecystectomy.

Ddt/mm

D:
T:

_____
Lisa Valhas, M.D.   Date

GODFREY REGIONAL HOSPITAL
123 Main Street • Aldon, FL 77714 • (407) 555-1234

EXERCISE 56

RADIOLOGY REPORT

MR#:
DOB:
Dr.

Clinical summary:

DIAGNOSIS:
F/U from previous study

PART TO BE EXAMINED:
Sacrum

Abdomen:

Conclusion:

AP AND LATERAL VIEWS SACRUM:
There is a symmetric, incomplete attempt at sacralization of L5 with enlarged left lateral aspect of the body of L5, which is articulating with the upper aspect of the left side of the sacrum. There is a 2 centimeter by 1 centimeter area of slightly increased density centrally on left side of this junction of the sacrum and transitional vertebra, which is unchanged from prior lumbar spine exam and most likely is related to arthritis or perhaps a bone island. If symptoms persist, might further evaluate with nuclear bone scan and/or CT exam.

Ddt/mm

D:
T:

_____
Lisa Valhas, M.D.   Date

GODFREY REGIONAL HOSPITAL
123 Main Street • Aldon, FL 77714 • (407) 555-1234

EXERCISE 57

RADIOLOGY REPORT

MR#:
DOB:
Dr.

Clinical summary:

DIAGNOSIS:
Cough

PART TO BE EXAMINED:
Chest

Abdomen:

Conclusion:

PA AND LATERAL CHEST:
Mild generalized cardiomegaly with the heart having increased one centimeter in size since prior study. Moderate prominence of the bronchovascular markings since the prior study and may be evidence of vascular congestion and/or interstitial inflammatory process. Little if any pleural fluid. Can't exclude mild circulatory failure. Correlate clinically. No localized infiltrate.

Ddt/mm

D:
T:

_____
Lisa Valhas, M.D.   Date

GODFREY REGIONAL HOSPITAL
123 Main Street • Aldon, FL 77714 • (407) 555-1234

EXERCISE 58

RADIOLOGY REPORT

MR#:
DOB:
Dr.

Clinical summary:

DIAGNOSIS:
Pain—no injury

PART TO BE EXAMINED:
L shoulder

Abdomen:

Conclusion:

TWO VIEWS LEFT SHOULDER:
Moderate degenerative changes at the left AC joint noted.

Ddt/mm

D:
T:

_____
Lisa Valhas, M.D.   Date

GODFREY REGIONAL HOSPITAL
123 Main Street • Aldon, FL 77714 • (407) 555-1234

EXERCISE 59

RADIOLOGY REPORT

MR#:
DOB:
Dr.

Clinical summary:

DIAGNOSIS:
Pain—injury

PART TO BE EXAMINED:
L knee

Abdomen:

Conclusion:

TWO VIEWS LEFT KNEE:
No abnormality evident.

Ddt/mm

D:
T:

_____
Lisa Valhas, M.D.   Date

GODFREY REGIONAL HOSPITAL
123 Main Street • Aldon, FL 77714 • (407) 555-1234

EXERCISE 60

RADIOLOGY REPORT

MR#:
DOB:
Dr.

Clinical summary:

DIAGNOSIS:
Pain

PART TO BE EXAMINED:
Rt ankle

Abdomen:

Conclusion:

THREE VIEWS RIGHT ANKLE:
Moderate amount of overlying soft tissue swelling. No fracture or subluxation. Localized area of radiolucency in the distal aspect of the fibula is noted on the oblique view and is most likely within normal limits and secondary to some normal thinning of the bone in that area, but if there are persisting symptoms over that area, might further evaluate with nuclear bone scan. No significant change in the appearance of the distal fibula compared to the prior study.

Ddt/mm

D:
T:

_____
Lisa Valhas, M.D.   Date

GODFREY REGIONAL HOSPITAL
123 Main Street • Aldon, FL 77714 • (407) 555-1234

EXERCISE 61

RADIOLOGY REPORT

MR#:
DOB:
Dr.

Clinical summary:

DIAGNOSIS:
Postpartum bleeding × 3 months

PART TO BE EXAMINED:
Pelvic US

Abdomen:

Conclusion:

PELVIC ULTRASOUND:
Patient is 3 months post partum and presents with vaginal bleeding. Anteverted uterus top normal in size. There is relative thickening and irregularity to the endometrium over a length of 2.9 centimeters and with a width of 1.2 centimeters; this is a nonspecific finding, but in view of the patient's history, abnormality such as some residual placenta or other products of gestation cannot be excluded. Both ovaries appear normal. No mass or abnormal fluid collection in the pelvis.

Ddt/mm

D:
T:

_____

Lisa Valhas, M.D.   Date

GODFREY REGIONAL HOSPITAL
123 Main Street • Aldon, FL 77714 • (407) 555-1234

EXERCISE 62

RADIOLOGY REPORT

MR#:
DOB:
Dr.

Clinical summary:

DIAGNOSIS:
Questionable fibroid

PART TO BE EXAMINED:
Pelvis

Abdomen:

Conclusion:

PELVIC ULTRASOUND EXAM:
The technologist performed the exam and hard-copy images are reviewed.

The uterus measures approximately 5 cm AP × 6 cm transverse diameter. Endometrial canal thickness is up to 0.39 cm, within normal limits.

There is an area of altered echogenicity within the parenchyma of the uterus posterior to the endometrium measuring 3.8 × 2.4 × 1.9 cm. Additionally, an area of altered echogenicity is present anterior to the endometrium, measuring 1.8 × 1.5 cm. These likely represent leiomyomas of the uterus. A malignancy of the uterus is much less likely but also included in the differential diagnosis.

Approximate ovarian measurements are right 2.2 × 2.3 cm. and left 2.7 × 2.3 cm. There are small follicular cysts within the left ovary, with the largest measuring up to 0.8 cm in diameter.

Ddt/mm

D:
T:

Lisa Valhas, M.D.   Date

GODFREY REGIONAL HOSPITAL
123 Main Street • Aldon, FL 77714 • (407) 555-1234

RADIOLOGY REPORT

MR#:
DOB:
Dr.

Clinical summary:

DIAGNOSIS:
Size, dates, and position

PART TO BE EXAMINED:
OB ultrasound

Abdomen:

Conclusion:

OB ULTRASOUND EXAM:
The technologist performed the exam and hard-copy images are reviewed.

Single intrauterine pregnancy with fetus in the breech position. Placenta is located posteriorly and to the left in the uterus and does not appear low-lying. Normal volume of amniotic fluid. Fetal cardiac motion observed by the technologist. Fetal anatomy appears within normal limits on the images provided. Average ultrasound age estimated to be 27 weeks 2 days. Refer to the OB worksheet for other measurements.

Ddt/mm

D:
T:

_____
Lisa Valhas, M.D.   Date

GODFREY REGIONAL HOSPITAL
123 Main Street • Aldon, FL 77714 • (407) 555-1234

EXERCISE 64

RADIOLOGY REPORT

MR#:
DOB:
Dr.

Clinical summary:

PROCEDURE:
Chest and abdominal CT

Abdomen:

Conclusion:

CHEST CT:
Exam performed both with and without IV contrast. There is a 2 cm × 1/2 cm × 11/2 cm nonspecific soft tissue mass on the anterior superior aspect of the right hilar area and cannot exclude small lung malignancy. No other mediastinal or hilar abnormality evident. No abnormality involving the main or segmental bronchi. Small amount of fibrosis at the posterior apex of the right lung. No pleural fluid.

ABDOMEN CT:
Exam performed both with and without IV contrast. Oral contrast also given. Liver is normal except for a 1-cm benign cyst anteriorly in the right lobe of the liver. The left adrenal gland is normal. There is a nonhomogeneous 4 cm × 3 1/2 cm × 3 1/2 cm partially cystic soft-tissue mass in the area of the right adrenal gland, which could represent metastasis, benign entity such as hyperplasia, or adenoma—or less likely—primary adrenal neoplasm. Spleen and pancreas are normal. Kidneys are normal except for several benign cysts in each kidney, with the largest cyst measuring 2 1/2 cm in size and located laterally in mid aspect of the right kidney. Gallbladder is normal with no biliary ductal dilatation. Abdominal aorta of normal size. No ascites or adenopathy.

Ddt/mm

D:
T:

_____
Lisa Valhas, M.D.   Date

GODFREY REGIONAL HOSPITAL
123 Main Street • Aldon, FL 77714 • (407) 555-1234

EXERCISE 65

RADIOLOGY REPORT

MR#:
DOB:
Dr.

Clinical summary:

EXAMINATION OF:
Elbow (2 views)

CLINICAL SYMPTOMS:
Left arm pain

Abdomen:

Conclusion:

LEFT ELBOW:
Two views were obtained. No effusion is seen. There are degenerative changes, both medially and laterally. No fracture, subluxation, or dislocation is identified.

CONCLUSION:
Degenerative changes. No acute abnormality is seen.

Ddt/mm

D:
T:

_____

Lisa Valhas, M.D.   Date

GODFREY REGIONAL HOSPITAL
123 Main Street • Aldon, FL 77714 • (407) 555-1234

EXERCISE 66

RADIOLOGY REPORT

MR#:
DOB:
Dr.

Clinical summary:

EXAMINATION OF:
Chest (PA or AP and lateral)

CLINICAL SYMPTOMS:
Chest pain

Abdomen:

Conclusion:

PA AND LATERAL CHEST:
The bony structures are demineralized. There are surgical sutures in the sternum. There are small pleural effusions on each side. The heart is enlarged. The aorta is tortuous. The pulmonary vessels are congested. No area of confluent infiltrate is seen.

CONCLUSION:
Cardiomegaly with evidence of congestive heart failure.

Ddt/mm

D:
T:

_____
Lisa Valhas, M.D.   Date

GODFREY REGIONAL HOSPITAL
123 Main Street • Aldon, FL 77714 • (407) 555-1234

ANSWERS

SECTION ONE: EVALUATION AND MANAGEMENT

	CPT-4 Code	ICD-9-CM Code
1.	99202	459.0, V13.5
2.	99284	786.3, V10.22
3.	99284	428.0, 413.9
4.	99213	782.0
5.	99213	729.5
6.	99214	523.8
7.	99213	716.96, 719.06
8.	99213-25, 30901	784.7
9.	99214	787.2
10.	99213	780.9
11.	99213	486, 491.21
12.	99213	816.01, E918
13.	99201	522.5
14.	99213	463, 462
15.	99282	298.9, 780.09
16.	99281-25, 92950	429.9
17.	99214	780.4
18.	99214	428.0
19.	99213	519.8, 491.21
20.	99213-25, 30901	784.7
21.	99213	681.00
22.	99203	346.90
23.	99283	251.2, 280.9
24.	99214	794.8
25.	99284	780.2
26.	99214	847.9
27.	99213	569.3
28.	99213-25, 12011	873.0, E888.9
29.	99213-25, 12052	873.42, E816.1
30.	99213	780.2, 724.5
31.	99202	719.46
32.	99203	455.4, 599.0
33.	99213	428.0
34.	99213	822.0, E885.9
35.	99202	599.7

36. 99202	727.51
37. 99213	490, 511.0
38. 99213-25, 29125-RT	813.42, E885.9
39. 99212-25, 29125-58	V54.8, 813.81
40. 99213	787.03
41. 99202	923.20, E917.9
42. 99213	996.76
43. 99214	786.59
44. 99213	782.1
45. 99214	729.81
46. 99202	924.11, 924.20, 910.0, E884.4
47. 99283/84-25, 32000	427.5, 827.1, 813.80, 812.20, 807.09, E917.9
48. 99282	794.8, 789.09
49. 99213	786.50
50. 99284	530.3
51. 99214	427.89, 496, 596.54, 718.90
52. 99283	429.9
53. 99283-25, 92953	426.11, E888.9
54. 99284-25, 29515	820.21, 821.20, 599.7, E812.0
55. 99213	786.05, 786.50
56. 99284	784.0, 782.0, 729.5
57. 99284	812.30, 813.93, 814.11, E884.9
58. 99283	491.21
59. 99213	724.5
60. 99282-25, 12002	890.0, E966
61. 99213	729.5, 782.3, 459.81, 250.41, 414.00
62. 99213	787.2
63. 99202	786.59, 496, 518.0
64. 99285	427.5, 410.10, 410.00, 427.41, 276.8
65. 99213	922.31, E884.9, E848
66. 99285-25, 92953, 92950	798.1
67. 99213	959.1, E917.0
68. 99282	786.05, 496
69. 99213/4	465.9, 490, 729.5, 719.45, E888.9
70. 99281-25, 16020	944.23, 944.11, E924.8

SECTION TWO: SURGERY

INTEGUMENTARY EXERCISES

CPT-4 Code	ICD-9-CM Code
1. 14060	173.3
2. 11646, 15120	173.2
3. 11602, 15220	195.5
4. 19125-RT (19290, 76942 Rad)	217
5. 58558, 11056-59	236.0, 238.2
6. 12051, 12013	873.43, 873.54, 873.69, E882
7. 19162-RT	174.9
8. 11440, 11400-51, 11400-76/51, 11040-51	709.9, 882.0
9. 19140-RT	611.1
10. 20240	707.15, 355.8
11. 11760-58, 11750	883.0, 816.02
12. 11600-58	172.8
13. 67961	238.2
14. 19182-RT, 11200-59	611.1, 701.9
15. 28505-T1, 11044-59	895.0, 893.0, 826.1

16.	13100	998.4, 682.9
17.	19120-RT	217
18.	11402, 11401-51, 12031-51	709.9
19.	11642, 15240	195.0
20.	14020, 11043	873.1
21.	14060	173.3, 210.4
22.	17000	141.9, 145.9
23.	17000, 17003	078.0
24.	99213-25	873.0, E885.9
	12001	873.0, E885.9
25.	99282	873.42, E920.8

MUSCULOSKELETAL EXERCISES

	CPT-4 Code	**ICD-9-CM Code**
1.	23410-RT, 23120-51-RT	840.4, 716.91
2.	27425-LT	719.46
3.	26746-F3, 11012-51, 26426-51, 26418-51, 76000 Rad	816.13, 842.19
4.	26540 F5, 26075-51-F5	815.00
5.	27696-LT	845.02, 845.09
6.	29877-LT	717.7, 719.26
7.	29873-RT, 29877-59-RT	717.7, 727.83, 727.89
8.	23410-RT, 29826-51-RT	840.4
9.	28289-LT	735.2
10.	26123, 26125 x3	728.6
11.	23450-LT	718.31, 755.59
12.	11752	730.27, 707.15
13.	26123	728.6
14.	26735-F9, 11010-51, 76000 Rad	816.11
15.	28820-T1, 28288-51, 15340-59	707.15, 838.09, 718.47
16.	28208 X2	735.8, 755.69
17.	23410-LT, 29826-51-LT	840.4
18.	24351-RT	726.32
19.	29881-LT, 29877-59-LT	836.0, 717.83, 727.09
20.	28285-T6	755.67, 735.4
21.	28296-RT	735.0
22.	23120-RT, 29826-51-RT	726.2
23.	25611-LT, 76000 Rad	813.42, 733.82
24.	25800-RT	716.13
25.	29880-RT	836.0, 836.1
26.	27870-LT	718.87
27.	29879-RT, 29881-51-RT	836.0, 738.8, 717.7, 715.96
28.	29887-RT	719.86
29.	25605-LT	813.83
30.	27899	998.59, 041.9
31.	29877-RT	717.9, 715.96
32.	25575-RT, 76000 Rad	733.81
33.	29880-LT, 29877-59-LT	717.83, 836.0, 717.7
34.	27675	845.09
35.	10060	682.7, V58.89
36.	29880-LT, 29877-59-LT, 29873-51-LT	836.1, 836.0, 717.7
37.	25116	727.05
38.	28104, 20680-51	V54.0, 729.5, 733.90
39.	26951, 26567 (Clarify which procedure is done on which finger: F7, F8)	883.2, E919.3
40.	25565-LT, 24655-51-LT, 12001-59, 76000 Rad	813.18

41.	28285-T8, 28285 T9	735.4, 755.66
42.	28116, 28208-51, 28118-51, 20900-51, 20902-51, 76000 Rad	755.67, 734
43.	28160	274.0
44.	29881-LT, 29876-51-LT	836.0, 727.09
45.	28296-LT, 28285 T1, 28285-T2, 28285-T3	735.1, 735.4
46.	26735 F4, 76000 Rad	816.01
47.	26055	727.03
48.	28296-RT, 28285-T6, 28285-T7, 28285-T8, 28280-51	735.8, 735.0, 727.1, 735.4
49.	29880-RT	836.1, 836.0
50.	29877-LT	717.0
51.	29848-LT	354.0
52.	28292-TA, 28285-T1	735.0, 735.4
53.	27570-RT, 20610-51	718.56, V43.65
54.	25605 LT, 20690, 76000 Rad	813.42
55.	29880-RT, 29877-51-RT	715.96, 836.1, 717.84
56.	27570-RT, 20610-51	719.56, V43.65
57.	26115	719.64
58.	25611-LT, 76000 Rad	813.42
59.	29877-LT, 29876-51-LT	717.83, 844.9
60.	29877-RT	717.7
61.	29292 TA, 28285 T1, 28285 T2	735.0, 735.4
62.	20680, 20612-51	996.77, 727.41, V54.0
63.	27509-LT, 76000 Rad	732.2, 820.01
64.	27385	844.9
65.	28113, 11040-59	707.15, 250.80
66.	25620-LT, 76000 Rad	813.42
67.	10120	915.6
68.	28030	355.6
69.	27766-LT, 20680-51	733.82, 996.78, 905.4, V54.0
70.	28810-52-LT	895.0
71.	99282-25	813.01, 881.00, E880.9
	29105-LT	813.01, E880.0
	12001	881.00, E880.9
72.	99282-25	923.3, E917.9
	29130	923.3, E917.0

RESPIRATORY EXERCISES

	CPT-4 Code	**ICD-9-CM Code**
1.	31256-LT, 31255-51-LT, 30130-51-LT	478.0, 473.2, 473.0
2.	31267-RT, 31254-51-RT	478.1
3.	30520, 30130-50	802.0, 470, 478.0
4.	31256-LT, 31255-50-51, 30130-50-51	384.20, 470, 471.9, 473.0, 733.90
5.	31267-LT, 31254-50, 30520-59	380.50, 389.00, 470, 471.9, 473.0, 473.2
6.	30520, 30630-51	738.0, 478.1
7.	60500	252.0, 226
8.	31256-50, 31254-50-51, 30520-59, 30130-50-51	470, 478.0, 473.8, 471.9, 478.1
9.	68420-RT	375.42
10.	31255-50	473.9, 471.9
11.	60220-RT	241.0, 382.9, 383.1
12.	30520	470, 478.1
13.	31267-51-RT, 31254-51-RT	473.0, 473.2
14.	31256-50, 31254-50-51, 30140-50-51	473.0, 473.2, 478.0, 470, 478.1
15.	31287-50, 31276-51, 31267-50-51, 31255-50	473.8, 471.8
16.	31255-50, 31267-51-LT, 30520-51, 30130-51-50	470, 478.1, 473.0, 473.2, 471.9, 733.90

	CPT-4 Code	ICD-9-CM Code
17.	31256-50, 31254-50-51, 31240-51	473.0, 473.2, 478.1
18.	32000	786.05, 511.9, V10.11
19.	31628	518.89
20.	31540	478.4
21.	32405, 76360	786.6
22.	32000	511.9, V10.3
23.	32002, 76934(Rad)	511.9
24.	32405, 76360(Rad)	518.89
25.	99282-25	784.7
	30901-50	

CARDIOVASCULAR EXERCISES

	CPT-4 Code	ICD-9-CM Code
1.	36561, 76000 Rad	197.5
2.	37607	996.73, 585.9
3.	36581, 76000 Rad	996.73
4.	37780-LT	454.9
5.	36569	996.73, 585.9
6.	36569 (if older than 2 years)	996.73, 585.9
7.	33233, 33208	V53.31
8.	37720	454.9

GASTROINTESTINAL EXERCISES

	CPT-4 Code	ICD-9-CM Code
1.	45380 only	787.91, V10.05
2.	49000	789.00
3.	45385, 45380-51	211.3
4.	43239	787.1, 783.21, 787.91
5.	45385, 45383-51, 43239-59	787.1, V16.0
6.	45380	578.1, 783.21
7.	41599	145.9
8.	42420, 15732-51	210.2
9.	43215	935.1, E915
10.	45385, 45383-51, 45382-51	747.61, 211.3, 562.10, 455.3
11.	43239	535.60, 535.50, 553.3, 211.1
12.	43215	935.1, E915
13.	45378	578.1
14.	45380	211.3
15.	42820	463, 519.8, 474.10
16.	40812	528.9
17.	45382, 45380-51	747.61, 211.3, 564.1, 455.0
18.	47000, 76942 Rad	794.8
19.	55060-RT	603.9
20.	47000-52	794.8
21.	49585 (if older than 5 years), 49580 (if younger than 5 years)	553.1
22.	42415, 38500-51	210.2
23.	42450	527.6
24.	46080	569.3
25.	47579	573.8
26.	49970	No dx given
27.	47562	574.10

GENITOURINARY EXERCISES

CPT-4 Code	ICD-9-CM Code
1. 52500	595.9
2. 54150	V50.2
3. 57120	618.3
4. 52332	788.0, 599.7, 593.89
5. 55700, 52000-59	790.93, 600.0
6. 99282-25, 51702	788.20, V13.09
7. 58120	627.8
8. 49322	614.6, 617.0, 620.2
9. 58662	625.9, 625.3, 617.9
10. 49321	783.21, 790.99, 614.6
11. 49320	628.9, 614.6
12. 54520-RT, 54600-LT	608.2
13. 58563, 58558-51	626.2
14. 49322	625.9, 614.6
15. 58120	627.1, 622.7
16. 58662, 58350-51	617.3, 617.2, 625.9
17. 52260	595.9, 599.7, 596.9, 596.8
18. 59812	634.91
19. 58670	614.9, V25.2
20. 57505-52	621.3, 622.4, 620.2
21. 58301	996.76
22. 58662, 58670-51, 58558-59	625.9, 626.9, 620.2
23. 52332	788.0, 788.9
24. 51040	788.20, 600.0, 596.0, 577.0
25. 52204	625.9, 788.9, V13.2
26. 56501	625.8, 078.10, 042.9
27. 10120	623.8, 998.11
28. 49322	625.9, 614.6, 620.2
29. 57000	V53.6
30. 52000	788.20
31. 52310, 74420	594.1, 594.2, 185, 599.7

NERVOUS SYSTEM EXERCISES

CPT-4 Code	ICD-9-CM Code
1. 63650, 76005 Rad	(none)
2. 62310, 20552, 76005 Rad	729.2, 784.0
3. 63650, 76005 Rad	724.5
4. 64721-RT, 64718-59-RT	354.2, 354.0
5. 62368	722.83, V58.89
6. 20552	729.1
7. 20552	729.1
8. 20605, 20605-76	719.43, 729.2
9. 64622, 64623 x4, 76003 Rad	724.8
10. 62290 x2	724.2
11. 64622 x2, 62287, 76005 Rad	722.10
12. 64622, 62287, 76005 Rad	724.2, 729.2
13. 62310	724.2, 729.2
14. 62362, 62350, 72265, 62311, 76005 Rad	722.83
15. 62362, 76005 Rad	V53.09
16. 62350, 62361, 72255, 76005 Rad	724.2

	CPT-4 Code	ICD-9-CM Code
17.	62361	724.5, 722.2
18.	64721-LT	354.0
19.	62311	724.2, 729.2
20.	64721-RT	354.0
21.	64510, 76005 Rad	729.5
22.	64622, 64623 x2	724.2
23.	64475, 64476 x3, 76005 Rad	724.2
24.	62350, 72265, 76005 Rad, 96530	996.2

EYE EXERCISES

	CPT-4 Code	ICD-9-CM Code
1.	68420-50-52	375.89
2.	67914-53-E2	374.14
3.	66170-LT	365.11
4.	66984-RT	366.9
5.	66986	996.79, 367.31
6.	68440-50, 67914-E2, 67914-E4	374.10, 375.52
7.	66250-LT	364.8
8.	67923-E2	374.10

EAR EXERCISES

	CPT-4 Code	ICD-9-CM Code
1.	69436-RT	381.4
2.	69210	380.4, 319
3.	69644-LT	382.9, 383.1
4.	69631-LT	380.50, 389.00
5.	69610-LT, 15732-51, 15120-51	384.20
6.	69210	380.4
	99212-25	
7.	69200	931
	99281-25	931
8.	69436-50	381.4

SECTION THREE: RADIOLOGY

	CPT-4 Code	ICD-9-CM Code
1.	70470	784.0
2.	74270	564.0
3.	76857	625.9, 789.00
4.	76700	787.02, 789.00
5.	74240	789.00, 787.02
6.	71020	783.21
7.	76815	646.83
8.	73090-RT	V54.8
9.	73560-LT	719.46, E888.9, V43.65
10.	76815	761.7
11.	74170, 72193	593.9
12.	72148	756.12, 724.00
13.	73721	836.0
14.	76857	621.6
15.	70547, 70551	None
16.	93925	443.9, 729.5
17.	74246	789.00, 787.02

#	CPT	ICD
18.	74160, 72193	789.04
19.	74249	789.00
20.	76857, 76938, 50390	620.2
21.	74020	789.00
22.	70450	780.79
23.	74415	596.8
24.	71270	574.20, 518.89
25.	76090-LT	793.8
26.	93880	433.10, V12.59
27.	71270	V10.11
28.	73130-RT	923.3
29.	73130-RT, 71020	959.4, 959.1, E888.9
30.	73110-LT	719.43
31.	71020	786.05
32.	78460	786.50
33.	78704	None
34.	74420	None
35.	73110-RT	719.43, E888.9
36.	71010, 76000	793.1
37.	76645-RT, 76090-RT	793.8
38.	71270	518.89, 511.0
39.	73565, 73560-50	719.46, E888.9
40.	73620-LT	959.7
41.	76075	627.2, 244.9, 174.9
42.	73030-RT	959.2
43.	76075	737.10
44.	73650-RT	719.47
45.	76700	575.9
46.	70390	527.2
47.	74410	599.0
48.	71100, 71020	V54.8
49.	74170	573.8
50.	70486	473.9
51.	70220, 71020	786.2
52.	76815	646.83
53.	74240, 76700	789.06, 789.01
54.	70486, 73030-RT	473.9, 719.41
55.	74240	786.50, V12.79
56.	72220-52	793.5
57.	71020	786.2
58.	73030-LT	719.41
59.	73560-LT	959.7
60.	73610-RT	719.47
61.	76857	666.24
62.	76857	620.2
63.	76815	646.83
64.	71270, 74170	573.8
65.	73070-LT	729.5
66.	71020	786.50